SITE-SPECIFIC CANCER SERIES

Pancreatic and Hepatobiliary Cancers

Edited by

Catherine M. Handy, PhD, RN, AOCN®, and Denise O'Dea, APRN-BC, OCN®

Oncology Nursing Society
Pittsburgh, Pennsylvania

ONS Publications Department

Executive Director, Professional Practice and Programs: Elizabeth M. Wertz Evans, RN, MPM, CPHQ, CPHIMS, FACMPE
Publisher and Director of Publications: Barbara Sigler, RN, MNEd
Managing Editor: Lisa M. George, BA
Technical Content Editor: Angela D. Klimaszewski, RN, MSN
Staff Editor II: Amy Nicoletti, BA
Copy Editor: Laura Pinchot, BA
Graphic Designer: Dany Sjoen

Library of Congress Cataloging-in-Publication Data

Pancreatic and hepatobiliary cancers / edited by Catherine M. Handy and Denise O'Dea.
    p. ; cm. -- (Site-specific cancer series)
  Includes bibliographical references.
  ISBN 978-1-935864-18-9 (alk. paper)
  I. Handy, Catherine M. II. O'Dea, Denise. III. Oncology Nursing Society. IV. Series: Site-specific cancer series.
  [DNLM: 1. Pancreatic Neoplasms. 2. Biliary Tract Neoplasms. 3. Liver Neoplasms. WI 810]
  LC Classification not assigned
  616.99'436--dc23
                                                                                    2012038596

Publisher's Note

This book is published by the Oncology Nursing Society (ONS). ONS neither represents nor guarantees that the practices described herein will, if followed, ensure safe and effective patient care. The recommendations contained in this book reflect ONS's judgment regarding the state of general knowledge and practice in the field as of the date of publication. The recommendations may not be appropriate for use in all circumstances. Those who use this book should make their own determinations regarding specific safe and appropriate patient-care practices, taking into account the personnel, equipment, and practices available at the hospital or other facility at which they are located. The editors and publisher cannot be held responsible for any liability incurred as a consequence from the use or application of any of the contents of this book. Figures and tables are used as examples only. They are not meant to be all-inclusive, nor do they represent endorsement of any particular institution by ONS. Mention of specific products and opinions related to those products do not indicate or imply endorsement by ONS. Web sites mentioned are provided for information only; the hosts are responsible for their own content and availability. Unless otherwise indicated, dollar amounts reflect U.S. dollars.

ONS publications are originally published in English. Publishers wishing to translate ONS publications must contact ONS about licensing arrangements. ONS publications cannot be translated without obtaining written permission from ONS. (Individual tables and figures that are reprinted or adapted require additional permission from the original source.) Because translations from English may not always be accurate or precise, ONS disclaims any responsibility for inaccuracies in words or meaning that may occur as a result of the translation. Readers relying on precise information should check the original English version.

Printed in the United States of America

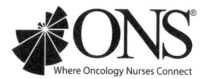

Oncology Nursing Society
Integrity • Innovation • Stewardship • Advocacy • Excellence • Inclusiveness

Contributors

Editors

Catherine M. Handy, PhD, RN, AOCN®
Oncology Clinical Nurse Specialist
New York Presbyterian Hospital/Weill Cornell Medical
    Center
New York, New York
Chapter 1. Overview

Denise O'Dea, APRN-BC, OCN®
Nurse Practitioner
NYU Cancer Institute
New York, New York
Chapter 1. Overview

Authors

Jamie Cairo, DNP, APRN-BC, AOCNP®
Nurse Practitioner Specializing in Hematology and Oncology
Aurora Cancer Care
Kenosha, Wisconsin
Chapter 6. Liver Metastases

Nicoletta Campagna, DNP, APRN-BC, AOCNP®
Nurse Practitioner—Medical Oncology
Cancer Treatment Centers of America–Midwestern
    Regional Medical Center
Zion, Illinois
Chapter 6. Liver Metastases

Elizabeth Cruz, RN, BSN, OCN®
Clinical Nurse III, Gastrointestinal Medical Oncology
Memorial Sloan-Kettering Cancer Center
New York, New York
Chapter 3. Pancreatic Endocrine Tumors

Gail W. Davidson, RN, BSN, OCN®
Regional Liver Therapy Disease Management Coordinator
Arthur G. James Cancer Hospital and Richard J. Solove
    Research Institute
Columbus, Ohio
Chapter 5. Primary Hepatocellular Carcinoma

Betty Ferrell, PhD, FAAN, MA, FPCN, CHPN
Research Scientist/Professor
Nursing Research and Education
Department of Population Sciences
City of Hope
Duarte, California
Chapter 7. Quality of Life and Symptom Management

Theresa Wicklin Gillespie, PhD, MA, RN
Associate Professor, Division of Surgical Oncology,
    Department of Surgery and Department of Hematology
    and Medical Oncology
Winship Cancer Institute
Emory University School of Medicine
Atlanta, Georgia
Chapter 2. Pancreatic Exocrine Tumors

Peter Miller, RN, BSN, PHN
Case Manager, Hospice
Butte Home Health and Hospice
Chico, California
Chapter 9. Advance Care Planning

Neal R. Niznan, MSW, LCSW
Social Worker
Department of Radiation Oncology/Roberts Proton Therapy
    Center
Penn Medicine
Philadelphia, Pennsylvania
Chapter 10. Economic and Social Challenges

Maria Petzel, RD, CSO, LD, CNSC
Senior Clinical Dietitian
The University of Texas MD Anderson Cancer Center
Houston, Texas
Chapter 8. Nutritional Challenges

Virginia Sun, RN, PhD
Assistant Professor
Nursing Research and Education, Department of Population
    Sciences
City of Hope
Duarte, California
Chapter 7. Quality of Life and Symptom Management

Lisa M. Wall, RN, PhD, AOCNS®
Clinical Nurse Specialist, Gastrointestinal Surgery
Memorial Sloan-Kettering Cancer Center
New York, New York
Chapter 3. Pancreatic Endocrine Tumors

Lyn Wooten, RN, MSN
Gastrointestinal Oncology Coordinator
WFU Baptist Medical Center
Winston-Salem, North Carolina
Chapter 5. Primary Hepatocellular Carcinoma

Alisa M. Yee, MSN, ACNP-BC, NP
GI Surgery Oncology Nurse Practitioner
Helen Diller Family Comprehensive Cancer Center
University of California, San Francisco
San Francisco, California
Chapter 4. Gallbladder and Bile Duct Tumors

Disclosure

Editors and authors of books and guidelines provided by the Oncology Nursing Society are expected to disclose to the readers any significant financial interest or other relationships with the manufacturer(s) of any commercial products.

A vested interest may be considered to exist if a contributor is affiliated with or has a financial interest in commercial organizations that may have a direct or indirect interest in the subject matter. A "financial interest" may include, but is not limited to, being a shareholder in the organization; being an employee of the commercial organization; serving on an organization's speakers bureau; or receiving research from the organization. An "affiliation" may be holding a position on an advisory board or some other role of benefit to the commercial organization. Vested interest statements appear in the front matter for each publication.

Contributors are expected to disclose any unlabeled or investigational use of products discussed in their content. This information is acknowledged solely for the information of the readers.

The contributors provided the following disclosure and vested interest information:

Catherine M. Handy, PhD, RN, AOCN®: Celgene, Cephalon, honoraria

Denise O'Dea, PhD, APRN-BC, OCN®: Celgene, Amgen Inc., honoraria

Contents

CHAPTER 1

Overview

Catherine M. Handy, PhD, RN, AOCN®, and Denise O'Dea, APRN-BC, OCN®

Introduction

Cancers of the liver and pancreas are challenging problems in oncology. The five-year survival rates remain dismal for both types of cancer. This book is designed to provide an updated overview of cancers of the liver, bile duct, and gallbladder and exocrine and endocrine tumors of the pancreas. Symptom management and nutrition, psychosocial, and economic challenges will be detailed as they relate to pancreatic and liver cancers.

Hepatocellular carcinoma (HCC) is the most common form of primary liver cancer, accounting for 80% of the reported cases. In 2012, the American Cancer Society estimated that the incidence of liver and intrahepatic bile duct cancers was 28,720 new cases, with 20,550 deaths from the disease estimated for the same time period (American Cancer Society, 2012). Overall, the five-year survival rate for liver cancer is 14%.

When referring to pancreatic cancer, we usually mean exocrine tumors of the pancreas. In 2012, the American Cancer Society estimated the incidence of pancreatic cancer to be 43,920 new cases, with 37,390 deaths from the disease estimated for the same period (American Cancer Society, 2012). Overall, the five-year survival rate for pancreatic cancer, for all stages, is 6%, and one-year survival is 26% (American Cancer Society, 2012).

Pancreatic endocrine tumors arising from endocrine tissue within the pancreas are much less common malignancies, accounting for 2% of all pancreatic cancers (Capelli et al., 2009).

According to the American Cancer Society's 2012 statistical projections, the number of new U.S. cases of gallbladder and other biliary cancers is estimated to be 9,810, with 3,200 deaths estimated to occur (American Cancer Society, 2012).

Signs and Symptoms

The signs and symptoms of liver and pancreatic cancers are similar and can include weight loss, poor appetite, abdominal pain, and jaundice. Patients with pancreatic cancer can sometimes develop glucose intolerance. Liver enlargement is the most common physical sign of liver cancer, occurring in 50%–90% of patients (American Cancer Society, 2012).

Nutrition

Malnutrition is a common problem in patients with cancer and has been associated with adverse outcomes, including poor quality of life and increased morbidity and mortality. A poor prognostic indicator in patients with cancer is weight loss. The National Cancer Institute (2011) reported that at diagnosis, 80% of patients with gastrointestinal cancers are malnourished.

Because of the anatomic location of the pancreatic and hepatobiliary systems, patients with cancer are at an especially high risk for nutrition problems. The incidence of malnutrition in patients with pancreatic or hepatobiliary cancers is more common than with many other types of cancer (Bruera, 1997). Nutritional status may be affected by cancer itself as well as the treatments for the cancer. Nutrient needs may be altered by the disease or treatment. At the same time, the disease or treatment can change the patient's ability to ingest, digest, and absorb the appropriate nutrients to meet these needs (Hurst & Gallagher, 2006).

Socioeconomics

The cost of cancer care is high in both dollars and human suffering. Because of the poor outcomes of patients with pancreatic and liver cancers, the costs are usually higher than with other cancers. Unfortunately, we know that disparities can exist in caring for patients with cancer. These disparities can be due to financial and geographic barriers, ineffective provider-patient communication, inadequate screening, and poor long-term follow-up, among other factors (National Institutes of Health, 2004).

During the course of diagnosis and treatment, patients experience many disruptions in their lives. Cancer symptoms and treatment side effects can interfere with patients' ability to carry on with a normal life. They may experience financial burdens, loss of work, and difficulties with interpersonal relationships.

The complicated health insurance systems can have an impact on any patient, regardless of socioeconomic status. Many patients find themselves underinsured or uninsured, leading to difficulties in managing their disease and finances. The role of the social worker in oncology is imperative to providing excellent patient care for all patients.

Summary

Liver and pancreatic cancers are complicated diseases of the gastrointestinal tract. They are, unfortunately, often met with poor outcomes. The nature of these diseases leads to complex treatment plans, complicated side effect management, poor nutrition, and challenges related to psychosocial and economic experiences.

This book seeks to provide an in-depth review of pancreatic and liver cancers. Caring for patients with liver and pancreatic cancers is difficult on many levels. A multidisciplinary approach is imperative for the care of these patients.

It is clear from the poor outcomes associated with liver and pancreatic cancers that additional research is needed in this area. Nurses can play an important role in the future research and outcomes of these patients.

References

American Cancer Society. (2012). Cancer facts and figures 2012. Retrieved from http://www.cancer.org/acs/groups/content/@epidemiologysurveilance/documents/document/acspc-031941.pdf

Bruera, E. (1997). ABC of palliative care. Anorexia, cachexia, and nutrition. *BMJ, 315,* 1219–1222.

Capelli, P., Martignoni, G., Pedica, F., Falconi, M., Antonello, D., Malpeli, G., & Scarpa, A. (2009). Endocrine neoplasms of the pancreas: Pathologic and genetic features. *Archives of Pathology and Laboratory Medicine, 133,* 350–364. doi:10.1043/1543-2165-133.3.350

Hurst, J.D., & Gallagher, A.L. (2006). Energy, macronutrient, micronutrient, and fluid requirements. In L. Elliott, L.L. Molseed, P.D. McCallum, & B. Grant (Eds.), *The clinical guide to oncology nutrition* (2nd ed., pp. 54–71). Chicago, IL: American Dietetic Association.

National Cancer Institute. (2011). Nutrition in cancer care (PDQ®) [Health professional version]. Retrieved from http://www.cancer.gov/cancertopics/pdq/supportivecare/nutrition/HealthProfessional

National Institutes of Health. (2004). Economic costs of cancer health disparities. Retrieved from http://crchd.cancer.gov/attachments/NCIeconomiccosts.pdf

CHAPTER 2

Pancreatic Exocrine Tumors

Theresa Wicklin Gillespie, PhD, MA, RN

Introduction

Epidemiology

Pancreatic cancer remains an extremely lethal disease; even when diagnosed at a localized stage, the five-year survival for these cases is only 23% (American Cancer Society [ACS], 2012). The unavailability of screening tests, coupled with lack of specific symptoms that would allow early diagnosis, means that the vast majority of pancreatic cancers are found at later stages, with only 8% of patients diagnosed at an early stage of disease (ACS, 2012). In 2012, ACS estimated the incidence of pancreatic cancer to be 43,920 new cases, with 37,390 deaths from the disease estimated for the same period. Overall, the five-year survival rate for pancreatic cancer, for all stages, is 6%, and one-year survival is 26% (ACS, 2012). Although the incidence is relatively small, pancreatic cancer ranks as the fourth leading cause of cancer deaths for both men and women.

References to pancreatic cancer in the literature primarily refer to the more common histologic type of pancreatic tumor, the exocrine, or ductal epithelial adenocarcinoma, type. The second type, endocrine or islet cell tumor, is much rarer, representing less than 5% of all pancreatic malignancies (Zhou et al., 2010). Epidemiologic studies using mainly Surveillance, Epidemiology, and End Results (SEER) data have demonstrated that the incidence of pancreatic neuroendocrine tumors has been increasing over time (Halfdanarson, Rabe, Rubin, & Petersen, 2008), with the rates rising by 106% for men and 125% for women during the period of 1977–2005 (Zhou et al., 2010). Conversely, the incidence rates of exocrine cancer of the pancreas have decreased during the same period, by 19% for men and by 5% for women.

Pancreatic cancer, in general, is a disease of older adults, with incidence increasing with age and median age at diagnosis occurring at age 65 years or older (Huggett & Pereira, 2011). For adults, the incidence rates for pancreatic exocrine

tumors were 14–28 times higher for those aged 60 years or older than for younger adults (p < 0.01) (Zhou et al., 2010). Pancreatic malignancies occur in pediatric populations as well; however, their incidence is very small (Perez et al., 2009). Analysis of SEER data over a 30-year period revealed only 58 cases of malignant pancreatic neoplasms in children up to age 19; more than 53% of the tumors were classified as exocrine.

When SEER data are examined by race or ethnicity, changes in incidence and mortality trends for exocrine tumors are observed over time. Based on SEER data for 1977–2005, the incidence rates for exocrine tumors decreased by 11% among Caucasians and 17% among African Americans (Zhou et al., 2010). Much smaller changes were found for other racial groups (e.g., Asian/Pacific Islander, American Indian/Alaska Native); incidence of exocrine tumors decreased by only 0.2%–3% during this period.

As opposed to incidence rates, mortality from pancreatic exocrine tumors has increased slightly overall, whereas survival has been essentially unchanged for the past 20 years (Zhou et al., 2010). When investigating mortality rates by race or ethnicity, both African American men and women have higher death rates associated with pancreatic cancer compared to their Caucasian counterparts. Among African American men, the death rate is 15.4 per 100,000 (age-adjusted to the U.S. standard population in 2000) versus 12.2 for Caucasian men; among women, the African American rate is 12.4 versus 9.1 for Caucasians (ACS, 2011). The reasons for these differences are unknown but may be associated with higher rates among African Americans of obesity, diabetes, or other potential risk factors for pancreatic cancer, including increased rates in African Americans of K-*ras* mutations, also an identified risk factor for pancreatic cancer (Pernick, Sarkar, & Philip, 2003).

Anatomically, nearly 80% of pancreatic exocrine tumors are found in the head of the pancreas (Sener, Fremgen, Menck, & Winchester, 1999), with the remainder apportioned between the tail and the body of the pancreas. Because symptoms at presentation depend on the tumor's anatomic location and the stage of disease, the majority of pancreatic exocrine cancers are associated with obstructive cholestasis, resulting in the appearance of jaundice that may aid in diagnosis.

Risk Factors

The etiology of pancreatic cancer is unclear, although certain risk factors have been identified. Among potential environmental exposures, the causative role of tobacco smoke is associated with the highest level of evidence. Case-control studies have demonstrated an increased risk of pancreatic cancer in smokers that is 2.5–3.6 times that of nonsmokers (Hassan et al., 2007). Like other tobacco-related cancers, the risk escalates as the use and duration of exposure to tobacco smoke increase. Tobacco exposure is thought to account for about 25% of pancreatic cancer cases (Lowenfels & Maisonneuve, 2004), and declines in smoking rates may explain some of the decreases in incidence over time.

Family history of pancreatic exocrine tumors is also a strong risk factor; about 5%–10% of patients with pancreatic cancer have relatives with previously diagnosed pancreatic cancer (Shi, Hruban, & Klein, 2009). For families who have four or more members affected with pancreatic cancer, the risk of having pancreatic cancer is 57 times higher than for those families with no affected member (Tersmette et al., 2001). Genetic disorders and syndromes have also been associated with pancreatic cancer risk (Zavoral, Minarikova, Zavada, Salek, & Minarik, 2011), such as Lynch syndrome (also known as *hereditary nonpolyposis colorectal cancer*), Peutz-Jeghers syndrome (characterized by the development of intestinal polyps), cystic fibrosis, hereditary pancreatitis, *BRCA2* carriers, and familial atypical multiple mole melanoma, pointing to a genetic link for pancreatic cancer.

Dietary risk factors have been explored but remain somewhat controversial as potential factors in pancreatic cancer. Dietary intake of alcohol, coffee, processed meats, high-fat and high-cholesterol foods, and aspirin, as well as obesity, have been examined as possibly contributing to the development of pancreatic cancer, with varying results (Hidalgo, 2010). Blood types A, B, and AB have been associated with cancers of the pancreas as well as other tumor types (Wolpin et al., 2009).

The potential causative role of diabetes in pancreatic cancer remains a subject of much study and debate. Many patients with pancreatic cancer may exhibit new-onset diabetes as a manifestation of their cancer (Hsu & Saif, 2011). Close to 80% of patients with pancreatic cancer also have confirmed diabetes or impaired glucose tolerance, with the diagnosis of diabetes often occurring at the same time or within two years prior to the cancer diagnosis (Gullo, Pezzilli, & Morselli-Labate, 1994; Permert et al., 1993). Pancreatic cancer has been associated only with type 2 diabetes, and family history of diabetes does not appear to have an impact (Sharma, El-tawil, Renfrew, Walsh, & Molinari, 2011). Several large stud-

ies have investigated the role of type 2 diabetes in pancreatic cancer, finding a relative risk of 2.1 for developing pancreatic cancer (Everhart & Wright, 1995; Wideroff et al., 1997). Gestational diabetes also has been associated with a high risk of pancreatic cancer (relative risk of 7.1), hypothesized to be due to insulin binding to the insulin-like growth factor-I and contributing to cancer cell growth (Gapstur et al., 2000). New-onset diabetes in individuals older than age 50 may be an early sign of pancreatic cancer, although only about 1% of such cases are linked to pancreatic cancer (Chari et al., 2005). However, no data to date have shown that screening of individuals with new-onset diabetes leads to earlier diagnosis of pancreatic cancer or to reduced mortality from malignancy (Ogawa et al., 2002).

The Role of Nursing in Prevention and Early Detection

Nurses in both oncology and primary care settings can contribute in key ways toward potential prevention and early detection of this almost universally lethal cancer. The known association of pancreatic cancer with tobacco smoke exposure and possible risks associated with diet, obesity, alcohol intake, and diabetes provide the basis for education of the public as well as family members of those diagnosed with pancreatic exocrine tumors. As for other cancers linked to tobacco, the diagnosis of a family member with a smoking-associated cancer may present the nurse with a compelling teachable moment for those family members who are considered at risk but not yet diagnosed.

Screening family members with relatives diagnosed with pancreatic cancer in order to facilitate earlier detection has proved to be challenging, in part because studies of hereditary factors for pancreatic cancer have been inconsistent. However, families with two or more known cases of pancreatic exocrine tumors may benefit from a more comprehensive assessment of risk, inclusion in registries for high-risk families, and familial studies of genetic mutations (Rieder et al., 2002; Shi et al., 2009). In an attempt to objectively evaluate risk factors and pedigree data from at-risk families, computerized assessment tools have been developed. PancPRO is an initial tool developed by Wang and colleagues (2007) for use as a model for risk prediction in individuals with familiar pancreatic cancer in order to identify those at highest risk for the disease. Nurses play a pivotal role in educating families about their increased risk of pancreatic cancer and facilitating the assessment and quantitative prediction of such risk.

Risk assessments and familial registries are anticipated ultimately to serve as tools to help diagnose pancreatic cancer early enough to influence survival rates. Specialized, comprehensive screening programs for high-risk individuals involve genetic testing, endoscopic ultrasound (EUS), and imaging with computed tomography (CT) or magnetic resonance imaging (MRI) (Hruban, Canto, & Yeo, 2001). Currently, such screening programs are considered investigational, including their cost-effectiveness. The lack of definitive technology to accomplish the goal of earlier detection creates extreme anxiety in many individuals from high-risk families. Nurses are essential to delivering interventions to reduce the risk of pancreatic cancer, including education about modifying lifestyle behaviors related to smoking, diet, and alcohol consumption, as well as providing referrals and offering emotional support to ameliorate the distress experienced by these individuals and the entire family unit.

Diagnosis

In the absence of effective screening for early detection, in most cases, diagnosis of pancreatic exocrine tumors depends on symptomatic assessment and differential diagnosis to rule out pancreatic cancer. Symptoms present at the time of diagnosis of pancreatic cancer depend mainly on the anatomic location of the tumor. As stated previously, tumors of the head of the pancreas may present as jaundice or signs of obstruction. Other anatomic locations may be manifested as abdominal or back pain but are more indicative of advanced disease. Earlier symptoms tend to be rather vague, such as weight loss, early satiety, or anorexia, and associated with multiple possible diagnoses (Krech & Walsh, 1991). Grahm and Andrén-Sandberg (1997) found, however, that 25% of patients eventually diagnosed with pancreatic cancer complained of upper abdominal symptoms up to six months prior to diagnosis, but clinicians did not pursue these symptoms.

Pancreatitis represents a situation where further workup should be performed to determine if a more serious condition underlies the presentation (Raimondi, Lowenfels, Morselli-Labate, Maisonneuve, & Pezzilli, 2010). Chronic pancreatitis, particularly hereditary pancreatitis, has been reported as a risk factor for pancreatic cancer, especially if the chronic condition persists for more than five to seven years (Farrow & Evers, 2002). Thus, chronic pancreatitis that continues for several years should be periodically evaluated as a possible risk factor for pancreatic cancer (Kudo, Kamisawa, Anjiki, Takuma, & Egawa, 2011). A diagnosis of acute pancreatitis may indicate obstruction of the pancreatic duct due to cancer, and pancreatic cancer should be a consideration in the assessment of acute pancreatitis (Bracci et al., 2009).

The search for serum biomarkers that might be used for screening for pancreatic exocrine tumors remains paramount. Among the many tumor markers applied to screening for and therapeutic monitoring of these cancers, carbohydrate antigen 19-9 (CA 19-9) has had the most widespread application in pancreatic cancer. Nevertheless, CA 19-9 is not specific to pancreatic cancer; levels are elevated in other cancers and conditions, including cholestasis (Hidalgo, 2010), and approximately 10% of patients, even with advanced disease,

will show undetectable levels due to an inability to generate CA 19-9. In addition, elevated serum bilirubin can cause a false increase in CA 19-9 in patients with jaundice, thus confounding a diagnosis of pancreatic cancer in these individuals (Boeck, Stieber, Holdenrieder, Wilkowski, & Heinemann, 2006). Combining CA 19-9 with other serum markers (e.g., carcinoembryonic antigen [known as CEA] and carbohydrate antigen 242 [CA 242]) has not resulted in greater specificity or sensitivity for pancreatic cancer. Neither of these markers is indicated as a single tumor marker for pancreatic cancer, although CA 242 has shown promise as an independent prognostic marker (Sharma et al., 2011).

Diagnostic workup of patients suspected of pancreatic exocrine tumors includes diagnosis of disease, staging in order to determine prognosis and resectability, and assessment of physical symptoms requiring intervention for management and palliation. A variety of imaging modalities may be employed for visualization of a mass and its anatomic location in a patient suspected of a diagnosis of pancreatic cancer.

Transabdominal ultrasound may be used as an initial screening technique to determine resectability but is less useful in smaller tumors (smaller than 3 cm). CT with IV contrast is deemed the imaging modality of choice and should be performed using well-defined pancreatic imaging protocols. Such techniques include use of thin slices and triphasic cross-sectional imaging. The use of thin cuts (approximately 3 mm) allows detailed visualization of the anatomy and vasculature critical to determination of resection and identification of smaller tumors and metastatic disease. With multiphase imaging, noncontrast is combined with contrast phases in order to carefully examine the arterial, portal venous, and pancreatic parenchyma. Newer pancreas protocols with MRI are also becoming more common. Such techniques are generally adequate with about 80%–90% accuracy to determine whether a mass exists, the other anatomic structures in its proximity, if the tumor might be surgically removed, or whether other management approaches are indicated (Miura et al., 2006). Positron-emission tomography (PET) scanning can also add to the diagnosis if the CT scan is thought to be equivocal.

EUS demonstrates even higher sensitivity to detection of pancreatic cancers (98%), even when small, versus a CT scan (86%) (DeWitt et al., 2004). EUS can be further enhanced with the addition of IV contrast agents. For obtaining tumor tissue for diagnosis, EUS is the optimal approach. EUS is considered superior to CT-directed fine-needle aspiration for biopsy because of its overall diagnostic yield, general safety, and lower risk of possible peritoneal seeding. However, EUS does have some associated disadvantages, including that it is an invasive technique and its success is largely dependent on the experience of the person performing the test. EUS has also been associated with a less than 1% risk of pancreatitis, bleeding, and perforation of the duodenum. The procedure is also quite costly. Alternatively, endoscopic retrograde cholangiopancreatography may be used to collect tissue for diagnosis through ductal brushing and lavage and may also serve to place a stent to relieve obstruction in patients who experience jaundice. If washings are found to be positive on cytology, the patient is considered to have metastatic (M1) disease and should be treated accordingly, regardless of whether the tumor was resected.

Unlike most other malignancies, a tissue diagnosis is not required prior to attempting surgical resection of suspected pancreatic exocrine tumors, although the anticipated surgery is associated with significant morbidity and mortality. A nondiagnostic biopsy is not considered justification for delaying surgical resection if the index of suspicion for pancreatic cancer is considered high (National Comprehensive Cancer Network, 2012). Histopathologic confirmation, however, is needed before chemotherapy or radiation therapy is initiated for treatment of documented pancreatic cancer.

Nursing Considerations of Pancreatic Cancer Diagnosis

Diagnostic workup, staging, and treatment planning based on the staging results all require careful preparation of the patient and education as to the planned interventions and interpretation of findings. Nurses, especially those in advanced practice settings, should be attentive to generalized or vague symptoms in patients, particularly ill-defined abdominal complaints, with cancer clearly considered in the differential. Both gastrointestinal and gynecologic cancers (e.g., ovarian cancer) may show similar, imprecise symptoms at early presentation.

Patient and family education is critical to ensure that the limitations of serum biomarkers are well understood and that findings are not misinterpreted. Other laboratory tests, such as liver function studies, also will likely be drawn, and the translation of these results in the context of the patient's complete physical presentation is commonly in the nurse's domain.

Preparing the patient for imaging studies, including EUS, will be important for the success of these interventions and reduction of any potential side effects. Explaining the need for staging of the tumor to determine if the cancer is able to be resected and the reasons why tissue for histologic diagnosis may not be pursued is crucial at this point in the patient's treatment planning. The results of the staging work-up, including whether the tumor is found to be unresectable, likewise will benefit from the nurse's careful explanation to the patient and family.

Current and Evolving Treatments for Management of Pancreatic Exocrine Tumors

Although overall survival for the majority of patients diagnosed with exocrine tumors of the pancreas has not changed

significantly for more than two decades, research and clinical trials to improve outcomes in these patients have been vigorously pursued during that period. Although definitive advances in therapy have been insufficient to impact overall mortality from this overwhelmingly fatal disease, progress in different therapeutic modalities and combinations of treatment approaches and the nursing role for each option are presented below.

Surgery

Surgery remains the foundation for therapy for pancreatic exocrine tumors. In cases where pancreatic malignancies are found at an early stage, surgical resection represents the only chance for cure, although only 15%–20% of patients meet the criteria for resection (Castellanos, Cardin, & Berlin, 2011). Thus, meticulous staging of disease to determine resectability is paramount. According to the *Expert Consensus Statement on Pretreatment Assessment of Resectable and Borderline Resectable Pancreatic Cancer* (Callery et al., 2009), exocrine tumors are considered unresectable if any of the following factors are present: (a) distant metastases, (b) aortic invasion or encasement, (c) encasement of more than half of the superior mesenteric vein, or (d) lymph node involvement beyond the field to be resected, among other findings. Some centers may perform staging laparoscopy prior to definitive resection, particularly for tumors involving the tail or body of the pancreas, in order to rule out metastatic deposits not seen on imaging tests. Staging laparoscopy might be an option if the patient is considered borderline resectable or has other indications to raise the index of suspicion for metastatic disease (e.g., high CA 19-9 level, large tumor seen on scans).

If the tumor is considered resectable, optimal outcomes following surgery are reported at institutions that routinely perform a higher volume of pancreatic cancer resections (Gooiker et al., 2011). Such a volume-outcome relationship has been reported for other cancers involving complex care that may be enhanced at centers that provide such care more frequently and have established processes and experienced multidisciplinary teams in place to support these complexities. A significant benefit was found for patients treated for pancreatic cancer at high-volume centers in terms of both postoperative mortality (odds ratio 0.32, 95% confidence interval 0.16–0.64) and survival (hazard ratio 0.79, confidence interval 0.70–0.89). Although advantages exist for patients to stay within their own community for treatment, including costs and psychosocial support, outcomes are definitely improved when surgical resection is performed at a high-volume center. If the patient is considered to have resectable disease, the nurse may serve to facilitate referral to a high-volume center if the patient and family prefer that option.

If the exocrine pancreatic tumor is resectable, the malignancy's location will dictate the optimal surgical procedure.

Cephalic pancreaticoduodenectomy (Whipple procedure), distal pancreatectomy, or total pancreatectomy may be performed (Hidalgo, 2010). Although a more extensive resection has not been shown to improve survival and increases postoperative morbidity, the surgery should attempt to produce negative (tumor-free) margins, if possible.

The question of lymph node resection has been debated more recently. Removal of at least 12–15 lymph nodes is recommended in exocrine tumors involving the head of the pancreas but not for the minority of tumors that are found in the body (15%) or tail (10%) (Pavlidis, Pavlidis, & Sakantamis, 2011). More extensive lymphadenectomy associated with tumor resections located in the body and tail of the pancreas has resulted in greater complications, including wound infections, fistula, and delayed gastric emptying, but not improved survival (Pavlidis et al., 2011).

The role of preoperative biliary decompression to relieve obstructive jaundice caused by tumors located in the head of the pancreas or periampullary area has proved to be controversial as well. Preoperative biliary drainage, intended to reduce mortality and complications in patients undergoing pancreaticoduodenectomy, has been associated with increased wound infections, sepsis, longer length of stay in the hospital, and higher postoperative mortality compared with patients who underwent surgery without delays caused by biliary decompression (van der Gaag et al., 2009, 2010).

The classic Whipple procedure has been part of the surgical approach to pancreatic exocrine tumors for nearly a century. In this surgery, the pancreatic head, duodenum, common bile duct, gallbladder, distal portion of the stomach, and nearby lymph nodes are removed in an en bloc resection (Trede, 1993). A newer approach, pylorus-preserving pancreaticoduodenectomy (PPPD), may be performed for cancer occurring in the pancreatic head. The goal of this surgery is to achieve better long-term gastrointestinal function by preserving the stomach along with the initial two centimeters of the duodenum (Loos, Kleeff, Friess, & Büchler, 2008). Although PPPD has been shown to reduce operative time and blood loss and improve postoperative weight gain and quality of life compared to the classic Whipple operation, other studies indicate PPPD is associated with a higher incidence of delayed gastric emptying, despite pylorus preservation (Park, Kim, Jang, Ahn, & Park, 2003).

Pancreatic fistula and leakage of secretions represent major complications of pancreatic resection, occurring in up to 20% of cases, even at high-volume centers (Bassi et al., 2001). Consequently, painstaking care must be taken in pancreatico-enteric reconstruction to prevent fistula formation. No surgical reconstruction technique has been proved to be superior in reducing postoperative complication rates or prevention of pancreatic fistulae.

A more recent entry in surgical therapy is laparoscopic pancreatic resection. Laparoscopic distal pancreatic resection is the most frequently performed laparoscopic pancreatic surgery and has been proved to be feasible and safe (Kooby et al., 2008). However, data regarding morbidity, mortality, and length of stay following surgery are similar between laparoscopic and open techniques.

Postoperative complications require knowledgeable, alert, and skilled nursing care to mitigate as much as possible the adverse events commonly associated with pancreatic cancer resection. The duration of some complications experienced following resection will depend on the type of surgery performed and whether sufficient, healthy pancreatic tissue remains postoperatively. Preoperative education of patients and their loved ones about potential complications is a crucial responsibility of the nurses caring for patients scheduled to undergo pancreatic resection for known or suspected pancreatic exocrine tumors. The list of possible adverse events associated with any type of pancreatic surgery is extensive, and the risk of serious morbidity as well as mortality is high. Thus, patient and family teaching prior to resection with reinforcement during the postoperative period is an essential component to achieving optimal outcomes in cases of exocrine tumors of the pancreas.

Complications of the Immediate Postoperative Period

One of the most common postoperative problems encountered following resection of exocrine tumors of the pancreas is pancreatic fistulae, occurring in both the early and late stages of postoperative recovery. Presenting symptoms of internal pancreatic fistulae include abdominal ascites and unilateral or bilateral pleural effusion. In the absence of preexisting liver dysfunction, abdominal ascites in the postoperative period should alert the nurse to the need for prompt follow-up (Morrison, 2010). Although postoperative pulmonary dysfunction may be associated with multiple causes, pancreatic fistulae should be high on the list of possible etiologies in these patients following pancreatic cancer resection. The patient may also exhibit fever, chest pain, and profuse amounts of fluid drainage. In addition to treating the symptoms, the care of fistulae may require another operation to repair the leak or insertion of an intra-abdominal drainage tube (Morrison, 2010).

Gastric ileus is a complication that may occur in the immediate postoperative period following pancreatic cancer resection. Although this problem may resolve on its own during postoperative healing, the use of opioid pain medications can exacerbate the ileus further and cause it to persist. The patient will generally present with symptoms such as nausea and vomiting, constipation, anorexia, early satiety, and decreased bowel sounds upon auscultation. The nurse can aid in the resolution of a gastric ileus by ensuring the patient receives a liquid diet and medications to promote gastric emptying. A nasogastric tube or similar intervention may be required to support gastric decompression.

Depending on the extent of surgery performed, the patient may be left with little or no healthy pancreatic tissue needed to perform the major physiologic roles of the pancreas:

- Exocrine function that carries out digestion through excretion of digestive enzymes. Dysfunction can lead to poor absorption of nutrients, inability to digest fats and other foods, malnutrition, and significant weight loss.
- Endocrine function that produces critical hormones such as insulin and glucagon that control blood glucose levels. Dysfunction of the endocrine system can result in permanent, insulin-dependent diabetes, although the patient may have already been dealing with diabetes prior to the diagnosis of pancreatic cancer.

Complications in both exocrine and endocrine functions can occur immediately after surgery and may continue without resolution for the remainder of the patient's life.

In the case of exocrine insufficiency, the patient may experience abdominal pain and diarrhea and may produce foul-smelling, fatty stools (steatorrhea) because of poor fat absorption and impaired digestion (Morrison, 2010). Consequently, the individual will be unable to gain weight and often loses a significant amount of weight. Poor nutrition and nutrient absorption results in inferior wound healing, severe diarrhea causes dehydration and electrolyte imbalance, and all these complications contribute to significant fatigue (Ellison, Chevlen, Still, & Dubagunta, 2002).

If the impairment of the exocrine function is caused by some intraoperative trauma to the pancreas that may repair itself over time, then this condition will resolve as the pancreas heals. However, if even after a recovery period insufficient healthy pancreatic tissue is available, then the exocrine insufficiency will require long-term treatment with digestive enzymes taken a few minutes before each meal (Kahl & Malferheiner, 2004).

If the endocrine function of the pancreas is damaged as a result of pancreatic resection, the patient will develop insulin-dependent diabetes. In many cases, the patient may have been diagnosed with new-onset diabetes prior to diagnosis because of tumor-associated pancreatic function impairment. Nearly all patients will be treated with insulin for glucose control in the immediate postoperative period because the surgery frequently causes endocrine dysfunction. Patients will require instruction during this period to self-monitor their glucose levels in preparation for discharge to home. During the weeks following surgery, blood glucose will be checked frequently because the levels are anticipated initially to be poorly controlled (Crippa et al., 2007). Depending on the residual pancreatic tissue, the patient may recover endocrine function during the first four to six postoperative weeks or may learn that permanent endocrine impairment has resulted from the surgery, and the individual will remain insulin dependent (Crippa et al., 2007).

Even if the patient undergoes a successful, "curative" resection of pancreatic exocrine cancer and is able to endure the myriad postoperative complications that commonly occur, five-year survival is still only 20% or less (Raut et al., 2007), with patients experiencing a high risk of locoregional failure as well as metastatic disease. Such findings suggest a systemic aspect to the disease regardless of localized treatment and indicate a need for adjuvant therapy consisting of radiation therapy, chemotherapy, or combination chemoradiation following surgery. In addition, neoadjuvant therapy is gaining greater popularity as a treatment option intended to either enhance resectability or reduce risk of recurrence (Gillen, Schuster, Meyer Zum Büschenfelde, Friess, & Kleeff, 2010).

Radiation

The role of adjuvant radiation therapy alone remains unclear because the suspected systemic nature of pancreatic cancer would seem to support the concept that external beam radiation therapy (EBRT) given on its own would not reduce the risk of dying from more widespread disease. Randomized trials of EBRT alone compared to EBRT plus chemotherapy demonstrated inferior outcomes, including survival outcomes, for patients who received EBRT alone. Randomized controlled trials, meta-analyses, and systematic reviews over many years have established the advantage of combination chemoradiation as opposed to radiation alone (Sultana et al., 2007). The effectiveness of these adjuvant approaches seems to focus on the contribution of chemotherapy, despite the added degree of toxicity experienced with cytotoxic chemotherapy.

Chemotherapy

Historically, 5-fluorouracil with or without leucovorin has been used as adjuvant therapy following pancreatic resection, with response rates up to 26% but no improvement in survival (Moertel, 1976). The important role of gemcitabine as adjuvant therapy in resected exocrine tumors of the pancreas was determined more than a decade ago through a randomized trial of gemcitabine versus 5-fluorouracil (Burris et al., 1997), which demonstrated a survival advantage with gemcitabine. Since that time, multiple agents have been tested but have not shown significant improvement in outcomes compared to gemcitabine.

Randomized controlled trials have evaluated the effectiveness of chemotherapy combined with radiation, including a Radiation Therapy Oncology Group study that compared adjuvant radiation plus continuous 5-fluorouracil to a similar chemoradiation regimen followed by gemcitabine. When the cancer is located in the head of the pancreas, superior median and overall three-year survival was reported for those patients randomized to receive gemcitabine (Crane et al., 2009). Those randomized to gemcitabine, however, also experienced significantly higher toxicity.

Chemotherapy is used in advanced disease as well as in the adjuvant setting. Gemcitabine has consistently served as the mainstay for systemic treatment of advanced pancreatic exocrine tumors. Erlotinib, a small molecule that inhibits epidermal growth factor receptor when combined with gemcitabine, has shown a statistically significant improvement in survival (Moore et al., 2007), but the combination of agents also exhibits far greater toxicity. The high incidence of *KRAS2* mutations among patients with pancreatic exocrine tumors and the inability of erlotinib to target tumors successfully that have such mutations further limit the value of the gemcitabine-erlotinib combination in advanced disease. Consequently, chemotherapy treatment for patients with advanced disease generally focuses on gemcitabine given alone or with a platinum agent, erlotinib in *KRAS* wild-type tumors, or a fluoropyrimidine (Heinemann, Boeck, Hinke, Labianca, & Louvet, 2008).

Multimodality Therapy

Questions regarding the optimal approach using chemotherapy, perhaps combined with radiation, led to the development of a randomized controlled trial comparing gemcitabine plus concurrent radiation therapy with gemcitabine alone for locally advanced unresectable disease. Close to 35% of patients are found with locally advanced disease at time of original presentation; therefore, the need for effective therapies focused on this stage of disease is critical. This randomized trial was led by the Eastern Cooperative Oncology Group (ECOG) but had to be stopped early because of poor accrual—only 74 patients of the planned 316 were enrolled. Despite this limitation of the small sample size, overall survival was found to be superior in the group randomized to receive chemoradiation compared to gemcitabine alone (11.1 months versus 9.2 months; p = 0.017) (Loehrer et al., 2011). Although increased rates of more severe toxicities were observed in the chemoradiation arm, overall toxicities and quality-of-life measures were not significantly different between the two groups, indicating that the combination regimen that produced the improved survival was also reasonably well tolerated.

Nursing Implications

The inability to answer a vital question related to optimal therapy for pancreatic cancer because of inadequate study enrollment, such as that which occurred with the ECOG trial, raises concerns about how best to address a fundamental gap in the literature. Nurses may encourage patients to identify and participate in clinical trials for which they are eligible that might directly benefit their own care, or care of others in the future, by stressing the importance of clinical trials designed to treat exocrine tumors of the pancreas.

Healthcare providers may need to keep in mind that the vast majority of patients diagnosed with and treated for exocrine tumors of the pancreas are relatively old. In addition to their age, these patients may be recovering from extensive surgical resection and may be dealing with multiple comorbid conditions, including diabetes, fatigue, digestion dysfunction, and some degree of frailty. Thus, the common side effects experienced with cytotoxic chemotherapy that are more readily tolerated by younger, healthier populations, particularly gastrointestinal toxicities (e.g., nausea, vomiting, diarrhea), may represent a huge challenge to patients who recently underwent a risky pancreatic resection and are coping with postoperative complications (Jacobs et al., 2009).

Nurses serve as the prime educators for patients and their families prior to initiating radiation therapy, chemotherapy, or combination chemoradiation therapy (Sun, 2010). The need for excellent communication among all care providers and patients is essential for accurate assessment of patients' status as these individuals attempt to navigate the physical and emotional difficulties resulting from treatment with surgery, chemotherapy, or chemoradiation. Some patients will have been recently diagnosed with diabetes and will be in the process of trying to manage this chronic, serious condition on top of the toxicity profile generated by chemotherapy or chemoradiation therapy (Coleman, 1996). Nurses should be particularly focused on appropriate referrals, if needed (e.g., to an endocrinologist for diabetes management).

Supportive and Palliative Care

Despite the best efforts in medical science to make advances in treating pancreatic exocrine tumors, the long-term outcomes in this disease remain dismal. Overall, less than 5% of patients will survive more than five years from the time of diagnosis. Thus, much of the nursing care directed toward patients with this diagnosis will be delivered as symptom management and palliative care (McEwen, Sanchez, Rosario, & Allen, 1996). In addition to the gastrointestinal symptoms previously discussed, patients diagnosed with pancreatic cancer also experience a high incidence of pain, fatigue, and mood disorders, including depression (Alter, 1996). Depression may be exhibited in this population at higher rates than found in other cancers and may be independent of pain or manifestations of other psychological distress. Patients' depression in the palliative care setting should be managed with pharmacologic interventions as well as with supportive psychotherapy.

Pain represents a common problem requiring symptom management in patients with pancreatic cancer, with incidence rates cited as high as 70%–80% at the time of diagnosis (Yan & Myers, 2007). Opioids are commonly given as first-line pain management, but their efficacy in pain control may vary, even with high doses (Michaels & Draganov,

2007). For opioid-resistant pancreatic cancer pain, more invasive techniques may be pursued. Celiac plexus block (CPB) and celiac plexus neurolysis (CPN) have been used for decades to reduce narcotic use, increase pain control, and improve quality of life (Gunaratnam, Sarma, Norton, & Wiersema, 2001). A CPB is a nerve block of the abdominal celiac plexus of nerves, generated through injection of a local anesthetic, occasionally accompanied by a steroid, epinephrine, or other compounds to prolong the CPB effects (Allen et al., 2011). With CPN, neurolytic substances, such as absolute alcohol, are injected into the area of the celiac ganglia, causing permanent ablation of neural tissue, thus controlling pain (Yan & Myers, 2007).

Earlier interventions used posterior percutaneous or intraoperative approaches to CPN, which were associated with a small but calculated risk of about 1% for serious complications, such as paralysis and paresthesia of the lower extremities (Eisenberg, Carr, & Chalmers, 1995). Currently, EUS-guided CPN (EUS-CPN) is more commonly used, and with this technique, the target nerves can be more accurately located, allowing for greater safety in delivery of neurolysis and reduced adverse events (Levy et al., 2008). A meta-analysis by Puli, Reddy, Bechtold, Antillon, and Brugge (2009) reported that CPN resulted in pain reduction in approximately 80% of the patients in the studies reviewed. A recent randomized, double-blind, controlled clinical trial of EUS-CPN performed at the time of diagnosis with early pain management compared to standard opioid pain management demonstrated that early use of EUS-CPN resulted in improved pain scores but did not affect overall quality of life or survival (Wyse, Carone, Paquin, Usatii, & Sahai, 2011).

In view of the high proportion of patients who will present with unresectable tumors or disease that is already systemic at the time of diagnosis, many individuals will benefit from hospice referral early in their care continuum. The median survival of patients with advanced metastatic disease is only about 10 weeks (Bruno, Haverkort, Tijssen, Tytgat, & van Leeuwen, 1998). Palliative care, although not necessarily extending survival, affects quality of life and can provide improved symptom management. Symptoms that may require intervention include gastric outlet obstruction, jaundice, pain, and weight loss.

Nutritional needs in the palliative care setting are particularly important for patients with advanced pancreatic cancer. About 90% of patients will have experienced significant weight loss by the time they are diagnosed. The many digestive problems that occur as a result of the tumor's anatomic location or resection of the cancer contribute further to weight loss concerns. Initial nutritional problems can lead to documented malignancy-associated cachexia, which in turn can result in death (Ellison et al., 2002). A careful nutritional assessment at baseline and during the course of the disease may aid in designing the optimal intervention for nutritional management. Although nutritional therapy is unlikely to extend survival, specific interventions (e.g., hyperalimentation, administration of nutritional supplements) may benefit patients with advanced pancreatic cancer by improving their quality of life.

Patients who have undergone pancreatectomy or who experience exocrine pancreatic insufficiency require pancreatic enzyme replacement therapy to assist with digestion and address nutritional insufficiencies (Dhanasekaran & Toskes, 2010). Although pancreatic enzymes had been previously exempted from U.S. Food and Drug Administration (FDA) review and were available for many years, the FDA set a deadline of April 2010 for the makers of all pancreatic enzyme products to distribute only FDA-approved products (Bobo, 2010). As of March 2012, the FDA had approved a total of five pancreatic enzyme products designed to aid in food digestion: (a) Ultresa® (2012), (b) Viokace® (2012), (c) Pancreaze® (2010), (d) Creon® (2009), and (e) Zenpep® (2009) (Yao, 2012). These pancrelipases, derived from porcine pancreatic extract, all contain lipases, proteases, and amylases needed for digestion (Giuliano, Dehoorne-Smith, & Kale-Pradhan, 2011).

Summary

Pancreatic exocrine tumors continue to represent an almost universally fatal disease, with very limited five-year survival even when found at an early stage. Multidisciplinary approaches to care of this disease have contributed significantly to progress in diagnosis and treatment, and nurses represent critical components of the multidisciplinary care team. Nursing plays an important role in assessment and recognition of imprecise symptoms at the time of initial presentation; in diagnosis and staging of disease; in the delivery of surgical, radiation, chemotherapy, and combined-modality therapies; and in evaluation of associated outcomes. Nurses are pivotal in the extensive patient and family caregiver education required for management of this complex disease and the symptoms that manifest because of cancer and its treatment. Nurses in varied settings provide crucial referrals to high-volume centers for optimal therapy at the time of initial diagnosis, to clinical trials as potential treatment options, or to palliative care teams or hospice programs early in the continuum of advanced disease.

Opportunities abound from which to make continued progress in the understanding of the underlying etiology of pancreatic exocrine tumors, to identify new biomarkers for early detection, to learn more about familial and genetic aspects of patients and families considered at high risk for the disease, to be able to predict pancreatic cancer risk and prognosis following specific interventions, and to participate in efforts to devise interventions that improve survival while also reducing toxicity. Nurses are in prime positions to reduce and control symptoms, offer palliative relief from pain and suffering, and provide expert counsel regarding nutritional support. Oncology nurses, in particular, are well poised to enhance quality of life throughout the entire continuum of care and improve important patient-centered outcomes in pancreatic exocrine tumors.

References

Allen, P.J., Chou, J., Janakos, M., Strong, V.E., Coit, D.G., & Brennan, M.F. (2011). Prospective evaluation of laparoscopic celiac plexus block in patients with unresectable pancreatic adenocarcinoma. *Annals of Surgical Oncology, 18,* 636–641. doi:10.1245/s10434-010-1372-x

Alter, C.L. (1996). Palliative and supportive care of patients with pancreatic cancer. *Seminars in Oncology, 23,* 229–240.

American Cancer Society. (2011). *Cancer facts and figures for African Americans 2011–2012.* Atlanta, GA: Author.

American Cancer Society. (2012). *Cancer facts and figures 2012.* Atlanta, GA: Author.

Bassi, C., Falconi, M., Salvia, R., Mascetta, G., Molinari, E., & Pederzoli, P. (2001). Management of complications after pancreaticoduodenectomy in a high volume centre: Results on 150 consecutive patients. *Digestive Surgery, 18,* 453–457. doi:10.1159/000050193

Bobo, E.G. (2010, April 12). FDA approves pancreatic enzyme product, Pancreaze [Press release]. Retrieved from http://www.fda.gov/NewsEvents/Newsroom/PressAnnouncements/2010/ucm208135.htm

Boeck, S., Stieber, P., Holdenrieder, S., Wilkowski, R., & Heinemann, V. (2006). Prognostic and therapeutic significance of carbohydrate antigen 19-9 as tumor marker in patients with pancreatic cancer. *Oncology, 70,* 255–264. doi:10.1159/000094888

Bracci, P.M., Wang, F., Hassan, M.M., Gupta, S., Li, D., & Holly, E.A. (2009). Pancreatitis and pancreatic cancer in two large pooled case-control studies. *Cancer Causes and Control, 20,* 1723–1731. doi:10.1007/s10552-009-9424-x

Bruno, M.J., Haverkort, E.B., Tijssen, G.P., Tytgat, G.N., & van Leeuwen, D.J. (1998). Placebo controlled trial of enteric coated pancreatin microsphere treatment in patients with unresectable cancer of the pancreas head region. *Gut, 42,* 92–96. doi:10.1136/gut.42.1.92

Burris, H.A., III, Moore, M.J., Andersen, J., Green, M.R., Rothenberg, M.L., Modiano, M.R., ... Von Hoff, D.D. (1997). Improvements in survival and clinical benefit with gemcitabine as first-line therapy for patients with advanced pancreas cancer: A randomized trial. *Journal of Clinical Oncology, 15,* 2403–2413.

Callery, M.P., Chang, K.J., Fishman, E.K., Talamonti, M.S., Traverso, L., & Linehan, D.C. (2009). Pretreatment assessment of resectable and borderline resectable pancreatic cancer: Expert consensus statement. *Annals of Surgical Oncology, 16,* 1727–1733. doi:10.1245/s10434-009-0408-6

Castellanos, E.H., Cardin, D.B., & Berlin, J.D. (2011). Treatment of early-stage pancreatic cancer. *Oncology, 25,* 182–189.

Chari, S.T., Leibson, C.L., Rabe, K.G., Ransom, J., de Andrade, M., & Petersen, G.M. (2005). Probability of pancreatic cancer following diabetes: A population-based study. *Gastroenterology, 129,* 504–511.

Coleman, J. (1996). Supportive management of the patient with pancreatic cancer: Role of the oncology nurse. *Oncology, 10*(Suppl. 9), 23–25.

Crane, C.H., Winter, K., Regine, W.F., Safran, H., Rich, T.A., Curran, W., ... Willett, C.G. (2009). Phase II study of bevacizumab with concurrent capecitabine and radiation followed by maintenance gemcitabine and bevacizumab for locally advanced pancreatic cancer. Radiation Therapy Oncology Group RTOG 0411. *Journal of Clinical Oncology, 27,* 4096–4102. doi:10.1200/JCO.2009.21.8529

Crippa, S., Bassi, C., Warshaw, A.L., Falconi, M., Partelli, S., Thayer, S.P., ... Fernández-del Castillo, C. (2007). Middle pancreatectomy: Indications, short- and long-term operative outcomes. *Annals of Surgery, 246,* 69–76. doi:10.1097/01.sla.0000262790.51512.57

DeWitt, J., Deereaux, B., Chriswell, M., McGreevey, K., Howard, T., Imperiale, T.F., ... Sherman, S. (2004). Comparison of endoscopic ultrasonography and multidetector computed tomography for detecting and staging pancreatic cancer. *Annals of Internal Medicine, 141,* 753–763.

Dhanasekaran, R., & Toskes, P.P. (2010). Pancrelipase for pancreatic disorders: An update. *Drugs Today, 46,* 855–866. doi:10.1358/dot.2010.46.11.1541553

Eisenberg, E., Carr, D.B., & Chalmers, T.C. (1995). Neurolytic celiac plexus block for treatment of cancer pain: A meta-analysis. *Anesthesia and Analgesia, 80,* 290–295. Retrieved from http://www.anesthesia-analgesia.org/content/80/2/290.long

Ellison, N.M., Chevlen, E., Still, C.D., & Dubagunta, S. (2002). Supportive care for patients with pancreatic adenocarcinoma: Symptom control and nutrition. *Hematology/Oncology Clinics of North America, 16,* 105–121. doi:10.1016/S0889-8588(01)00006-5

Everhart, J., & Wright, D. (1995). Diabetes mellitus as a risk factor for pancreatic cancer. A meta-analysis. *JAMA, 273,* 1605–1609. doi:10.1001/jama.1995.03520440059037

Farrow, B., & Evers, B.M. (2002). Inflammation and the development of pancreatic cancer. *Surgical Oncology, 10,* 153–169. doi:10.1016/S0960-7404(02)00015-4

Gapstur, S.M., Gann, P.H., Lowe, W., Liu, K., Colangelo, L., & Dyer, A. (2000). Abnormal glucose metabolism and pancreatic cancer mortality. *JAMA, 283,* 2552–2558. doi:10.1001/jama.283.19.2552

Gillen, S., Schuster, T., Meyer Zum Büschenfelde, C., Friess, H., & Kleeff, J. (2010). Preoperative/neoadjuvant therapy in pancreatic cancer: A systematic review and meta-analysis of response and resection percentages. *PLOS Medicine, 7,* e1000267. doi:10.1371/journal.pmed.1000267

Giuliano, C.A., Dehoorne-Smith, M.L., & Kale-Pradhan, P.B. (2011). Pancreatic enzyme products: Digesting the changes. *Annals of Pharmacotherapy, 45,* 658–666. doi:10.1345/aph.1P770

Gooiker, G.A., van Gijn, W., Wouters, M.W., Post, P.N., van de Velde, C.J., Tollenaar, R.A., & Signalling Committee Cancer of the Dutch Cancer Society. (2011). Systematic review and meta-analysis of the volume-outcome relationship in pancreatic surgery. *British Journal of Surgery, 98,* 485–494. doi:10.1002/bjs.7413

Grahm, A.L., & Andrén-Sandberg, A. (1997). Prospective evaluation of pain in exocrine pancreatic cancer. *Digestion, 58,* 542–549.

Gullo, L., Pezzilli, R., & Morselli-Labate, A.M. (1994). Diabetes and the risk of pancreatic cancer. *New England Journal of Medicine, 331,* 81–84. doi:10.1056/NEJM199407143310203

Gunaratnam, N.T., Sarma, A.V., Norton, I.D., & Wiersema, M.J. (2001). A prospective study of EUS-guided celiac plexus neurolysis for pancreatic cancer pain. *Gastrointestinal Endoscopy, 54,* 316–324.

Halfdanarson, T.R., Rabe, K.G., Rubin, J., & Petersen, G.M. (2008). Pancreatic neuroendocrine tumors (PNETs): Incidence, prognosis and recent trend toward improved survival. *Annals of Oncology, 19,* 1727–1733. doi:10.1093/annonc/mdn351

Hassan, M.M., Bondy, M.L., Wolff, R.A., Abbruzzese, J.L., Vauthey, J.N., Pisters, P.W., ... Li, D. (2007). Risk factors for pancreatic cancer: Case-control study. *American Journal of Gastroenterology, 102,* 2696–2707. doi:10.1111/j.1572-0241.2007.01510.x

Heinemann, V., Boeck, S., Hinke, A., Labianca, R., & Louvet, C. (2008). Meta-analysis of randomized trials: Evaluation of benefit from gemcitabine-based combination chemotherapy applied in advanced pancreatic cancer. *BMC Cancer, 8,* 82–92. doi:10.1186/1471-2407-8-82

Hidalgo, M. (2010). Pancreatic cancer. *New England Journal of Medicine, 362,* 1605–1617. doi:10.1056/NEJMra0901557

Hruban, R.H., Canto, M.I., & Yeo, C.J. (2001). Prevention of pancreatic cancer and strategies for management of familial pancreatic cancer. *Digestive Diseases, 19,* 76–84. doi:10.1159/000050656

Hsu, C., & Saif, M.W. (2011). Diabetes and pancreatic cancer. Highlights from the 2011 ASCO Annual Meeting. Chicago, IL, USA; June 3–7, 2011. *JOP: Journal of the Pancreas, 12,* 330–333. Retrieved from http://www.joplink.net/prev/201107/28.html

Huggett, M.T., & Pereira, S.P. (2011). Diagnosing and managing pancreatic cancer. *Practitioner, 255,* 21–25.

Jacobs, N.L., Que, F.G., Miller, R.C., Vege, S.S., Farnell, M.B., & Jatoi, A. (2009). Cumulative morbidity and late mortality in long-term survivors of exocrine pancreas cancer. *Journal of Gastrointestinal Cancer, 40,* 45–50. doi:10.1007/s12029-009-9082-y

Kahl, S., & Malferheiner, P. (2004). Exocrine and endocrine pancreatic insufficiency after pancreatic surgery. *Best Practice and Research Clinical Gastroenterology, 18,* 947–955. doi:10.1016/j.bpg.2004.06.028

Kooby, D.A., Gillespie, T.W., Bentrem, D., Nakeeb, A., Schmidt, M.C., Merchant, N.B., ... Hawkins, W.G. (2008). Left-sided pancreatectomy: A multicenter comparison of laparoscopic and open approaches. *Annals of Surgery, 248,* 438–446. doi:10.1097/SLA.0b013e318185a990

Krech, R.L., & Walsh, D. (1991). Symptoms of pancreatic cancer. *Journal of Pain and Symptom Management, 6,* 360–367. doi:10.1016/0885-3924(91)90027-2

Kudo, Y., Kamisawa, T., Anjiki, H., Takuma, K., & Egawa, N. (2011). Incidence of and risk factors for developing pancreatic cancer in patients with chronic pancreatitis. *Hepato-Gastroenterology, 58,* 609–611.

Levy, M.J., Topazian, M.D., Wiersema, M.J., Clain, J.E., Rajan, E., Wang, K.K., ... Chari, S.T. (2008). Initial evaluation of the efficacy and safety of endoscopic ultrasound-guided direct ganglia neurolysis and block. *American Journal of Gastroenterology, 103,* 98–103. doi:10.1111/j.1572-0241.2007.01607.x

Loehrer, P.H., Sr., Feng, Y., Cardenes, H., Wagner, L., Brell, J.M., Cella, D., ... Benson, A.B., III. (2011). Gemcitabine alone versus gemcitabine plus radiotherapy in patients with locally advanced pancreatic cancer: An Eastern Cooperative Oncology Group trial. *Journal of Clinical Oncology, 29,* 4105–4112. doi:10.1200/JCO.2011.34.8904

Loos, M., Kleeff, J., Friess, H., & Büchler, M.W. (2008). Surgical treatment of pancreatic cancer. *Annals of the New York Academy of Sciences, 1138,* 169–180. doi:10.1196/annals.1414.024

Lowenfels, A.B., & Maisonneuve, P. (2004). Epidemiology and prevention of pancreatic cancer. *Journal of Clinical Oncology, 34,* 238–244.

McEwen, D.R., Sanchez, M.M., Rosario, A., & Allen, W.E. (1996). Managing patients with pancreatic cancer. *AORN Journal, 64,* 716–735. doi:10.1016/S0001-2092(06)63261-4

Michaels, A.J., & Draganov, P.V. (2007). Endoscopic ultrasonography guided celiac plexus neurolysis and celiac plexus block in the management of pain due to pancreatic cancer and chronic pancreatitis. *World Journal of Gastroenterology, 13,* 3575–3580. Retrieved from http://www.wjgnet.com/1007-9327/full/v13/i26/3575.htm

Miura, F., Takada, T., Amano, H., Yoshida, M., Furui, S., & Takeshita, K. (2006). Diagnosis of pancreatic cancer. *HPB, 8,* 337–342. doi:10.1080/13651820500540949

Moertel, C.C. (1976). Chemotherapy of gastrointestinal cancer. *Clinical Gastroenterology, 5,* 777–793.

Moore, M.J., Goldstein, D., Hamm, J., Figer, A., Hecht, J.R., Gallinger, S., ... Parulekar, W. (2007). Erlotinib plus gemcitabine compared with gemcitabine alone in patients with advanced pancreatic cancer: A phase III trial of the National Cancer Institute of Canada Clinical Trials Group. *Journal of Clinical Oncology, 25,* 1960–1966. doi:10.1200/JCO.2006.07.9525

Morrison, M. (2010). Post-pancreatic resection. General overview and unique complications. *Dimensions of Critical Care Nursing, 29,* 157–162. doi:10.1097/DCC.0b013e3181de95dc

National Comprehensive Cancer Network. (2012). *NCCN Clinical Practice Guidelines in Oncology: Pancreatic adenocarcinoma* [v. 2.2012]. Retrieved from http://www.nccn.org/professionals/physician_gls/pdf/pancreatic.pdf

Ogawa, Y., Tanaka, M., Inoue, K., Yamaguchi, K., Chijiiwa, K., Mizumoto, K., ... Nakamura, Y. (2002). A prospective pancreatographic study of the prevalence of pancreatic carcinoma in patients with diabetes mellitus. *Cancer, 94,* 2344–2349. doi:10.1002/cncr.10493

Park, Y.C., Kim, S.W., Jang, J.Y., Ahn, Y.J., & Park, Y.H. (2003). Factors influencing delayed gastric emptying after pylorus-preserving pancreaticoduodenectomy. *Journal of the American College of Surgeons, 196,* 859–865. doi:10.1016/S1072-7515(03)00127-3

Pavlidis, T.E., Pavlidis, E.T., & Sakantamis, A.K. (2011). Current opinion on lymphadenectomy in pancreatic cancer surgery. *Hepatobiliary and Pancreatic Diseases International, 10,* 21–25. doi:10.1016/S1499-3872(11)60002-7

Perez, E.A., Gutierrez, J.C., Koniaris, L.G., Neville, H.L., Thompson, W.R., & Sola, J.E. (2009). Malignant pancreatic tumors: Incidence and outcome in 58 pediatric patients. *Journal of Pediatric Surgery, 44,* 197–203. doi:10.1016/j.jpedsurg.2008.10.039

Permert, J., Ihse, I., Jorfeldt, L., von Schenck, H., Arnqvist, H.J., & Larsson, J. (1993). Pancreatic cancer is associated with impaired glucose metabolism. *European Journal of Surgery, 159,* 101–107.

Pernick, N.L., Sarkar, F.H., & Philip, P.A. (2003). Clinicopatholgic analysis of pancreatic adenocarcinoma in African Americans and Caucasians. *Pancreas, 26,* 28–32. doi:10.1097/00006676-200301000-00006

Puli, S.R., Reddy, J.B., Bechtold, M.L., Antillon, M.R., & Brugge, W.R. (2009). EUS-guided celiac plexus neurolysis for pain due to chronic pancreatitis or pancreatic cancer pain: A meta-analysis and systematic review. *Digestive Diseases and Sciences, 54,* 2330–2337. doi:10.1007/s10620-008-0651-x

Raimondi, S., Lowenfels, A.B., Morselli-Labate, A.M., Maisonneuve, P., & Pezzilli, R. (2010). Pancreatic cancer in chronic pancreatitis: Aetiology, incidence, and early detection. *Best Practice and Research Clinical Gastroenterology, 24,* 349–358. doi:10.1016/j.bpg.2010.02.007

Raut, C.P., Tseng, J.F., Sun, C.C., Wang, H., Wolff, R.A., Crane, C.H., ... Evans, D.B. (2007). Impact of resection status on pattern of failure and survival after pancreaticoduodenectomy for pancreatic adenocarcinoma. *Annals of Surgery, 246,* 52–60. doi:10.1097/01.sla.0000259391.84304.2b

Rieder, H., Sina-Frey, M., Ziegler, A., Hahn, S.A., Przypadlo, E., Kress, R., ... Bartsch, D.K. (2002). German national case collection of familial pancreatic cancer—Clinical-genetic analysis of the first 21 families. *Onkologie, 25,* 262–266. doi:10.1159/000064320

Sener, S.F., Fremgen, A., Menck, H.R., & Winchester, D.P. (1999). Pancreatic cancer: A report of treatment and survival trends for 100,313 patients diagnosed from 1985–1995, using the National Cancer Database. *Journal of the American College of Surgeons, 189,* 1–7. doi:10.1016/S1072-7515(99)00075-7

Sharma, C., Eltawil, K.M., Renfrew, P.D., Walsh, M.J., & Molinari, M. (2011). Advances in diagnosis, treatment and palliation of pancreatic carcinoma: 1990–2010. *World Journal of Gastroenterology, 17,* 867–897. doi:10.3748/wjg.v17.i7.867

Shi, C., Hruban, R.H., & Klein, A.P. (2009). Familial pancreatic cancer. *Archives of Pathology and Laboratory Medicine, 133,* 365–374.

Sultana, A., Smith, C., Cunningham, D., Starling, N., Tait, D., Neoptolemos, J.P., & Ghaneh, P. (2007). Systematic review, including meta-analyses, on the management of locally advanced pancreatic cancer using radiation/combined modality therapy. *British Journal of Cancer, 96,* 1183–1190. doi:10.1038/sj.bjc.6603719

Sun, V. (2010). Update on pancreatic cancer treatment. *Nurse Practitioner, 25,* 16–22. doi:10.1097/01.NPR.0000383949.48853.8f

Tersmette, A.C., Petersen, G.M., Offerhaus, G.J., Falatko, F.C., Brune, K.A., Goggins, M., ... Hruban, R.H. (2001). Increased risk of incident pancreatic cancer among first-degree relatives of patients with familiar pancreatic cancer. *Clinical Cancer Research, 7,* 738–744.

Trede, M. (1993). *Surgery of the pancreas.* Edinburgh, Scotland: Churchill Livingstone.

van der Gaag, N.A., Klock, J.J., de Castro, S.M., Busch, O.R., van Gulik, T.M., & Gouma, D.J. (2009). Preoperative biliary drainage in patients with obstructive jaundice: History and current status. *Journal of Gastrointestinal Surgery, 13,* 814–820. doi:10.1007/s11605-008-0618-4

van der Gaag, N.A., Rauws, E.A., van Eijck, C.H., Bruno, M.J., van der Harst, E., Kubben, F.J., ... Gouma, D.J. (2010). Preoperative biliary drainage for cancer of the head of the pancreas. *New England Journal of Medicine, 362,* 129–137. doi:10.1056/NEJMoa0903230

Wang, W., Chen, S., Brune, K.A., Hruban, R.H., Parigiani, G., & Klein, A.P. (2007). PancPRO: Risk assessment for individuals with a family history of pancreatic cancer. *Journal of Clinical Oncology, 25,* 1417–1422. doi:10.1200/JCO.2006.09.2452

Wideroff, L., Gridle, G., Mellemkjaer, L., Chow, W.H., Linet, M., Keehn, S., ... Olsen, J.H. (1997). Cancer incidence in a population-based cohort of patients hospitalized with diabetes mellitus in Denmark. *Journal of the National Cancer Institute, 89,* 1360–1365. doi:10.1093/jnci/89.18.1360

Wolpin, B.M., Chan, A.T., Hartge, P., Chanock, S.J., Kraft, P., Hunter, D.J., ... Fuchs, C.S. (2009). ABO blood group and the risk of pancreatic cancer. *Journal of the National Cancer Institute, 18,* 424–431. doi:10.1093/jnci/djp020

Wyse, J.M., Carone, M., Paquin, S.C., Usatii, M., & Sahai, A.V. (2011). Randomized, double-blind, controlled trial of early endoscopic ultrasound-guided celiac plexus neurolysis to prevent pain progression in patients with newly diagnosed, painful, inoperable pancreatic cancer. *Journal of Clinical Oncology, 29,* 3541–3546. doi:10.1200/JCO.2010.32.2750

Yan, B.M., & Myers, R.P. (2007). Neurolytic celiac plexus block for pain control in unresectable pancreatic cancer. *American Journal of Gastroenterology, 102,* 430–438. doi:10.1111/j.1572-0241.2006.00967.x

Yao, S. (2012, March 1). FDA approves two new pancreatic enzyme products to aid food digestion [Press release]. Retrieved from http://www.fda.gov/NewsEvents/Newsroom/PressAnnouncements/ucm294143.htm

Zavoral, M., Minarikova, P., Zavada, F., Salek, C., & Minarik, M. (2011). Molecular biology of pancreatic cancer. *World Journal of Gastroenterology, 17,* 2897–2908. doi:10.3748/wjg.v17.i24.2897

Zhou, J., Eneworld, L., Stojadinovic, A., Clifton, G.T., Potter, J.F., Peoples, G.E., & Zhu, K. (2010). Incidence rates of exocrine and endocrine pancreatic cancers in the United States. *Cancer Causes and Control, 21,* 853–861. doi:10.1007/s10552-010-9512-y

CHAPTER 3

Pancreatic Endocrine Tumors

Lisa M. Wall, RN, PhD, AOCNS®, and Elizabeth Cruz, RN, BSN, OCN®

Introduction

As the eighth most frequent cause of cancer death worldwide, cancers of the pancreas claim the lives of approximately 227,000 individuals each year (Jemal et al., 2011). Almost 85% of pancreatic cancers develop from the ductal cells and manifest as ductal adenocarcinomas (Morgan & Adams, 2010). These tumors are aggressive in nature and account for the dismal overall survival rates. Pancreatic endocrine tumor (PET) is by far a less common cancer that arises from different cells known as islet cells. They make up approximately 2%–3% of all cancers of the pancreas (Capelli et al., 2009). Most PETs progress slowly and have a more favorable prognosis when compared to the more aggressive adenocarcinoma. PETs affect both men and women with a slight female predominance and present most commonly in adults between the ages of 40 and 60 years old (Klöppel & Heitz, 1988). They can occur sporadically or be hereditary. Sporadic PETs usually present as a solitary lesion, whereas those related to hereditary syndromes are frequently multifocal. Hereditary forms are very rare and part of hereditary syndromes, such as the multiple endocrine neoplasia type 1 (known as MEN-1) or von Hippel-Lindau syndrome (Capelli et al., 2009). There are no other known environmental risk factors.

Classification Systems

PETs can grow in any part of the pancreas. They usually present as solid, solitary, round masses that are 1–5 cm in size and tend to be vascular in nature. Because PETs are rare and heterogeneous tumors, different systems are used to categorize them to better define prognosis and treatment. The World Health Organization (WHO) defines malignant PETs by their histologic features as either well-differentiated neoplasms or poorly differentiated carcinomas (Solcia, Klöppel, & Sobin, 2000). More than 90% of PETs are well-differentiated tumors and are classified as low or intermediate grade. Well-differentiated PETs grow slowly over years and respond well to some treatments; patients can often live for years even in the setting of bulky metastatic disease. In contrast, poorly differentiated tumors are high-grade cancers that are aggressive, progress rapidly, and are generally managed with platinum chemotherapy (Klimstra et al., 2010).

Endocrine neoplasms of the digestive system vary biologically depending on the anatomic site of origin. A variety of different organ-specific systems have been developed for nomenclature, grading, and staging of neuroendocrine tumors (NETs), causing much confusion. Recently, however, a new proposal for grading and staging NETs has been published (Klimstra et al., 2010; Rindi et al., 2006). The updated WHO classification is one that proposes staging NETs as follows: well-differentiated (either low or intermediate grade) and poorly differentiated neuroendocrine carcinoma. Low grade is defined as less than 2 mitoses/10 high-power field (HPF) or a Ki-67 protein score less than 3%. Intermediate grade is defined as 2–20 mitoses/10 HPF or a Ki-67 score of 3%–20% (Klimstra et al., 2010).

PETs are also classified as "functioning" or "nonfunctioning" depending on the presence or absence of clinical symptoms related to hormone hypersecretion. Tumors can express hormones excreted by the pancreas (e.g., insulin, glucagon, somatostatin) or hormones produced by other organs (e.g., gastrin, adrenocorticotropic hormone) (Ekeblad, 2010). Although these hormones can be debilitating, they are not incorporated into the staging system.

Survival rates vary greatly depending on the tumor, node, metastasis (TNM) stage and grade of the tumor. In their retrospective study of 274 consecutive patients who underwent surgical resection of PETs, Scarpa and colleagues (2010) reported a 10-year survival rate of 91% for small and localized tumors, whereas node-positive and metastatic disease yielded 10-year survival rates of 20% or less. Casadei and colleagues (2009) examined the value of the WHO and

TNM classification systems for patients with PETs. They followed 76 patients and found that patients with tumors smaller than 4 cm had better survival compared with patients with tumors larger than 4 cm ($p = 0.024$). Increased risk of death was associated with T4 tumors or those that invaded adjacent structures ($p < 0.001$), tumors with positive nodal status (N1) ($p = 0.005$), and those with distant metastasis (M1) ($p < 0.001$). In using the WHO classification system, Casadei and colleagues (2009) reported increased risk of death in patients with poorly differentiated neoplasms compared to those with well-differentiated neoplasms ($p < 0.001$). Finally, they found overall survival rates of 79.5%, 69.4%, and 63.5% at 5, 10, and 15 years, respectively, with a mean overall survival of 19.2 ± 1.5 years.

Types of Pancreatic Endocrine Tumors and Clinical Presentation

The incidence of nonfunctional (i.e., non–hormone producing) endocrine tumors was originally thought to be less than 30%; however, the incidence is greatly increasing, in part because of increased imaging and surveillance endoscopy (Jani, Moser, & Khalid, 2007; Yao, Phan, & Chang, 2007). Most nonfunctional PETs are found incidentally because their presenting symptoms are nonspecific, such as nausea and abdominal pain, and they tend to be larger than functional tumors (4–10 cm). Functional tumors are commonly associated with a clinical syndrome or symptoms related to the hormone emitted by the tumor. The most common type of PET functional tumor is the insulinoma, which secretes insulin or proinsulin and causes hypoglycemia (Capelli et al., 2009; Ekeblad, 2010). Symptoms of hypoglycemic syndrome include confusion, blurred or double vision, agitation, seizures, tachycardia, and coma. Symptoms frequently appear during fasting or exercise, and patients are commonly obese. Insulinomas are benign 90% of the time and usually present as solitary tumors. The second most frequent type of functional PET is the gastrinoma (Capelli et al., 2009; Ekeblad, 2010). The anatomic area near the common bile duct, duodenum, and pancreatic head is the most common location for gastrinomas. In about 80% of cases, these tumors are malignant and frequently present with liver metastases. Because these tumors produce gastrin, symptoms include gastroesophageal reflux disease, diarrhea, malabsorption, and peptic ulcers. Patients with gastrinoma need to be screened carefully for a family history of other endocrine cancers or a personal history of other endocrinopathies because they are at high risk for the hereditary MEN-1 syndrome. Other types of functional PETs are glucagonomas, VIPomas (tumors that secrete vasoactive intestinal peptide), somatostatinomas, and ectopic hormone-producing PETs (Capelli et al., 2009) (see Table 3-1).

Diagnostic Testing

Biochemical and Tissue Markers

Tumor markers are substances that are produced and released by tumor cells and are reflective of tumor activity. Depending on the PET type, tumors release certain proteins or hormones that may be helpful in the diagnosis and evaluation of the disease. Their value as tumor markers is usually measured by their sensitivity and specificity. *Sensitivity* refers to the percent of time an abnormal result correlates to the disease, and *specificity* refers to the percent of time a normal result accurately reflects the absence of disease.

The two most common markers for endocrine carcinomas are chromogranin A (CgA) and 5-hydroxy-indol acetic acid (5-HIAA) (Arnold et al., 2009; Capelli et al., 2009) (see Table 3-2). CgA is a protein found in the plasma and is a reflection of tumor mass and spread. Laboratory values for CgA may also be used to assess the rate of tumor growth and are useful in patients with functional and nonfunctional endocrine tumors. Normal CgA blood levels are less than 39 ng/L and can rise into the thousands in cases with great tumor burden. The sensitivity of the CgA test is about 80%, and its specificity is about 95% (Capelli et al., 2009). Serotonin is a hormone released by endocrine tumors and can be detected in urine using the 5-HIAA 24-hour urine test. High levels of 5-HIAA are most commonly associated with endocrine tumors that occur outside the pancreas (carcinoid tumors). The 5-HIAA urine test can positively detect carcinoid tumors that have metastasized to the liver more than 70% of the time. Diet, medications, and comorbidities can affect both markers and produce a false-positive test result. For example, CgA may be elevated in patients with renal insufficiency and in patients who are taking proton pump inhibitors. Similarly, 5-HIAA may be altered by the intake of certain types of foods, such as caffeine, alcohol, bananas, and tomatoes (Joy, Walsh, Tokmakejian, & Van Uum, 2008). Patients should be given instructions regarding the foods and medicines they should avoid before testing for these markers, and clinicians must consider influential factors that may alter results (see Table 3-2).

High levels of serum hormones as identified in Table 3-1 are related to functional PETs and can be used as tumor markers. Nonfunctional PETs also release hormones whose levels increase in relation to tumor activity. PETs may also express trypsin, a marker of acinar differentiation, which is helpful in diagnosing a mixed acinar-endocrine carcinoma (Capelli et al., 2009). Neuron-specific enolase and pancreatic polypeptide are two other markers that are investigational. Higher levels may be associated with a more aggressive PET.

Table 3-1. Types and Characteristics of Functional Pancreatic Endocrine Tumors			
Type	**Hormone**	**Symptoms**	**Characteristics**
Insulinoma	Insulin	Hunger, confusion, agitation, blurred vision, tachycardia, seizures, coma	Most common functional pancreatic endocrine tumor Small in size Benign in 90% of cases
Gastrinoma	Gastrin	Abdominal pain due to peptic ulcer, diarrhea and reflux esophagitis	Malignant in 80% of cases Most frequently in head of pancreas
Glucagonoma	Glucagon	Weight loss, muscle wasting, diabetes, dermatitis, deep vein thrombosis, depression	Usually malignant Rarest of pancreatic endocrine tumors Most frequently in tail of pancreas Large in size More than 50% have liver metastases at presentation
VIPoma	Vasoactive intestinal polypeptide	Massive and watery diarrhea, hypokalemia, achlorhydria	Malignant tumor Most frequently found in tail of pancreas Large in size
Somatostatinoma	Somatostatin	Hyperglycemia, weight loss, diarrhea, anemia, cholelithiasis, malabsorption	More than 50% present with liver metastases Large in size Five-year survival 60%
Ectopic hormone-producing pancreatic endocrine tumors	Adrenocorticotropic hormone	Cushing syndrome	Usually malignant Large in size
	Corticotrophin-releasing factor	Acromegaly	
	Parathyroid hormone	Hypercalcemia	

Note. Based on information from Capelli et al., 2009; Ekeblad, 2010.

Imaging Tools for Endocrine Tumors

The most common tools used to diagnose and assess PETs are high-resolution multiphase (also known as "triple-phase") computed tomography (CT) scan, magnetic resonance imaging (MRI), somatostatin-receptor scintigraphy (also known as octreotide scan), endoscopic ultrasound (EUS), and endoscopic retrograde cholangiopancreatography (ERCP) (Arnold, Benning, Neuhaus, Rolwage, & Trautmann, 1993; Kennedy et al., 2008; Scarpa et al., 2010). An abdominal CT scan using a pancreatic protocol is the test of choice to detect tumors in the pancreas. CT scan can identify small tumors in the pancreas and determine their relationship to nearby blood vessels and organs. Because the density of NETs is similar to that of the liver, all CT scans should be done with triple-phase technique to be able to detect metastases in the liver. MRI has similar sensitivity and resolution as the triple-phase CT. A magnetic resonance cholangiopancreatography (MRCP) helps to visualize pancreatic and biliary cancers. The MRI and MRCP use magnetic fields rather than radiation to obtain images, so they may be safer for the patient. The octreotide scan detects tumors that overexpress the somatostatin receptor. This scan is not helpful for detecting tumors that do not express the so-

matostatin receptor. Tumors that are found to be "octreotide negative" by octreotide scan tend to be more aggressive. Approximately 90% of nonpancreatic endocrine tumors (carcinoid tumors) express somatostatin receptors (Morgan & Adams, 2010).

EUS is performed under sedation. An endoscope is passed from the mouth into the stomach and small intestine that lay next to the pancreas. At the end of the scope is an ultrasound that produces images of any lesions in the pancreas. Samples of tissue or fluid from the lesions can be obtained for biopsy. An endoscope is also used to perform an ERCP, which is good at evaluating and treating obstructions in the bile duct. Dye is injected through the endoscope into the biliary tree, and x-rays are obtained. Brush biopsies can be performed at the site of the stricture to help with diagnosis. If a biliary obstruction is identified, a stent may be placed to open the blockage (Krishna & Lee, 2011; Lee & Conwell, 2012).

Nursing Considerations for Diagnostic Tests

For patients who are undergoing testing to diagnose new or potentially progressing disease, patient education is essential to optimize test performance, prevent complications,

Table 3-2. Comparison of Two Endocrine Tumor Markers: Chromogranin A (CgA) and 5-Hydroxyindol Acetic Acid (5-HIAA)

Test	Purpose	Specimen	Normal Range	Usefulness	Factors That May Affect Accurate Measurement
CgA	Measures the concentration of CgA in the plasma. CgA is a glycoprotein expressed by endocrine tumors. Elevated levels reflect increased tumor burden.	Single blood test	< 39 ng/L	Functional and nonfunctional pancreatic and nonpancreatic endocrine tumors	Renal impairment Hypergastrinemia Corticotherapy Proton pump inhibitors
5-HIAA	Measures the amount of 5-HIAA in urine. 5-HIAA is the primary metabolite of serotonin, a hormone commonly expressed by endocrine tumors.	24-hour urine test	3–15 mg per 24 hours	Endocrine tumors outside the pancreas	Foods (i.e., avocado, banana, eggplant, pineapple, tomato, plum, kiwi, walnuts) Drugs that can increase 5-HIAA measurements include acetaminophen, caffeine, ephedrine, diazepam, nicotine, glyceryl guaiacolate (an ingredient found in some cough medicines), and phenobarbital. Drugs that can decrease 5-HIAA measurements include aspirin, ethyl alcohol, imipramine, levodopa, monoamine oxidase inhibitors, heparin, isoniazid, methyldopa, and tricyclic antidepressants.

Note. Based on information from Arnold et al., 2009; Capelli et al., 2009; Joy et al., 2008.

and reduce anxiety. Patients also need to be assessed for risk factors related to the diagnostic test and collaborate with the physician to ensure the test is performed safely. CT and MRI scans use contrast to evaluate the pancreas; therefore, patients undergoing these scans should be assessed for allergies to dye contrast. CT contrast allergies are more common than those related to the gadolinium used in MRI. In some cases, premedication with prednisone and diphenhydramine may allow patients with an allergy to safely obtain the scan. Patients also need to be assessed for renal insufficiency and encouraged to increase fluids after the scan. Patients who are on certain medications (e.g., Glucophage® for diabetes) may have to stop their medication around the time of the scan to minimize side effects related to renal function.

Patients undergoing EUS or ERCP require sedation and should not eat or drink fluids before this test. Patients should arrange for someone to take them home, as they should not drive after sedation. Because these are invasive tests, medications that may place the patient at risk for bleeding (e.g., anticoagulants) may need to be placed on hold prior to the procedure. After the procedure is completed, the nurse plays an important role in assessing the patient for potential complications. Although rare, complications can include bleeding, infection, perforation, or pancreatitis from these procedures. Signs or symptoms of a complication may include abdominal pain or fever.

Current Treatments

The clinical course and outcomes of patients with PETs are variable. In a patient with localized disease, surgery remains the treatment of choice and is the only chance for cure. In patients with metastatic disease, some patients will have indolent tumors and will remain symptom-free for years, whereas others experience symptoms requiring therapy related to their diagnosis, either from tumor burden or hormone hypersecretion. Similarly, although patients' survival with metastatic PET is often measured in years, once the PET progresses or becomes symptomatic, the prognosis is poor (Zhou, Zhang, Zheng, & Zhu, 2012). An important challenge is to distinguish those who will die early from their disease from those who will have a more indolent course so that the appropriate level of care can be delivered. Reliable genetic predictors could provide significant advancements in prognosis and treatment; however, such markers are currently unavailable. It is imperative that the therapy decided upon is tailored to improve the patient's quality of life by managing symptoms caused by the tumor as well as treatment for cure or progression control. An algorithm for the diagnosis and treatment of PETs is outlined in Figure 3-1.

Localized Treatments for Primary Tumor

Surgical resection is the treatment of choice for PETs and the only therapy that offers a potential for cure (Capelli et al., 2009; Falconi et al., 2006; Scarpa et al., 2010). The type of pancreatic resection depends on the location of the tumor (see Figure 3-2). For tumors that are at the head of the pancreas, a pancreaticoduodenectomy or Whipple procedure is indicated. This procedure involves removing the head of the pancreas along with the duodenum, gallbladder, part of the common bile duct, and part of the stomach. The pancreas, bile duct, stomach, and intestines are then reconnected (Sauerland, Engelking, Wickham, & Pearlstone, 2009). Recovery from this procedure takes about six to eight weeks. Nutrition counseling is an important part of patient care. Most patients will return to normal eating patterns over time; however, patients experience decreased appetite for the first month after surgery and should be encouraged to eat six to eight small meals a day in order to consume adequate calories. Most patients will lose about 15 pounds in the first few weeks after

surgery. Weight stabilization should occur by three weeks postoperatively. Patients may experience difficulties digesting fats due to injury to the pancreatic duct. This can be short or long term. Fat malabsorption manifests as frequent, loose, greasy-appearing stools and can be treated with pancreatic enzymes during meals. Nurses play an important role in assessing patients' nutritional status and collaborating with a dietitian to help patients plan their diet.

For tumors at the tail of the pancreas, a distal pancreatectomy is performed. Most often, this procedure can be done laparoscopically and may include the removal of the spleen depending on the location of the tumor in relation to the splenic vasculature. Pancreatic resections can be performed on the central part of the pancreas, thereby preserving the head and tail of the pancreas. This procedure is less common. In both of these procedures, patients can experience fat malabsorption; however, this is more common after pancreaticoduodenectomy. Diabetes may develop as a result of any pancreatic resection but usually occurs in patients already at high risk for diabetes. Diabetes may worsen in patients who already have the disease. In certain cases where there is a single, small PET, enucleation of the tumor can be performed. This surgical procedure involves removing the tumor without resecting or cutting into the pancreatic tissue and minimizes long-term side effects related to resection (Sauerland et al., 2009).

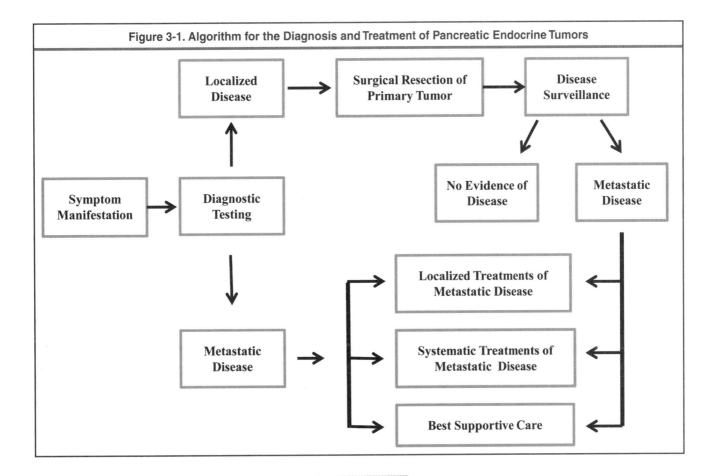

Figure 3-1. Algorithm for the Diagnosis and Treatment of Pancreatic Endocrine Tumors

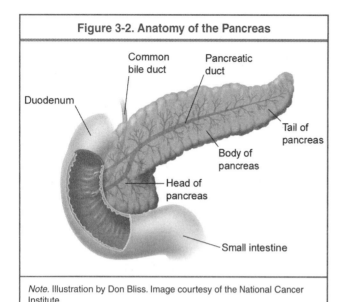

Figure 3-2. Anatomy of the Pancreas

Common bile duct

Pancreatic duct

Duodenum

Tail of pancreas

Body of pancreas

Head of pancreas

Small intestine

Note. Illustration by Don Bliss. Image courtesy of the National Cancer Institute.

Aside from compromised nutritional status resulting in weight loss, common side effects of these procedures are pain and fatigue. Mobilizing patients early and providing adequate pain management regimens are key to preventing or minimizing these symptoms. Complications associated with pancreatic resection include pancreatic leak, delayed gastric emptying, and infection. The pancreas is a sponge-like organ that can leak pancreatic juices postoperatively. This occurs in about 20% of resections; in most cases, leaks seal up over time without intervention (Sauerland et al., 2009). For those that do not, a drain may need to be placed until the leak seals up. Delayed gastric emptying occurs when the stomach takes too long to empty its content into the small intestine. Symptoms related to this include abdominal distention, pain and bloating, nausea and vomiting of undigested food, and early satiety. In most cases, this is a short-term problem that resolves with conservative intervention. Patients should be educated on dietary modifications. They should be advised to eat small, frequent meals and to avoid lying down within two hours of eating. A low-fat diet and the avoidance of fresh fruits and raw vegetables may also help, as these foods require effective gastric motility. Medications may also be prescribed to promote gastric emptying.

Localized Treatments for Metastatic Endocrine Disease

Low-grade PETs grow slowly over time and often take years or even decades to metastasize. The most common place for PETs to metastasize is the liver. Approximately 60% of patients with nonfunctioning PETs and 50% of patients with gastrinomas present with liver metastases (Falconi et al., 2006). In some cases, resecting the primary tumor and metastatic

disease is an effective option. Falconi et al. (2006) suggested that only one of five patients meets criteria for this approach, but when this treatment is applicable, the five-year survival rate is 73%. Surgical debulking of metastatic disease is used primarily to control symptoms because of the hypersecretion of hormones or the direct impact of the mass on anatomic structures. Debulking may be used in combination with other therapies to control disease.

Patients who develop metastatic disease in the liver alone may be eligible for other localized treatments such as hepatic arterial embolization, radioembolization, or percutaneous ablation of their tumors (Casadei et al., 2010; Kennedy et al., 2008). Endocrine tumors are vascular in nature. Hepatic arterial embolization is a procedure in which an interventional radiologist performs an arteriogram to identify the arteries feeding the tumor and blocks them off with tiny pellets. When the pellets are coated with chemotherapy, the procedure is referred to as *chemoembolization*. Embolization performed without chemotherapy is called *bland embolization*. In both cases, the primary goal of embolization is to kill tumor cells by blocking the blood supply. Bland embolization can be repeated as many times as appropriate and as tolerated.

Radioembolization is internal radiotherapy (Kennedy et al., 2008). Similar to hepatic arterial embolization, an arteriogram is performed to map vessels for treatment delivery, and radioactive seeds, such as yttrium-90 microspheres, are inserted into the appropriate arteries to deliver high doses of radiation directly into the tumors. Unlike hepatic arterial embolization, this treatment is not meant to block blood supply because maximal response from radiation requires oxygenation of the tumor cells (Kennedy et al., 2008). Radioembolization has benefit over traditional forms of radiation therapy, such as external beam radiotherapy, because it is designed to target specific tumors with high-dose radiation with minimal effect to the surrounding healthy liver.

Radiofrequency ablation (RFA) is another localized treatment of metastatic PETs. RFA uses thermal energy to destroy metastatic tumors and is used to treat metastatic endocrine disease in the liver, lung, and bone. This procedure can be done percutaneously under radiologic guidance imaging or in an open surgical setting. Tumor ablation is limited to tumors that are less than 4 cm in circumference. Care must be taken to avoid injury to nearby structures (Cheng & Doherty, 2010).

Nurses play an important role in preparing patients for these procedures and assessing them after the procedure. Patients and family caregivers require education about how to prepare for the procedure and self-care after the procedure. Nurses need to identify preprocedure risk factors and assess post-procedure symptoms. For example, radiology-guided imaging often requires dye contrast to identify the location and vasculature of tumors during these procedures. Patients who have an allergy to CT contrast dye need to be premedicated to avoid a reaction or may not be eligible for this procedure.

Renal insufficiency is a major concern for patients undergoing these procedures. The combination of dye contrast and sedation often causes patients to become nauseated after the procedure and renders them unable to hydrate themselves adequately and flush out the contrast. In particular, patients with renal dysfunction are at high risk for dehydration after the procedure and should be hydrated prophylactically afterward.

Fever and pain are common post-procedure symptoms. Nurses need to educate patients and family caregivers about the importance of reporting temperatures greater than 100.5°F. Fever can be related to infection at the site of treatment or an outcome of tumor lysis. Pain may also be a sign of infection or abscess and can be localized at the site of treatment or vague by description.

Systemic Treatments

Medical treatments for PETs include biotherapy, such as somatostatin analogs and interferon alfa, and chemotherapy (Oberg, Akerström, Rindi, & Jelic, 2010). Drug regimens can be used in combination with localized treatments or as a primary treatment modality to palliate symptoms and control disease.

Biotherapy

Somatostatin is a 14-amino-acid peptide that inhibits secretion of a wide range of hormones (e.g., growth hormone, insulin, glucagon, gastrin) that a PET can produce (Reichlin, 1983). It acts by attaching itself to somatostatin receptors, which are expressed by approximately 80% of endocrine tumors (Eriksson, 2010; Reubi et al., 1990). Somatostatin analogs decrease symptom distress and reduce biochemical markers in 60% of patients but have little effect in reducing tumor burden (Eriksson, 2010).

Octreotide is an eight-amino-acid synthetic analog of somatostatin designed to bind with the somatostatin receptor and has a longer half-life than somatostatin. It is highly effective in controlling symptoms associated with PETs. A depot long-acting release (LAR) preparation is now available for once-monthly dosing and is currently the most common form of octreotide administration (di Bartolomeo et al., 1996; Novartis Pharmaceuticals, 2011). Disease stabilization has been reported in some patients with progressive NET disease of the small bowel when treated with octreotide or lanreotide, which is a similar drug (Faiss et al., 2003). Tumor shrinkage is extremely rare with less than 5% of patients showing regression (Arnold et al., 2009; Saltz et al., 1993).

Disease stabilization was recently shown in the PROMID (Placebo Randomized Octreotide Midgut) study (Rinke et al., 2009). In this study of 85 patients with locally advanced or metastatic endocrine disease in the midgut, the effect of octreotide LAR on controlling tumor growth was examined. Patients were randomly assigned to receive octreo-tide LAR 30 mg via deep intramuscular injection (a higher dose than the recommended starting dose of 20 mg) or a placebo dose (Rinke et al., 2009). The results demonstrated an antitumor benefit for octreotide LAR 30 mg. Median time to tumor progression was 14.3 months with octreotide LAR 30 mg versus 6.0 months with placebo, which was a 66% improvement (hazard ratio [HR] = 0.34; p < 0.001). There was no difference in overall survival; however, this may have been a result of treatment crossover. Because this trial only examined patients with endocrine tumors originating in the midgut, it is unclear whether the same benefit can be extrapolated to PETs.

The starting dose of octreotide LAR depot is 20 mg via deep intramuscular injection once a month. Octreotide LAR is usually initiated after a brief trial of a short-acting formulation of octreotide, with gradual dose changes as deemed necessary for best symptom control (Novartis Pharmaceuticals, 2011). Precise preparation of octreotide LAR is essential for adequate delivery of medication. This injection is administered into the gluteus muscle with rotation of sites to avoid tissue scarring and hardening of muscle that will prevent proper absorption of medication.

Lanreotide is another common somatostatin analog that has the same effects in managing symptoms as octreotide LAR and is available internationally (O'Toole et al., 2000). Although well tolerated overall, common side effects of somatostatin analogs are mild nausea, abdominal discomfort, bloating, and loose stools, which tend to dissipate over time. Sandostatin® LAR has been associated with ileus, and up to 24% of patients develop asymptomatic gallstones within the first 18 months of therapy (Newman et al., 1995).

Interferon (IFN) alfa are proteins made and released by lymphocytes and generally have the ability to fight off viruses, bacteria, and tumor cells. The ability of IFN alfa to stimulate T-cell function and to control the secretion of tumor products led to its initial use in patients with carcinoid syndrome (Moertel, Rubin, & Kvols, 1989; Oberg, 1996). Early reports on the use of IFN alfa in patients with PET reported combined biologic response (i.e., a decrease in hormone production) with objective response (i.e., tumor shrinkage). In a study from the Mayo Clinic, 9 million units of IFN alfa were administered to patients three times per week and showed a high degree of toxicity and minimal evidence of activity (Moertel et al., 1989). The researchers concluded that IFN alfa was not effective in treating PETs. In a subsequent clinical study, Saltz, Kemeny, Schwartz, and Kelsen (1994) found modest tumor activity when IFN alfa was combined with 5-fluorouracil (5-FU); however, it was not much different than findings from using 5-FU alone. A recent review of the available studies by Plöckinger and Wiedenmann (2007) estimated that approximately 10% of patients with endocrine tumors achieved some degree, however modest, of actual tumor regression. Overall, findings suggest that although IFN alfa may stabilize disease, the side effects often outweigh the benefits, as patients are quite symptomatic with fatigue, fever, and anorexia (Faiss et al., 2003; Valimaki et al., 1991). Therefore, these effects should be carefully considered before using these agents.

Regarding biotherapy options, it appears that somatostatin analogs are more effective than IFN alfa in controlling symptoms related to hormone hypersecretion. Somatostatin therapy has revolutionized the care of patients with hormonal-related symptoms; however, it rarely results in tumor regression. In contrast, IFN alfa has been shown to have some effect, although modest, in tumor regression but can result in side effects that outweigh the benefit of treatment. Patient performance status and quality of life should be considered when determining the best course of treatment.

Chemotherapy

The rarity of PETs and their heterogeneous nature have made it difficult to evaluate the efficacy of drug regimens because different criteria have been employed when evaluating disease response. Agents are given alone or in combination with other chemotherapies. Findings from older studies showed high response rates to some chemotherapy in patients with PETs; however, results were evaluated without the benefit of modern standards of response assessment and must be interpreted with caution. The lack of formal objective criteria for declaring an objective response and the frequent use of unreliable measures, such as perceived changes in physical examination or a drop in hormone level, account for the wide range of reported responses. However, more recent data suggest that PETs are more responsive to conventional chemotherapy as opposed to endocrine tumors outside of the pancreas.

The most common drugs given to treat patients with PETs are streptozocin, doxorubicin, 5-FU, and dacarbazine (Zhou et al., 2012). As single agents, each is responsible for low response rates ranging 7%–25%. Various combinations of these drugs have shown improved response rates (Kouvaraki et al., 2004; Moertel, Lefkopoulo, Lipsitz, Hahn, & Klaassen, 1992). Kouvaraki et al. (2004) found a high response rate for patients with PETs treated with the combination of streptozocin and fluorouracil. In a follow-up study, the Eastern Cooperative Oncology Group (ECOG) randomized 105 patients with advanced PETs to streptozocin plus doxorubicin, streptozocin and fluorouracil, or chlorozotocin alone (Moertel et al., 1992). The reported response rate was 69% for the streptozocin and doxorubicin combination, 33% for streptozocin and fluorouracil, and 30% for chlorozotocin alone. These findings led to the widespread impression that PETs were highly responsive to chemotherapy. Clinical experience, however, suggested otherwise. In a retrospective review of 16 consecutive patients with PETs treated with streptozocin and doxorubicin, Cheng and Saltz (1999) reported that only one patient had a major response, while the others showed no tumor shrinkage. Retrospective analysis of the Methods section of

Moertel and colleagues' (1992) study revealed that the 69% response rate was defined by either a 50% reduction on CT or liver-spleen scan, a 30% decrease in liver span on physical examination, or a 50% reduction in hormone secretion. They did not report how many patients actually had CT-documented regressions. Therefore, the 69% response rate is now acknowledged to be a gross overstatement of the degree of activity that can be expected from streptozocin-based therapy. To further support this conclusion, other studies have reported lower response rates that range from 6% to 39% (Kouvaraki et al., 2004; Rivera & Ajani, 1998). In a retrospective review examining objective tumor response rates and duration of progression-free survival in 84 patients with locally advanced or metastatic PETs treated with the combination of fluorouracil, streptozocin, and doxorubicin, Kouvaraki et al. (2004) found an overall response rate of 39%. Median time between the first cycle of chemotherapy and tumor response was 3.9 months, suggesting that PETs might respond slowly to chemotherapy. A second retrospective review examined the role of 5-FU, folinic acid, and streptozocin in patients with PETs (Gonzalez, Biswas, Clifton, & Corrie, 2003). Of the 15 evaluable patients, one patient had a complete response and seven patients had a partial response with no grade 3 or 4 toxicities reported as assessed using the WHO criteria.

Other studies examined the effect of dacarbazine and its "sister" oral compound temozolomide on endocrine tumors. Dacarbazine and temozolomide are alkylating agents that seem to be more active in PETs than in endocrine tumors outside the pancreas. In a phase II study conducted by ECOG examining the effect of dacarbazine on PETs, 14 of the 42 patients (33%) were reported to have had a partial or complete response (Ramanathan, Cnaan, Hahn, Carbone, & Haller, 2001). In another study conducted by the Southwest Oncology Group of 56 patients with metastatic endocrine disease receiving dacarbazine, a response rate of 16% was reported (Bukowski et al., 1994). This study is weakened by the lack of clearly defined response criteria, which makes it difficult to interpret results. In another phase II–III ECOG study, 249 patients with advanced carcinoid disease were randomized to either doxorubicin with fluorouracil or streptozocin with fluorouracil. Patients whose disease progressed on their first-line regimen were crossed over to dacarbazine. No difference in response rates and progression-free survival were found between the two first-line regimens. Patients who received dacarbazine after progression of disease on streptozocin-based therapy achieved a modest overall response rate of 8%; however, toxicity was considerable (Sun, Lipsitz, Catalano, Mailliard, & Haller, 2005).

Kulke et al. (2006) tested the combination of temozolomide and thalidomide in 29 patients with metastatic endocrine tumors. Patients received temozolomide at a dose of 150 mg/m^2 for seven days every two weeks plus daily thalidomide (dose range 50–400 mg). The overall response rate was approximately 25%, 45% for those with PETs, and only

7% for those with tumors outside the pancreas, further demonstrating the increased sensitivity of PETs to chemotherapy as compared to other endocrine tumors. Side effects were significant. Grades 3 and 4 lymphopenia were noted in 70% of patients, with 10% developing opportunistic infections, particularly pneumococcus pneumonia, a known side effect of temozolomide. A retrospective review of 18 patients with endocrine tumors (5 pancreatic, 13 nonpancreatic) showed that temozolomide was active in approximately 14% of patients, whereas a single phase II study examining the effect of thalidomide showed no antitumor activity (Ekeblad et al., 2007; Varker, Campbell, & Shah, 2008). These findings suggest that the active drug in this combination may be temozolomide. In another temozolomide-based study of 33 patients with newly diagnosed metastatic PETs, 67% of patients who received combination therapy of capecitabine and temozolomide experienced a partial response to this regimen and experienced minimal side effects (Strosberg, Choi, Gardner, & Kvols, 2008). Although this study used a small sample, findings illustrate promising antitumor activity with this combined therapy with relatively manageable side effects, such as fatigue, nausea and vomiting, and diarrhea after prolonged use.

Because of the modest response rates and significant toxicities, systemic chemotherapy rarely plays a role in the early management of metastatic low-grade PETs. It is usually reserved for patients with symptoms related to increased tumor burden and uncontrollable hormone secretion or in patients with rapidly progressing disease. A list of commonly used agents and common adverse effects appears in Table 3-3.

Targeted Therapy

Molecularly targeted therapy is a relatively new treatment choice that targets specific molecular abnormalities in endocrine tumors. In May 2011, sunitinib received U.S. Food and Drug Administration (FDA) approval for the treatment of PETs (FDA, 2011). Sunitinib is a multitargeted oral agent that blocks the vascular endothelial growth factor (VEGF) receptor as well as platelet-derived growth factor receptor-beta, KIT, and RET. A phase II study of 109 patients with advanced endocrine tumors received 50 mg sunitinib for four weeks followed by a two-week break. Of the patients with PETs, 17% (11 of 66) achieved a confirmed partial response compared with 2% (1 of 41) of patients with nonpancreatic endocrine tumors (Kulke et al., 2008). These positive results in PETs led to a randomized phase III trial. Patients with disease progression were randomly assigned to receive either 37.5 mg daily of sunitinib or a placebo. The dosage was administered at 37.5 mg daily (as opposed to the 50 mg dose in the phase II study) because of the increased rate of grade 3 fatigue discussed previously (Raymond et al., 2011). Although the original proposed study was designed to enroll 340 patients, the study was stopped prematurely by the independent Data Monitoring Committee, before the first pre-

planned interim efficacy analysis, because of an increased number of deaths in the placebo arm and based on a higher adverse rate in the placebo arm. The median progression-free survival in 171 patients enrolled was significantly longer with sunitinib (11.4 months versus 5.5 months). There were eight objective responses with sunitinib (an overall response rate of 9.3% versus none in the placebo group), two of which were described as complete. The size, location, and

Table 3-3. Commonly Used Chemotherapy Agents for Pancreatic Endocrine Tumors

Drug	Category	Selected Adverse Effects
Dacarbazine	Alkylating agent	Hematologic: leukopenia, thrombocytopenia Gastrointestinal: nausea, vomiting Other: photosensitivity
Doxorubicin	Anthracycline antineoplastic antibiotic	Hematologic: leukopenia, anemia, thrombocytopenia Gastrointestinal: nausea, vomiting, diarrhea, mucositis Cardiac: cardiomyopathy, arrhythmias Other: alopecia
5-fluorouracil	Antimetabolite	Hematologic: leukopenia, anemia, thrombocytopenia Gastrointestinal: anorexia, nausea, vomiting, diarrhea, mucositis, metallic taste
Streptozocin	Alkylating agent	Hematologic: leukopenia, anemia, thrombocytopenia Gastrointestinal: nausea, vomiting, diarrhea Endocrine: hypo- and hyperglycemia Hepatic: elevated bilirubin, liver function tests Neurologic: confusion and lethargy Renal: proteinuria, renal insufficiency
Temozolomide	Alkylating agent	Hematologic: neutropenia, thrombocytopenia Gastrointestinal: nausea, vomiting, diarrhea Neurologic: headache, fatigue Other: alopecia

Note. Based on information from Chu & DeVita, 2012.

number of lesions involved in the complete responses were unclear; this information could have strengthened this finding.

The most common adverse events associated with sunitinib included diarrhea (59%) as well as nausea (45%), asthenia (34%), vomiting (34%), fatigue (32%), anorexia (22%), stomatitis (22%), dysgeusia (20%), and epistaxis (20%). Hand-foot syndrome and hypertension of any grade occurred in 23% and 26% of patients receiving sunitinib, respectively. The most common grade 3 or 4 adverse events in this group were neutropenia (12%) and hypertension (10%). As noted in the RADIANT-2 trial discussed in the next section, information regarding the duration of each of these toxicities has not been reported, and this information would be clinically relevant. For example, grade 2 hand-foot syndrome would have a very different impact on a patient if it lasts for three days versus if it lasts for three weeks. Despite these side effects, there were no differences in the quality-of-life index with sunitinib. Sunitinib is also FDA approved for progressive PETs.

Mammalian Target of Rapamycin Inhibitors: Temsirolimus and Everolimus

The mammalian target of rapamycin (mTOR) is a serine-threonine kinase that has a central role in the regulation of cellular function and mediates downstream signaling from a number of signaling pathways, including VEGF and insulin-like growth factor, signals that have been implicated as critical pathways in endocrine tumor growth. In a phase II trial, 36 patients with documented progression of disease (15 patients with PETs, 21 patients with nonpancreatic endocrine tumors) were treated with 25 mg IV weekly doses of temsirolimus with an overall response rate of 5.6% and a six-month median time to progression (Duran et al., 2006). This is in contrast to a phase II trial of another mTOR inhibitor, everolimus, which was administered in 5 mg or 10 mg doses to 60 patients, combined with 30 mg octreotide (Yao, Phan, Chang, et al., 2008). In this study, 22% of patients had a partial response, 70% had stable disease, and 8% had disease progression.

This trial led to the pivotal phase III trial known as RADIANT-2. This trial was a randomized, double-blind, placebo-controlled, phase III study evaluating 10 mg/day oral everolimus with 30 mg intramuscular octreotide LAR every 28 days (n = 216) versus placebo with octreotide (n = 213). The primary end point was progression-free survival. The median progression-free survival of the everolimus group was 16.4 months as compared to 11.3 months for the placebo group (HR = 0.77, 95% CI 0.59–1.00; one-sided log rank test p = 0.026). The side effects associated with everolimus were greater than those experienced in the placebo group and consisted of stomatitis (62% versus 14%), rash (37% versus 12%), diarrhea (27% versus 16%), and fatigue (31% versus 23%). Everolimus plus octreotide LAR significantly improved survival in patients with advanced neuroendocrine disease and is now FDA approved for progressive PETs.

Patient Education Related to Chemotherapy and Biotherapy Regimens

Patient and family education regarding the administration of drug regimens and the management of symptoms related to drug therapies is essential in maximizing their effectiveness and minimizing their adverse effects. Temozolomide is an oral medication that patients self-administer. Providing patients with a written medication schedule on a calendar is a highly effective way to facilitate patient adherence to the correct self-medicating schedule, which optimizes the efficacy of treatment. In addition, patients receiving temozolomide must be on prophylactic Bactrim® three days a week to prevent pneumocystis pneumonia. This regimen should also be included in the drug calendar.

Gastrointestinal symptoms are common with most of the chemotherapeutic agents and the targeted therapies sunitinib and rapamycin and must be controlled in order to minimize or prevent weight loss, fatigue, dehydration, and immunosuppression. Patient education and frequent assessment throughout treatment are imperative to manage symptoms and maintain patients' quality of life while on treatment. Antiemetics, such as a 5-HT$_3$ receptor antagonist, should be given prior to the infusion or oral intake of drugs and as needed afterward to minimize nausea and vomiting. It is also important to remember that medications used for symptom management may also have side effects, and patients need to be educated regarding these issues as well. For example, 5-HT$_3$ receptor antagonist antiemetics can cause severe constipation. An aggressive bowel regimen should be initiated when taking this drug.

Low blood counts are another common side effect, which may make patients more susceptible to infection and injury. Patients should be instructed to report fever, chills, mouth sores, and falls. Similarly, patients need to be educated to report increased fatigue and shortness of breath, as these symptoms may indicate anemia.

Emerging Therapies for Pancreatic Endocrine Tumors

Continuous questioning as to the efficiency of currently available treatments has raised interest in exploring novel therapeutic approaches. Various studies have examined the expression of cellular growth factors and their receptors in PETs, and the elevated expression of some growth factors and receptors has been noted in patients with PETs. Some growth factor receptors that also function as tyrosine kinases provide promising therapies that target receptors such as VEGF. Studies examining targeted therapies have led to the addition of sunitinib as a treatment. Others, such as monoclonal antibodies that attack VEGF receptors (e.g., bevacizumab), are still under investigation.

Vascular Endothelial Growth Factor Inhibitors

Endocrine neoplasms are tumors that are highly vascular and extensively express VEGF; however, no trial has involved patients with PETs and bevacizumab. Bevacizumab was tested in a phase II trial in which 44 patients with advanced or metastatic endocrine tumors were randomly assigned to receive either bevacizumab (15 mg/kg every three weeks) or pegylated IFN alfa-2b (Yao, Phan, Hoff, et al., 2008). An 18% (4 of 22) partial response rate was reported in the bevacizumab group compared with 0% in the IFN alfa-2b group. At 18 weeks, 95% of the patients treated with bevacizumab remained progression free compared with 68% of patients treated with IFN alfa-2b. Grade 3 or 4 hypertension occurred in 53% of patients.

Radiolabeled Somatostatin Analog Therapy

In single-center trials, radionuclide somatostatin analog therapy for patients with advanced, unresectable indium-111 (^{111}In) pentetreotide-positive endocrine tumors has been reported to have some efficacy with acceptable toxicity (Waldherr et al., 2002; Waldherr, Pless, Maecke, Haldemann, & Mueller-Brand, 2001). Several radioisotopes linked to a somatostatin analog have been used and include ^{111}In, yttrium-90 (^{90}Y), and lutetium-177 (^{177}Lu). Studies of the ^{90}Y-labeled somatostatin analog, a high-energy beta-particle emitter, reported response rates of up to 27% (Waldherr et al., 2001, 2002). A European multicenter trial known as MAURITIUS evaluated 39 patients with endocrine tumors using ^{90}Y lanreotide (Virgolini et al., 2002). Minor tumor regression was seen in 20% of patients, with 44% of patients achieving stable disease. Adverse effects associated with ^{90}Y octreotide include renal and hematologic toxicities (Valkema et al., 2006).

An analysis of 504 patients with metastatic endocrine tumors receiving ^{177}Lu octreotate was reported (Kwekkeboom et al., 2005, 2008). Complete remission occurred in 2% of patients, partial remission in 28% of patients, and minor remission (decrease of greater than 25% and less than 50%) in 16% of patients. Only 20% of patients had disease progression three months after administration of ^{177}Lu octreotate. The median time to progression was approximately 40 months overall; however, only 43% of patients had documented disease progression before therapy was initiated. Serious toxicity was seen in three patients who developed myelodysplastic syndrome and two patients who developed nonfatal liver toxicity. Radiolabeled somatostatin analogs may have promise as an active treatment. The degree of activity and toxicity that patients can expect from this treatment has not yet been adequately defined, and this approach remains investigational.

Summary

PETs are a rare group of cancers that pose many challenges to patients and caregivers. Although surgery remains the only treatment with the opportunity for cure, patients can live for many years even with metastatic disease. Advances in medical treatment are directed toward controlling the disease and its symptoms. Nurses play an important role in educating and supporting patients and families through these complex and often multimodality treatments. They also have an opportunity to contribute to the evaluation of these new treatments with regard to quality of life and symptom control through research and make recommendations to enhance nursing practice.

References

Arnold, R., Benning, R., Neuhaus, C., Rolwage, M., & Trautmann, M.E. (1993). Gastroenteropancreatic endocrine tumours: Effect of Sandostatin on tumour growth. *Digestion, 54*(Suppl. 1), 72–75. doi:10.1159/000201081

Arnold, R., Chen, Y.J., Costa, F., Falconi, M., Gross, D., Grossman, A.B., … Plökinger, U. (2009). ENETS Consensus Guidelines for the Standards of Care in Neuroendocrine Tumors: Follow-up and documentation. *Neuroendocrinology, 90*, 227–233. doi:10.1159/000225952

Bukowski, R.M., Tangen, C.M., Peterson, R.F., Fleming, T.R., Taylor, S.A., Rinehart, J.J., … Macdonald, J.S. (1994). Phase II trial of dimethyltriazenoimidazole carboxamide in patients with metastatic carcinoid. *Cancer, 73*, 1505–1508. doi:10.1002/1097-0142(19940301)73:5<1505::AID-CNCR2820730530>3.0.CO;2-V

Capelli, P., Martignoni, G., Pedica, F., Falconi, M., Antonello, D., Malpeli, G., & Scarpa, A. (2009). Endocrine neoplasms of the pancreas: Pathologic and genetic features. *Archives of Pathology and Laboratory Medicine, 133*, 350–364. doi:10.1043/1543-2165-133.3.350

Casadei, R., Ricci, C., Pezzilli, R., Campana, D., Tomassetti, P., Calulli, L., … Minni, F. (2009). Value of both WHO and TNM classification systems for patients with pancreatic endocrine tumors: Results of a single-center series. *World Journal of Surgery, 33*, 2458–2463.

Casadei, R., Ricci, C., Pezzilli, R., Serra, C., Calculli, L., Morselli-Labate, A.M., … Minni, F. (2010). A prospective study on radiofrequency ablation locally advanced pancreatic cancer. *Hepatobiliary and Pancreatic Diseases International, 9*, 306–311. Retrieved from http://www.hbpdint.com/text.asp?id=1365

Cheng, S.P., & Doherty, G.M. (2010). Rare neuroendocrine tumors of the pancreas. *Cancer Treatment and Research, 153*, 253–270. doi:10.1007/978-1-4419-0857-5_14

Cheng, P.N., & Saltz, L.B. (1999). Failure to confirm major objective antitumor activity for streptozocin and doxorubicin in the treatment of patients with advanced islet cell carcinoma. *Cancer, 86*, 944–948. doi:10.1002/(SICI)1097-0142(19990915)86:6<944::AID-CNCR8>3.0.CO;2-P

Chu, E., & DeVita, V.T. (2012). *Physicians' cancer chemotherapy drug manual 2012*. Burlington, MA: Jones and Bartlett.

di Bartolomeo, M., Bajetta, E., Buzzoni, R., Mariani, L., Carnaghi, C., Somma, L., … Di Leo, A. (1996). Clinical efficacy of octreotide in the treatment of metastatic neuroendocrine tumors. A study by the Italian Trials in Medical Oncology Group. *Cancer, 77*, 402–408.

doi:10.1002/(SICI)1097-0142(19960115)77:2<402::AID-CNCR25>
3.0.CO;2-4

Duran, I., Kortmansky, J., Singh, D., Hirte, H., Kocha, W., Goss, G., ... Siu, L.L. (2006). A phase II clinical and pharmacodynamic study of temsirolimus in advanced neuroendocrine carcinomas. *British Journal of Cancer, 95,* 1148–1154. doi:10.1038/sj.bjc.6603419

Ekeblad, S. (2010). Islet cell tumours. *Advances in Experimental Medicine and Biology, 654,* 771–789. doi:10.1007/978-90-481-3271-3_34

Ekeblad, S., Sundin, A., Janson, E.T., Welin, S., Granberg, D., Kindmark, H., ... Skogseid, B. (2007). Temozolomide as monotherapy is effective in treatment of advanced malignant neuroendocrine tumors. *Clinical Cancer Research, 13,* 2986–2991. doi:10.1158/1078 -0432.CCR-06-2053

Eriksson, B. (2010). New drugs in neuroendocrine tumors: Rising of new therapeutic philosophies? *Current Opinion in Oncology, 22,* 381–386. doi:10.1097/CCO.0b013e32833adee2

Faiss, S., Pape, U.-F., Böhmig, M., Dörffel, Y., Mansmann, U., Golder, W., ... Wiedenmann, B. (2003). Prospective, randomized, multicenter trial on the antiproliferative effect of lanreotide, interferon alfa, and their combination for therapy of metastatic neuroendocrine gastroenteropancreatic tumors—The International Lanreotide and Interferon Alfa Study Group. *Journal of Clinical Oncology, 21,* 2689–2696. doi:10.1200/JCO.2003.12.142

Falconi, M., Bettini, R., Boninsegna, L., Crippa, S., Butturini, G., & Pederzoli, P. (2006). Surgical strategy in the treatment of pancreatic neuroendocrine tumors. *JOP: Journal of the Pancreas, 7*(Suppl. 1), 150–156. Retrieved from http://www.joplink.net/prev/200601/41. html

Gonzalez, M.A., Biswas, S., Clifton, L., & Corrie, P.G. (2003). Treatment of neuroendocrine tumours with infusional 5-fluorouracil, folinic acid and streptozocin. *British Journal of Cancer, 89,* 455–456. doi:10.1038/sj.bjc.6601167

Jani, N., Moser, A.J., & Khalid, A. (2007). Pancreatic endocrine tumors. *Gastroenterology Clinics of North America, 36,* 431–439, x–xi. doi:10.1016/j.gtc.2007.03.002

Jemal, A., Bray, F., Center, M.M., Ferlay, J., Ward, E., & Forman, D. (2011). Global cancer statistics. *CA: A Cancer Journal for Clinicians, 61,* 69–90. doi:10.3322/caac.20107

Joy, T., Walsh, G., Tokmakejian, S., & Van Uum, S.H. (2008). Increase of urinary 5-hydroxyindoleacetic acid excretion but not serum chromogranin A following over-the-counter 5-hydroxytryptophan intake. *Canadian Journal of Gastroenterology, 22,* 49–53. Retrieved from http://www.pulsus.com/journals/abstract.jsp?HCtype=Consumer&sCurrPg =journal&jnlKy=2&atlKy=7768&isuKy=761&isArt=t&

Kennedy, A.S., Dezarn, W.A., McNeillie, P., Coldwell, D., Nutting, C., Carter, D., ... Salem, R. (2008). Radioembolization for unresectable neuroendocrine hepatic metastases using resin 90Y-microspheres: Early results in 148 patients. *American Journal of Clinical Oncology, 31,* 271–279. doi:10.1097/COC.0b013e31815e4557

Klimstra, D.S., Modlin, I.R., Adsay, N.V., Chetty, R., Deshpande, V., Gonen, M., ... Yeo, J. (2010). Pathology reporting of neuroendocrine tumors: Application of the Delphic consensus process to the development of a minimum pathology data set. *American Journal of Surgical Pathology, 34,* 300–313. doi:10.1097/PAS.0b013e3181ce1447

Klöppel, G., & Heitz, P.U. (1988). Pancreatic endocrine tumors. *Pathology—Research and Practice, 183,* 155–168. doi:10.1016/S0344 -0338(88)80043-8

Kouvaraki, M.A., Ajani, J.A., Hoff, P., Wolff, R., Evans, D.B., Lozano, R., & Yao, J.C. (2004). Fluorouracil, doxorubicin, and streptozocin in the treatment of patients with locally advanced and metastatic pancreatic endocrine carcinomas. *Journal of Clinical Oncology, 22,* 4762–4771. doi:10.1200/JCO.2004.04.024

Krishna, S.G., & Lee, J.H. (2011). Endosonography in solid and cystic pancreatic tumors. *Journal of Interventional Gastroenterology, 1,* 193–201. doi:10.4161/jig.1.4.19971

Kulke, M.H., Lenz, H.J., Meropol, N.J., Posey, J., Ryan, D.P., Picus, J., ... Fuchs, C.S. (2008). Activity of sunitinib in patients with advanced

neuroendocrine tumors. *Journal of Clinical Oncology, 26,* 3403–3410. doi:10.1200/JCO.2007.15.9020

Kulke, M.H., Stuart, K., Enzinger, P.C., Ryan, D.P., Clark, J.W., Muzikansky, A., ... Fuchs, C.S. (2006). Phase II study of temozolomide and thalidomide in patients with metastatic neuroendocrine tumors. *Journal of Clinical Oncology, 24,* 401–406. doi:10.1200/ JCO.2005.03.6046

Kwekkeboom, D.J., de Herder, W.W., Kam, B.L., van Eijck, C.H., van Essen, M., Kooij, P.P., ... Krenning, E.P. (2008). Treatment with the radiolabeled somatostatin analog [¹⁷⁷Lu-DOTA⁰,Tyr³] octreotate: Toxicity, efficacy, and survival. *Journal of Clinical Oncology, 26,* 2124–2130. doi:10.1200/JCO.2007.15.2553

Kwekkeboom, D.J., Teunissen, J.J., Bakker, W.H., Kooij, P.P., de Herder, W.W., Feelders, R.A., ... Krenning, E.P. (2005). Radiolabeled somatostatin analog [¹⁷⁷Lu-DOTA⁰,Tyr³]octreotate in patients with endocrine gastroenteropancreatic tumors. *Journal of Clinical Oncology, 23,* 2754–2762. doi:10.1200/JCO.2005.08.066

Lee, L.S., & Conwell, D.L. (2012). Update on advanced endoscopic techniques for the pancreas: Endoscopic retrograde cholangiopancreatography, drainage and biopsy, and endoscopic ultrasound. *Radiologic Clinics of North America, 50,* 547–561. doi:10.1016/j. rcl.2012.03.002

Moertel, C.G., Lefkopoulo, M., Lipsitz, S., Hahn, R.G., & Klaassen, D. (1992). Streptozocin-doxorubicin, streptozocin-fluorouracil or chlorozotocin in the treatment of advanced islet-cell carcinoma. *New England Journal of Medicine, 326,* 519–523. doi:10.1056/ NEJM199202203260804

Moertel, C.G., Rubin, J., & Kvols, L.K. (1989). Therapy of metastatic carcinoid tumor and the malignant carcinoid syndrome with recombinant leukocyte A interferon. *Journal of Clinical Oncology, 7,* 865–868.

Morgan, K.A., & Adams, D.B. (2010). Solid tumors of the body and tail of the pancreas. *Surgical Clinics of North America, 90,* 287–307. doi:10.1016/j.suc.2009.12.009

Newman, C.B., Melmed, S., Snyder, P.J., Young, W.F., Boyajy, L.D., Levy, R., ... Gagel, R.F. (1995). Safety and efficacy of long-term octreotide therapy of acromegaly: Results of a multicenter trial in 103 patients—A clinical research center study. *Journal of Clinical Endocrinology and Metabolism, 80,* 2768–2775. doi:10.1210/jc.80.9.2768

Novartis Pharmaceuticals. (2011, September). *Sandostatin LAR® Depot* [Package insert]. Retrieved from http://www.pharma.us.novartis.com/ product/pi/pdf/sandostatin_lar.pdf

O'Toole, D., Ducreux, M., Bommelaer, G., Wemeau, J.L., Bouché, O., Catus, F., ... Ruszniewski, P. (2000). Treatment of carcinoid syndrome: A prospective crossover evaluation of lanreotide versus octreotide in terms of efficacy, patient acceptability, and tolerance. *Cancer, 88,* 770–776. doi:10.1002/(SICI)1097-0142(20000215)88:4<770::AID -CNCR6>3.0.CO;2-0

Oberg, K. (1996). Neuroendocrine gastrointestinal tumours. *Annals of Oncology, 7,* 453–463. doi:10.1093/oxfordjournals.annonc.a010633

Oberg, K., Akerström, G., Rindi, G., & Jelic, S. (2010). Neuroendocrine gastroenteropancreatic tumours: ESMO Clinical Practice Guidelines for diagnosis, treatment and follow-up. *Annals of Oncology, 21*(Suppl. 5), v223–v227. doi:10.1093/annonc/mdq192

Plöckinger, U., & Wiedenmann, B. (2007). Neuroendocrine tumors: Biotherapy. *Best Practice and Research: Clinical Endocrinology and Metabolism, 21,* 145–162. doi:10.1016/j.beem.2007.01.002

Ramanathan, R.K., Cnaan, A., Hahn, R.G., Carbone, P.P., & Haller, D.G. (2001). Phase II trial of dacarbazine (DTIC) in advanced pancreatic islet cell carcinoma: Study of the Eastern Cooperative Oncology Group-E6282. *Annals of Oncology, 12,* 1139–1143. doi:10.1023/A:1011632713360

Raymond, E., Dahan, L., Raoul, J.L., Bang, Y.J., Borbath, I., Lombard-Bohas, C., ... Ruszniewski, P. (2011). Sunitinib malate for the treatment of pancreatic neuroendocrine tumors. *New England Journal of Medicine, 364,* 501–513. doi:10.1056/NEJMoa1003825

Reichlin, S. (1983). Somatostatin. *New England Journal of Medicine, 309,* 1495–1501. doi:10.1056/NEJM198312153092406

Reubi, J.C., Kvols, L.K., Waser, B., Nagorney, D.M., Heitz, P.U., Charboneau, J.W., ... Moertel, C. (1990). Detection of somatostatin receptors in surgical and percutaneous needle biopsy samples of carcinoids and islet cell carcinomas. *Cancer Research, 50,* 5969–5977. Retrieved from http://cancerres.aacrjournals.org/content/50/18/5969.long

Rindi, G., Klöppel, G., Alhman, H., Caplin, M., Couvelard, A., de Herder, W.W., ... Wiedenmann, B. (2006). TNM staging of foregut (neuro)endocrine tumors: A consensus proposal including a grading system. *Virchows Archiv, 449,* 395–401. doi:10.1007/s00428-006-0250-1

Rinke, A., Müller, H.H., Schade-Brittinger, C., Klose, K.-J., Barth, P., Wied, M., ... Arnold, R. (2009). Placebo-controlled, double-blind, prospective, randomized study on the effect of octreotide LAR in the control of tumor growth in patients with metastatic neuroendocrine midgut tumors: A report from the PROMID Study Group. *Journal of Clinical Oncology, 27,* 4656–4663. doi:10.1200/JCO.2009.22.8510

Rivera, E., & Ajani, J.A. (1998). Doxorubicin, streptozocin, and 5-fluorouracil chemotherapy for patients with metastatic islet-cell carcinoma. *American Journal of Clinical Oncology, 21,* 36–38. doi:10.1097/00000421-199802000-00008

Saltz, L., Kemeny, N., Schwartz, G., & Kelsen, D. (1994). A phase II trial of alpha-interferon and 5-fluorouracil in patients with advanced carcinoid and islet cell tumors. *Cancer, 74,* 958–961.

Saltz, L., Trochanowski, B., Buckley, M., Heffernan, B., Niedzwiecki, D., Tao, Y., & Kelsen, D. (1993). Octreotide as an antineoplastic agent in the treatment of functional and nonfunctional neuroendocrine tumors. *Cancer, 72,* 244–248. doi:10.1002/1097-0142(19930701)72:1<244::AID-CNCR2820720143>3.0.CO;2-Q

Sauerland, C., Engelking, C., Wickham, R., & Pearlstone, D.B. (2009). Cancers of the pancreas and hepatobiliary system. *Seminars in Oncology Nursing, 25,* 76–92. doi:10.1016/j.soncn.2008.10.006

Scarpa, A., Mantovani, W., Capelli, P., Beghelli, S., Boninsegna, L., Bettini, R., ... Falconi, M. (2010). Pancreatic endocrine tumors: Improved TNM staging and histopathological grading permit a clinically efficient prognostic stratification of patients. *Modern Pathology, 23,* 824–833. doi:10.1038/modpathol.2010.58

Solcia, E., Klöppel, G., & Sobin, L. (Eds.). (2000). *Histological typing of endocrine tumours* (2nd ed.). Berlin, Germany: Springer.

Strosberg, J., Choi, J., Gardner, N., & Kvols, L. (2008). First-line treatment of metastatic pancreatic endocrine carcinomas with capecitabine and temozolomide [Abstract]. *Journal of Clinical Oncology, 26*(Suppl.), 4612. Retrieved from http://www.asco.org/ASCOv2/Meetings/Abstracts?&vmview=abst_detail_view&confID=55&abstractID=32319

Sun, W., Lipsitz, S., Catalano, P., Mailliard, J.A., & Haller, D.G. (2005). Phase II/III study of doxorubicin with fluorouracil compared with streptozocin with fluorouracil or dacarbazine in the treatment of advanced carcinoid tumors: Eastern Cooperative Oncology Group Study E1281. *Journal of Clinical Oncology, 23,* 4897–4904. doi:10.1200/JCO.2005.03.616

U.S. Food and Drug Administration. (2011, May 20). FDA approves Sutent for rare type of pancreatic cancer [Press release]. Retrieved from http://www.fda.gov/NewsEvents/Newsroom/PressAnnouncements/ucm256237.htm

Valimaki, M., Jarvinen, H., Salmela, P., Sane, T., Sjoblom, S.M., & Pelkonen, R. (1991). Is the treatment of metastatic carcinoid tumor with interferon not as successful as suggested? *Cancer, 67,* 547–549. doi:10.1002/1097-0142(19910201)67:3<547::AID-CNCR2820670302>3.0.CO;2-J

Valkema, R., Pauwels, S., Kvols, L.K., Barone, R., Jamar, F., Bakker, W.H., ... Krenning, E.P. (2006). Survival and response after peptide receptor radionuclide therapy with [^{90}Y-DOTA^0,Tyr^3]octreotide in patients with advanced gastroenteropancreatic neuroendocrine tumors. *Seminars in Nuclear Medicine, 36,* 147–156. doi:10.1053/j.semnuclmed.2006.01.001

Varker, K.A., Campbell, J., & Shah, M.H. (2008). Phase II study of thalidomide in patients with metastatic carcinoid and islet cell tumors. *Cancer Chemotherapy and Pharmacology, 61,* 661–668. doi:10.1007/s00280-007-0521-9

Virgolini, I., Britton, K., Buscombe, J., Moncayo, R., Paganelli, G., & Riva, P. (2002). In- and Y-DOTA-lanreotide: Results and implications of the MAURITIUS trial. *Seminars in Nuclear Medicine, 32,* 148–155. doi:10.1053/snuc.2002.31565

Waldherr, C., Pless, M., Maecke, H.R., Haldemann, A., & Mueller-Brand, J. (2001). The clinical value of [^{90}Y-DOTA]-D-Phe^1-Tyr^3-octreotide (^{90}Y-DOTATOC) in the treatment of neuroendocrine tumours: A clinical phase II study. *Annals of Oncology, 12,* 941–945. doi:10.1023/A:1011160913619

Waldherr, C., Pless, M., Maecke, H.R., Schumacher, T., Crazzolara, A., Nitzsche, E.U., ... Mueller-Brand, J. (2002). Tumor response and clinical benefit in neuroendocrine tumors after 7.4 GBq ^{90}Y-DOTATOC. *Journal of Nuclear Medicine, 43,* 610–616. Retrieved from http://jnm.snmjournals.org/content/43/5/610.full.pdf+html

Yao, J.C., Phan, A.T., Chang, D.Z., Wolff, R.A., Hess, K., Gupta, S., ... Meric-Bernstam, F. (2008). Efficacy of RAD001 (everolimus) and octreotide LAR in advanced low- to intermediate-grade neuroendocrine tumors: Results of a phase II study. *Journal of Clinical Oncology, 26,* 4311–4318. doi:10.1200/JCO.2008.16.7858

Yao, J.C., Phan, A., Hoff, P.M., Chen, H.X., Charnsangavej, C., Yeung, S.C., ... Ajani, J.A. (2008). Targeting vascular endothelial growth factor in advanced carcinoid tumor: A random assignment phase II study of depot octreotide with bevacizumab and pegylated interferon alpha-2b. *Journal of Clinical Oncology, 26,* 1316–1323. doi:10.1200/JCO.2007.13.6374

Yao, J., Phan, A., & Chang, D. (2007). Phase II study of RAD001 and depot octreotide (Sandostatin LAR) in advanced low grade neuroendocrine carcinoma (LGNET) [Abstract]. *Journal of Clinical Oncology, 25*(Suppl. 18S), 4503. Retrieved from http://www.asco.org/ASCOv2/Meetings/Abstracts?&vmview=abst_detail_view&confID=47&abstractID=33414

Zhou, C., Zhang, J., Zheng, Y., & Zhu, Z. (2012). Pancreatic neuroendocrine tumors: A comprehensive review. *International Journal of Cancer, 131,* 1013–1022. doi:10.1002/ijc.27543

CHAPTER 4

Gallbladder and Bile Duct Tumors

Alisa M. Yee, MSN, ACNP-BC, NP

Introduction

Despite gallbladder cancer first being described more than two centuries ago, little progress has been made in early diagnostics, prognosis, and effective treatment. It is considered a rare form of cancer, but it is the most common malignancy of the biliary tract. Gallbladder cancer is in general a late-presenting disease, and it does not show defined or specific signs and symptoms. Although less than half of the cases are resectable, surgery to remove the primary tumor and its local involvement is the most effective treatment.

Similar to gallbladder cancer, cancer of the bile duct (cholangiocarcinoma) is rare. It can occur anywhere in the biliary tree, but unlike gallbladder cancer, more than 90% of the patients present with the specific sign of jaundice when the tumor is located in the extrahepatic bile ducts. Stenting provides effective palliation for the jaundice, but surgery remains the principal treatment modality and only potential for cure. Although some overlap exists in the diagnosis and treatment of these two cancers, they are distinct enough to require separate discussions.

Gallbladder Cancer

The gallbladder is a pear-shaped sac attached to the undersurface of the liver, at the division of the right and left lobes (see Figure 4-1). Both the liver and the gallbladder are protected by the right lower ribs. The size of the gallbladder is usually 10 cm by 4 cm and has a fundus, body, and neck. The wall thickness is 1–2 mm. The gallbladder concentrates and stores bile made by the liver and contains approximately 30–50 ml of bile, but it can distend and hold up to 300 ml. Cholecystokinin, a gastrointestinal hormone, causes the gallbladder to contract and release bile (usually 500–1,000 ml/day) through the cystic duct. The cystic duct connects with the hepatic duct to form the common bile duct that empties into the small intestine (Huether, 2009).

After surgical removal of the gallbladder (cholecystectomy) for reasons such as gallstones (cholelithiasis), inflammation or infection (cholecystitis), or cancer, many people live without symptoms (Fenster, Lonborg, Thirlby, & Traverso, 1995). Its absence does not impair the production of needed bile but only affects its concentration and timed release into the small intestine.

Incidence

Gallbladder cancer was first described by Maximilian Stoll in 1777 on the basis of three cases seen on autopsy. Currently, it is the fifth most common gastrointestinal malignancy in the United States; however, it is the most common malignant tumor of the biliary tract worldwide (Lai & Lau, 2008). The incidence of gallbladder cancer is highly variable by racial-ethnic groups and geographical regions. The highest incidence rates worldwide were reported for women in Delhi, India (21.5/100,000), South Karachi, Pakistan (13.8/100,000), and Quito, Ecuador (12.9/100,000). High incidence was found in Korea and Japan and some central and eastern European countries (Randi, Franceschi, & La Vecchia, 2006).

In the United States, gallbladder cancer is two times more common in women than in men (American Cancer Society [ACS], 2012b). According to ACS's 2012 statistical projections, the number of new U.S. cases of gallbladder and other biliary cancers is predicted to be 4,480 in men and 5,330 in women (ACS, 2012b). A review of research published between 1983 and 2009 investigated the possible association of estrogen and progesterone hormone receptor expression with tumor differentiation, and findings were contradictory at best (Barreto, Haga, & Shukla, 2009). The incidence of gallbladder cancer increases progressively with age, with most patients typically receiving the diagnosis in the seventh decade of life (Randi et al., 2006).

Figure 4-1. Gallbladder, Liver, and Duct Anatomy

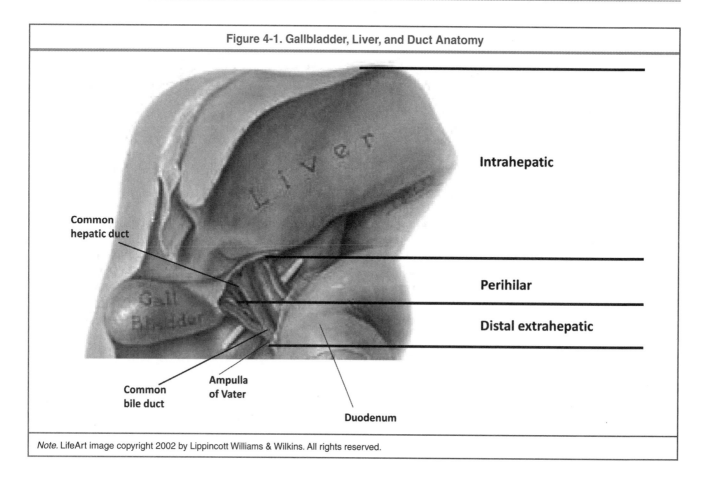

Risk Factors

Gallstones (cholelithiasis) are the most common risk factor for gallbladder cancer (Miller & Jarnagin, 2008). Up to 95% of gallbladder cancers are associated with gallstones (Serra et al., 1996). Although gallstones can range in size from a grain of sand (0.05–2 mm) to a golf ball (42 mm), it has been suggested that patients with gallstones greater than 30 mm in diameter have a 10-fold greater risk of developing gallbladder cancer than patients with gallstones smaller than 10 mm in diameter (Diehl, 1983). One possible explanation for the higher risk of gallbladder cancer with larger gallstones is reflected by the greater duration and intensity of epithelial irritation (Csendes, Becerra, Rojas, & Medina, 2000).

Abnormal anatomy present at birth such as choledocal cysts and anomalous pancreatic duct–biliary duct junction increases the likelihood of developing gallbladder cancer later in life (Benjamin, 2003; Hu, Gong, & Zhou, 2003). The cells that line the sacs of the choledocal cysts can be abnormal and occasionally show precancerous changes (Benjamin, 2003). It is still uncertain whether the increased risk of gallbladder cancer is associated with irritation from the pancreatic digestive juices or from bile not being able to flow easily through the bile ducts.

Porcelain gallbladder, a condition in which the wall of the gallbladder becomes covered with calcium deposits, has been associated with gallbladder cancer. Stippled calcification of the mucosa is thought to carry a higher risk of gallbladder cancer than generalized calcification of the gallbladder wall. On the basis of these associations, chronic inflammation is postulated to be involved in the pathogenesis of gallbladder cancer (Kwon et al., 2004; Stephen & Berger, 2001).

A family history of gallbladder cancer seems to increase a person's chance of developing the disease. Studies show that people with a first-degree relative (i.e., parent, sibling) with gallbladder cancer are five times more likely to develop gallbladder cancer than people who do not (Yasuhito, 2006). Heredity syndromes, including Gardner syndrome, neurofibromatosis type 1, and hereditary nonpolyposis cancer, are associated with increased incidence of gallbladder cancer (Hsing, Rashid, Devesa, & Fraumeni, 2006). Also, people who are typhoid carriers and chronically infected with salmonella (the bacterium that causes typhoid) are more likely to develop gallbladder cancer than those not infected (Randi et al., 2006).

It is not clear if exposure to certain chemicals present in the environment increases the risk of gallbladder cancer. One study suggested that workers in the rubber, paper mill, and petroleum industries may have a higher incidence of gallbladder cancers than the general public (Mancuso & Brennan, 1970).

Methylcholanthrene, O-aminoazotoluene, and nitrosamines were shown to cause gallbladder carcinoma in experimental animals (Albores-Saavedra & Henson, 1986). Because nitrosamines are found in many foodstuffs, such as meat and cheese products preserved with nitrite pickling salt, the U.S. government has established limits on the amount of nitrites used in meat products in order to decrease cancer risk (Department of Health, Education, and Welfare, 1973). A diet high in fresh fruits and vegetables seems to reduce the risk of many cancers, including gallbladder cancer, perhaps because these foods contain high levels of the antioxidant vitamins A, C, and E and other antioxidant chemicals (Ames & Gold, 1998).

Clinical Presentation

Patients with early-stage gallbladder cancer usually are asymptomatic. The lack of symptoms precludes early diagnosis of the disease, and when patients do have symptoms, they are often nonspecific and mimic biliary colic or chronic cholecystitis. Persistent right upper quadrant epigastric pain is the most common symptom, with other symptoms being nausea and vomiting, intolerance of fatty foods, chills, and fever (Ahrendt & Pitt, 2001; Pitt, Dooley, Yeo, & Cameron, 1995). Jaundice, anorexia, and weight loss are symptoms associated with advanced disease.

Preoperative diagnosis of gallbladder cancer is difficult. In one study, carcinoma of the gallbladder was correctly diagnosed preoperatively in only 8% of 53 patients. The most common misdiagnoses included chronic cholecystitis (28%), pancreatic cancer (13%), acute cholecystitis (9%), choledocolithiasis (8%), and gallbladder hydrops (8%) (White, Kraybill, & Lopez, 1988).

Assessment

Patient and Family History

The patient may have no previous specific symptoms but may have vague chronic complaints of right upper quadrant abdominal pain. A change in the pattern of pain may prompt the patient to seek medical attention. Other symptoms of concern are malaise, abdominal distention, and pruritus. Patients with risk factors for gallbladder cancer or a family history of gallbladder disease should be evaluated as follows (Hodgin, 2011).

Physical Examination

The physical examination should focus on the abdomen to check for masses, hepatomegaly, tenderness, or ascites. A palpable mass in the right upper quadrant may be caused by an enlarged gallbladder, known as the Courvoisier sign. A palpable mass in the umbilicus area may represent periumbilical lymphadenopathy, known as Sister Mary Joseph nodes. The skin and the sclera should be inspected for signs of jaundice. Because gallbladder cancer spreads to lymph nodes, the examination should include palpation above the collarbone for any enlarged lymph nodes, known as Virchow nodes (Mizutani, Nawata, Hirai, Murakami, & Kimura, 2005).

Diagnostic Evaluation

Laboratory studies include serum tests for carcinoembryonic antigen (CEA), carbohydrate antigen (CA 19-9), and cancer antigen 125 (CA 125), although these tumor markers are not specific for gallbladder cancer (Bartlett, Ramanthan, & Ben-Josef, 2008). No fasting is required for these blood tests, and the results should be available within one to eight days, depending upon the standards of the healthcare facility and the associated laboratory. Elevated alkaline phosphatase and bilirubin levels may reflect impaired hepatic reserve and are often found with advanced gallbladder cancer. Blood urea nitrogen (BUN), creatinine, and urinalysis should be performed to assess renal function before a patient undergoes a contrast-enhanced computed tomography (CT) scan. Complete blood count (CBC) may show anemia, which may also be an indicator of advanced gallbladder cancer. Prothrombin time (PT), partial thromboplastin time (PTT), and international normalized ratio (INR), if abnormal, may reflect liver failure (Pagana & Pagana, 1997).

Imaging studies include ultrasonography and a chest radiograph as standard initial imaging procedures in patients with right upper quadrant pain. The sensitivity of ultrasonography for detecting gallbladder cancer is 70%–100% (Nakeeb et al., 1996). Ultrasonography is used to identify a thickened gallbladder wall, a mass protruding into the gallbladder, tumor invasion of the liver, or porta hepatis and may reveal adjacent adenopathy. A dilated biliary tree and hepatic metastasis may also be identified by ultrasound (Levy, Murakata, & Rohrmann, 2001). No fasting is required for abdominal ultrasound unless a biopsy procedure is anticipated.

CT scans can demonstrate tumor invasion outside of the gallbladder and identify metastatic disease elsewhere in the abdomen or pelvis. The overall accuracy of CT scans for staging gallbladder cancers was reported as 71%–93% (Kim et al., 2002). Liver invasion occurs in 65% of cases, and the combination of CT scan and ultrasonography or magnetic resonance imaging (MRI) provides accurate details of disease extension (Levy et al., 2001). Before IV contrast is used, allergy to the contrast agent should be assessed, and patients should be premedicated as needed (Namasivayam, Kalra, Torres, & Small, 2006).

MRI has been useful in examining the abdomen for disease extension into other tissues or metastatic disease in the liver. It can provide details of the vasculature for preoperative planning via magnetic resonance angiogram (MRA) and bile duct passages via magnetic resonance cholangiopancreatography (MRCP). Several studies have reported the sensitivity and specificity of MRI with MRA for bile duct invasion (100% sensitive, 89% specific), liver invasion (67% sensitive, 89% specific), and vascular invasion (100% sensitive, 87% specific) (Kaza, Gulati, Wig, & Chawla, 2006; Kim et al., 2002).

Cholangiography (imaging of the bile ducts) via a percutaneous route or endoscopic retrograde cholangiopancreatography (ERCP) may establish the diagnosis of gallbladder cancer by bile cytology (see Figure 4-2). Palliative stenting to re-

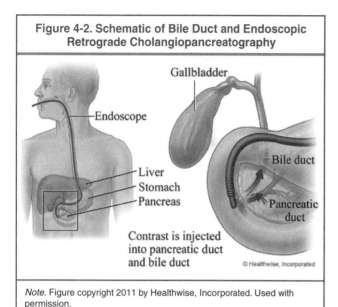

Figure 4-2. Schematic of Bile Duct and Endoscopic Retrograde Cholangiopancreatography

Endoscope

Gallbladder

Liver
Stomach
Pancreas

Bile duct

Pancreatic duct

Contrast is injected into pancreatic duct and bile duct

© Healthwise, Incorporated

Note. Figure copyright 2011 by Healthwise, Incorporated. Used with permission.

lieve biliary obstruction can be performed at the time of the evaluation (Stern & Sturgess, 2008).

Endoscopic ultrasonography (EUS) can be useful to assess regional lymphadenopathy and the depth of tumor invasion into the wall of the gallbladder. In conjunction with other imaging modalities, EUS can provide a means of obtaining bile for cytologic analysis, which has a diagnostic accuracy of 80% for the diagnosis of gallbladder cancer (Muguruma et al., 2001).

The usefulness of positron-emission tomography (PET) scanning has not been established in the evaluation of patients with gallbladder cancer. However, some evidence indicates that PET is useful for detecting the presence of distant metastatic disease in patients with otherwise potentially resectable disease (Corvera et al., 2008; Petrowsky et al., 2006).

Generally, needle biopsy is contraindicated if a patient is thought to have resectable gallbladder cancer because this cancer has a great propensity to spread in needle tracks, a laparoscopic port site, surgical wounds, and the peritoneal cavity (Fong, Brennan, Turnbull, Colt, & Blumgart, 1993; Merz, Dodge, Abellera, & Kisken, 1993). Therefore, needle biopsy is not indicated if surgical exploration is otherwise appropriate.

Gallbladder Cancer Staging

Cellular Characteristics

Gallbladder cancer can originate from the fundus (60%), body (30%), or neck (10%) of the gallbladder (Lai & Lau, 2008). Adenocarcinomas account for 80%–85% of gallbladder cancers. The histologic subtypes include papillary, nodular, and infiltrative (Bartlett et al., 2008; Duffy et al., 2008). The papillary subtype is less aggressive and more often localized and has a better prognosis than the other subtypes. Other rare histologic types of gallbladder cancer are squamous cell

cancer, sarcoma, carcinoid, lymphoma, and melanoma. Histologic grades of gallbladder carcinoma include well differentiated, moderately differentiated, poorly differentiated, and undifferentiated (Levin, 1999). Levin (1999) noted that the higher the histologic grade, the greater the association with advanced stage and rapid disease progression.

Gallbladder cancer generally disseminates by all four routes of tumor spread: (a) local invasion to liver or adjacent organs, (b) lymphatic spread, (c) peritoneal dissemination, and (d) hematogenous spread. The propensity for local invasion and lymphatic spread is the major concern. Because the gallbladder veins drain directly to the adjacent liver, gallbladder cancer often involves the liver (Lai & Lau, 2008).

Tumor, Node, Metastasis Classification

Gallbladder cancers are staged according to the depth of invasion and extent of spread to surrounding structures and lymph nodes, using the American Joint Committee on Cancer (AJCC) tumor, node, metastasis (TNM) classification (Edge et al., 2010) (see Figure 4-3). T stage describes the relative invasion of tumor through the layers of the gallbladder wall and into adjacent structures and is a primary factor in dictating appropriate treatment and predicting outcome. Accurate N staging requires that a minimum of three regional lymph nodes are histologically examined. Regional lymph nodes include hilar, celiac, paraduodenal, peripancreatic, and superior mesenteric nodes. If the gallbladder cancer metastasizes (M), then it typically spreads to the peritoneum and liver and occasionally to the lungs and pleura.

Gallbladder cancers categorized as stage I or II are potentially resectable with curative intent. Stage III generally indicates locally unresectable disease as a consequence of vascular invasion or involvement of multiple adjacent organs, and stage IV represents unresectable disease as a consequence of distant metastases (Miller & Jarnagin, 2008).

Treatment Options

Surgery

Surgery remains the only curative modality for gallbladder cancer (Benson et al., 2009). Removal of the gallbladder (cholecystectomy) via a laparoscopic technique is absolutely contraindicated when gallbladder cancer is known or suspected preoperatively. Patients with a preoperative suspicion of gallbladder cancer should undergo open exploration and cholecystectomy after proper preoperative assessment. The goal for surgical resection is complete tumor removal with negative histologic margins (2 cm around the tumor) because this is the most important factor for predicting long-term survival. The type of operation ranges from cholecystectomy to combined partial hepatectomy with regional lymph node dissection (Lai & Lau, 2008).

During the operative procedure, if the cancer is found to be unresectable because of involvement of adjacent organs,

Figure 4-3. American Joint Committee on Cancer Tumor, Node, Metastasis (TNM) Staging System for Gallbladder Cancer

Primary Tumor (T)

TX	Primary tumor cannot be assessed
T0	No evidence of primary tumor
Tis	Carcinoma in situ
T1	Tumor invades lamina propria or muscular layer
T1a	Tumor invades lamina propria
T1b	Tumor invades muscular layer
T2	Tumor invades perimuscular connective tissue; no extension beyond serosa or into liver
T3	Tumor perforates the serosa (visceral peritoneum) and/or directly invades the liver and/or one other adjacent organ or structure, such as the stomach, duodenum, colon, pancreas, omentum, or extrahepatic bile ducts
T4	Tumor invades main portal vein or hepatic artery or invades two or more extrahepatic organs or structures

Regional Lymph Nodes (N)

NX	Regional lymph nodes cannot be assessed
N0	No regional lymph node metastasis
N1	Metastasis to nodes along the cystic duct, common bile duct, hepatic artery or portal vein
N2	Metastasis to periaortic, pericaval, superior mesenteric artery, and/or celiac artery lymph node

Distant Metastasis (M)—carcinoma of gallbladder and cystic duct

M0	No distant metastasis
M1	Distant metastasis

Stage Grouping—carcinoma of gallbladder

0	Tis N0 M0
I	T1 N0 M0
II	T2 N0 M0
IIIA	T3 N0 M0
IIIB	T1–3 N1 M0
IVA	T4 N0–1 M0
IVB	Any T N2 M0
	Any T Any N M1

Histologic Grade (G)

GX	Grade cannot be assessed
G1	Well differentiated
G2	Moderately differentiated
G3	Poorly differentiated
G4	Undifferentiated

Note. From *AJCC Cancer Staging Manual* (7th ed., pp. 213–214), by S.B. Edge, D.R. Byrd, C.C. Compton, A.G. Fritz, F.L. Greene, and A. Trotti III (Eds.), 2010, New York, NY: Springer, www.springer.com. Copyright 2010 by American Joint Committee on Cancer. Adapted with permission.

then palliative surgery might be indicated to prevent or treat obstructive jaundice or gastric outlet obstruction. This would include internal biliary bypass or intestinal bypass. In addition, radiopaque clips can be placed at the tumor margins if external beam radiation is being considered (Hodgin, 2011). Intraoperative radiation has been used, but the benefit of using it together with a resection or external beam radiation has not been proved (Lindell et al., 2003).

If gallbladder cancer is confirmed on pathologic review after laparoscopic cholecystectomy, for patients with Tis or T1a disease with clear resection margins, no further surgical intervention is needed. For patients with T2 or advanced gallbladder cancer, a second radical operation is the only chance for long-term survival. The goal of the radical operation is to avoid cutting through the tumor, but the extent of the operation includes combined partial hepatectomy (wedge resection, segment IVb and V resection, right hepatectomy or extended right hepatectomy), and regional lymph node dissection. The extent of resection is at least partly dependent on the extent of the tumor. The extrahepatic bile duct should be excised whenever the tumor involves the cystic duct margin or the extrahepatic biliary tree. However, the extent of hepatic and lymph node resection, the need for resection of the extrahepatic bile duct in patients without biliary obstruction, the role of vascular resection, and the advisability of hepatopancreaticoduodenectomy remain matters of debate. Before any additional surgery, the patient should be adequately staged with preoperative imaging (Lai & Lau, 2008).

Nonsurgical Palliative Therapy

When surgery is contraindicated and a diagnosis needs to be established, percutaneous fine-needle biopsy with ultrasound or CT guidance may be considered. Palliative therapy in patients with unresectable or metastatic gallbladder cancer includes providing pain relief and preventing or treating sepsis (Hodgin, 2011). Biliary drainage for obstructive jaundice is an appropriate palliative procedure and should be done with an endoscopic biliary stent or a percutaneous transhepatic biliary stent before chemotherapy if technically feasible.

Chemotherapy has not shown significant activity against gallbladder cancer. Typically, 5-fluorouracil (5-FU) has been used in advanced disease with low efficacy (Yee, Sheppard, Domreis, & Blanke, 2002). Gemcitabine has shown activity in gallbladder cancer. Early-phase studies show an increased response rate with gemcitabine combination therapy over historical treatment response rates with 5-FU alone (Gebbia et al., 2001). A phase 3 trial found that patients with advanced gallbladder cancer treated with cisplatin plus gemcitabine lived an average of 3.6 months longer than those treated with gemcitabine alone (Valle et al., 2010).

A radiation oncologist should be a part of the multidisciplinary team because in unresectable gallbladder cancer, external beam radiation has been used to relieve pain or biliary obstruction. Although this cancer is usually considered to be radioresistant and consequently has no proven survival advantage with external beam radiation, some studies have reported improvement in five-year survival. This cancer's rarity and the fact that the majority of cases present at an advanced stage limit the ability to conduct prospective, randomized studies for targeted or combined chemotherapy and radiation therapies (Hodgin, 2011; Lai & Lau, 2008).

Prognosis and Surveillance

Survival in patients with gallbladder cancer is influenced strongly by the pathologic stage of the disease at presentation. A review of about 2,500 patients with gallbladder cancer from hospital cancer registries throughout the United States revealed five-year survival rates of 60%, 39%, 15%, 5%, and 1% for patients with stage 0–IV disease, respectively (Donohue, Stewart, & Menck, 1998). Results from a recent retrospective single-center analysis showed a 10.3-month median survival for the overall population of patients diagnosed with gallbladder cancer (Duffy et al., 2008). Median survival was 12.0 months for stage Ia–III disease and 5.8 months for those with stage IV disease (Duffy et al., 2008). Because patients with advanced disease usually have short survival times, close follow-up with or without imaging and hospice referral are essential to preserve the best quality of life.

No data currently support aggressive surveillance after resection of gallbladder cancer; thus, determining an appropriate follow-up schedule for visits and imaging should be based on a careful discussion between the patient and healthcare provider. Imaging studies every six months for two years should be considered (Benson et al., 2009).

Oncology Nursing Implications

Nursing care for patients with early-stage gallbladder cancer focuses on support during treatment decision making, attentive care before and after surgery, and symptom management. Nursing care of patients with advanced disease concentrates on palliation of symptoms and end-of-life care.

Symptom Management

Nursing interventions in the care of patients who have had abdominal surgery address acute pain related to the incision and drains; alteration in nutrition related to anorexia and nausea; ineffective airway clearance related to impaired physical mobility, ineffective cough, or sedation; and risk for infection related to the abdominal incision and indwelling catheters (Hodgin, 2011).

Because advanced disease usually involves the liver and biliary tree, potential complications include obstructive jaundice, liver abscess, and liver failure. Symptoms related to these potential complications are decreased appetite, persistent pain, fever, chills, and weight loss. Liver failure can have symptoms of increased abdominal girth and dyspnea, both related to ascites. Supportive measures for these symptoms include proper body positioning, sodium restriction, and diuretic therapy. Alternatively, the patient may be eligible for therapeutic abdominal paracentesis to provide temporary relief of abdominal distention and dyspnea (Hodgin, 2011).

Pain management should consist of a combination of opioid and nonopioid analgesics using the World Health Organization's three-step ladder approach. This approach was developed to manage cancer-induced pain and, when used correctly, provides adequate relief for approximately 75%–90% of patients (Hanks et al., 2001; Jacox, Carr, & Payne, 1994). An additional option for patients with intra-abdominal malignancies is an intervention called neurolytic celiac plexus block. Although the exact pain mechanism of intra-abdominal malignancies is not well understood, neurolytic celiac plexus blocks are commonly utilized to disrupt pain transmission from progressing to high central nervous system pain centers. The first neurolytic celiac plexus block was described in 1914 and has since been shown to offer both short- and long-term analgesia for patients with intra-abdominal cancers (Halpert & Erdek, 2008).

Recent research has identified higher depressive symptoms in patients with hepatobiliary malignancies, including gallbladder cancer, than in patients with other chronic illnesses, including other malignancies (Sun et al., 2008). Factors that may explain depression in these patients are associated with poor prognosis, the distress of having an advanced disease, and possible disruption of neuroendocrine and immune system markers. Possible interventions for depression include a combination of pharmacologic and nonpharmacologic methods (e.g., cognitive behavioral interventions, brief psychotherapy) (Sauerland, Engelking, Wickham, & Pearlstone, 2009).

Patient and Family Education

A patient may require right and left biliary stents to drain both lobes of the liver if the tumor is obstructing the bifurcation of the biliary tree into the liver. Patients with stents need to be taught how to care for and flush the stent, as it may be left in place for the remainder of the patient's life. Daily cleansing of the stent site is required, as is flushing the stent twice a day with sterile normal saline to maintain patency. Signs and symptoms of complications related to the stent, such as fever, chills, leakage, and inability to flush the stent, must be reviewed with the patient and family so that they understand to notify the clinician promptly to avoid problems and unnecessary hospitalization (Hodgin, 2011).

As the cancer progresses, liver failure will typically dominate the patient's clinical course. Nurses are instrumental in educating patients and families about the progression of liver failure, what to expect, and how to manage symptoms of decreased appetite, changes in taste, weight loss, lethargy, encephalopathy, and hepatic coma (Hodgin, 2011). Some useful tips are eating small, frequent snacks and possibly adding spices to prepared foods. Also, taking short naps and maintaining regular sleep patterns may help the patient to conserve energy (Pack, O'Connor, & O'Hagan, 2001).

Palliative care should be started early, including transition to hospice care, because most patients with gallbladder cancer present with advanced disease and survival is typically six months or less. Communication between the inpatient or outpatient nurse and the homecare or hospice clinician is important in providing quality care to these patients with rapidly changing conditions.

Nursing Research

A literature search of PubMed and CINAHL using *gallbladder cancer* as the search term and spanning the years 1990–2009 yielded very few published nursing studies on gallbladder cancer. Most of the studies focused on description and symptom management of hepatobiliary cancers and not on gallbladder cancer as its own distinct diagnosis. Nurse researchers are in an ideal position to advance the scientific knowledge of the symptom experience and quality of life of patients with gallbladder cancer. Because patients with hepatobiliary cancers have multiple symptoms, there are many avenues to explore in symptom management.

Future Considerations

Research

Early detection and aggressive surgical approaches are currently the most effective ways to increase survival for patients with gallbladder cancer. Research on the cytogenetic and molecular pathways of this disease has revealed multiple genetic alternations. There is suggestion that more than one pathway is involved in the initiation and progression of the cancer. Currently there are few diagnostic and prognostic markers (Singh et al., 2012).

Oncology nurses are in an ideal position to encourage patients and their families to participate in clinical trials. Clinical trials allow patients with a good performance status to have a more active role in their own health care, gain access to new research treatments before they are widely available, obtain expert medical care at leading healthcare facilities during the trial, and help others by contributing to medical research.

For a list of U.S. clinical trials accepting patients with gallbladder cancer, consult the National Cancer Institute Clinical Trials Registry (www.cancer.gov/clinicaltrials). The registry list can be further narrowed by location, drug, intervention, and other criteria.

Advocacy for Patients and Caregivers

First and foremost, oncology nurses should be advocates for their patients, but they should also recognize that when advocacy and support are given to the caregiver, both the patient and the healthcare team benefit. Caregivers are essential to continuity of care, particularly at the end of life. However, caregivers face significant challenges with considerable psychological and physical consequences (Glajchen, 2004). Caregivers, similar to the patients in their care, are faced with life-changing effects of this disease and its treatment. Oncology nurses are advocates for both patient and caregiver because they can anticipate and implement needed supportive care.

Bile Duct Tumors

Cholangiocarcinoma is a cancer of the bile ducts. Bile ducts are thin tubes, approximately four to five inches long, that drain bile from the liver into the small intestine (ACS, 2012a). Bile is required for the digestion of the fats in food. The liver excretes it into passages toward the hepatic duct, which joins with the cystic duct (carrying bile to and from the gallbladder) to form the common bile duct, which opens into the intestine. The biliary tree is a network of various-sized ducts branching through the liver.

Because cholangiocarcinomas can be located throughout the biliary tree, the cancer is broadly classified as either intrahepatic or extrahepatic cholangiocarcinoma (see Figure 4-1). Intrahepatic cholangiocarcinomas are also called *peripheral cholangiocarcinomas* and arise from the bile ducts inside the liver. Extrahepatic cholangiocarcinomas arise from bile ducts outside the liver and terminate at the ampulla of Vater (Lake, 1993). When the extrahepatic cholangiocarcinoma specifically is located at the junction of right and left hepatic ducts, it is called *hilar cholangiocarcinoma*, or *Klatskin tumor*. Klatskin tumors are the most common type of extrahepatic cholangiocarcinoma. When the tumor is located in the periampullar region, it is called *distal cholangiocarcinoma*. Extrahepatic cholangiocarcinomas are more common than intrahepatic cholangiocarcinomas (Nakeeb et al., 1996).

Incidence

Cancer of the biliary tree has been recognized for more than 100 years. In 1889, 18 cases of primary extrahepatic cholangiocarcinoma were reported in the literature (Musser, 1889). Currently, approximately 2,500 new cases of cholangiocarcinoma are diagnosed annually in the United States, compared to 5,000 cases of gallbladder cancer and 15,000 cases of hepatocellular cancer (Darwin, Kennedy, & Bonheur, 2012). Average incidence is 1–2 cases per 100,000 people, so it is considered a rare tumor and represents approximately 3% of all gastrointestinal cancers (Carriaga & Henson, 1995). The incidence in most Western countries is 2–6 cases per 100,000 people per year (Darwin et al., 2012). Native Americans have the highest annual incidence in North America, at 6.5 cases per 100,000 people, which is about six times higher than the rate among non–Native American populations (Darwin et al., 2012). The annual incidence is also high in Japan (5.5 cases per 100,000 people) and in Israel (7.3 cases per 100,000 people) (Darwin et al., 2012).

The increased prevalence of cholangiocarcinoma in Asian populations is associated with endemic parasitic infection within the bile duct (Darwin et al., 2012).

Although bile duct cancer can occur in younger patients, it mainly affects older people. According to ACS, at least two out of three people with bile duct cancer are older than age 65 at the time of diagnosis. The male-to-female ratio for cholangiocarcinoma is 1:2.5 in patients in their 60s and 70s and 1:15 in patients younger than 40 years (Darwin et al., 2012).

Risk Factors

Unlike in gallbladder cancer, cholelithiasis is not thought to be closely linked with the etiology of cholangiocarcinomas (Bartlett et al., 2008). Approximately 90% of patients diagnosed with cholangiocarcinoma do not have a recognized risk factor for the malignancy (Ben-Menachem, 2007). There is evidence of many risk factors that may be associated with the disease, including presence of chronic inflammation such as inflammatory bowel disease and primary sclerosing cholangitis (Fong et al., 1993; Fong, Kemeny, & Lawrence, 2001). Primary sclerosing cholangitis is an idiopathic disease characterized by multiple intrahepatic and extrahepatic inflammatory bile duct strictures that cannot be attributed to specific causes. These patients have a 10%–20% higher lifetime risk for developing cholangiocarcinoma than those without inflammatory bowel disease or primary sclerosing cholangitis. When cholangiocarcinoma occurs in these patients, it usually occurs in their fifth decade of life, approximately 20 years earlier than in individuals without these risk factors (Molmenti et al., 1999).

Chronic calculi of the bile duct and congenital diseases of the biliary tree (such as choledocal cysts) have been associated with bile duct cancer (Vogt, 1988). Certain chemical exposures to dioxins have been implicated primarily in workers in the aircraft, rubber, and wood-finishing industries (Fong et al., 2001). A radioactive contrast agent used for x-rays until the 1950s called Thorotrast® (thorium dioxide) can lead to bile duct cancer in individuals an average of 35 years after exposure (Lipshutz, Brennan, & Warren, 2002). This agent is no longer used because of its carcinogenicity.

In some Asian countries, infections by liver flukes (which are food- or waterborne parasitic worms that invade the bile duct) tend to be associated with bile duct cancers (Patel, 2006; Rajagopalan, Daines, Grossbard, & Kozuch, 2004). Liver fluke infection causes chronic inflammation and enhances the susceptibility of bile duct epithelium to carcinogens and free radicals, leading to genetic and epigenetic damage in cells. The types of liver fluke most closely related to bile duct cancer risk are *Clonorchis sinensis* and *Opisthorchis viverrini*. Hepatitis C infection has been associated with intrahepatic cholangiocarcinoma, but the relationship has not been fully established (Yamamoto et al., 2004).

Little is known about the molecular development of cholangiocarcinoma. Some of the more prevalent genetic altera-

tions (by microRNA expression) and epigenetic changes (hypermethylation of specific gene promoters thought to contribute to the carcinogenic process in cholangiocarcinoma) have been reviewed (Stutes, Tran, & DeMorrow, 2007).

Clinical Presentation

To some extent, the symptoms of cholangiocarcinoma depend on tumor location. Patients with cholangiocarcinoma in the extrahepatic bile ducts are more likely to have jaundice (90%), whereas those with intrahepatic tumors of the bile ducts often are asymptomatic in the early stages (Nakeeb et al., 1996). When patients do present with signs and symptoms of clay-colored stools, tea-colored urine, and pruritus, it is not until the later stages. When bile duct cancer causes symptoms it is usually because the bile duct is blocked, and the constellation of symptoms is very similar to that of other noncancerous diseases such as gallstones and hepatitis. In the late stages of intrahepatic cholangiocarcinoma, the patient may have vague abdominal pain and other nonspecific symptoms such as fever, fatigue, and weight loss (ACS, 2012a).

Assessment

Patient and Family History

All patients should be asked if they have any conditions or family history that predisposes them to cholangiocarcinoma. An assessment of other symptoms before jaundice is evident should include asking about pruritus, clay-colored stools, and tea-colored urine. Lack of appetite and subtle weight loss, malaise, and indigestion may accompany bile duct cancer (Hodgin, 2011).

Physical Examination

The physical examination is usually normal except for jaundice, icteric sclera, and multiple excoriations of the skin from pruritus. A mass may be palpable or the liver may be enlarged with intrahepatic biliary tumors. A distended gallbladder may be palpable with extrahepatic cholangiocarcinoma (Hodgin, 2011).

Diagnostic Evaluation

Laboratory tests include serum tests for CEA, CA 19-9, and CA 125, although these tumor markers are not specific for bile duct cancer (Bartlett et al., 2008). No fasting is required, and the results should be available within one to eight days depending on the laboratory and clinical facilities. Aspartate aminotransferase and alanine aminotransferase concentrations may be normal or minimally elevated. Because it is of biliary origin, alkaline phosphatase concentration usually rises in conjunction with bilirubin concentration. Elevated alkaline phosphatase and bilirubin concentrations may reflect impaired hepatic reserve and are often associated with more advanced disease. The levels of CA 19-9 seem to correlate with the stage of the disease. One study reported that the sensitivity of CA 19-9 above 100 U/ml for the diagnosis of cholangiocarcinoma in patients with resectable tumors was 33% compared to 72% in patients with unresectable tumors. Several new markers are currently being investigated. The human mucin 5, subtypes A and C (MUC5AC) are the most promising for future clinical use (Aljiffry, Walsh, & Molinari, 2009).

BUN, creatinine, and urinalysis should be performed to assess renal function before a patient undergoes a contrast-enhanced CT scan. CBC may show anemia, which may be an indicator of advanced disease. PT, PTT, and INR may reflect liver failure if abnormal. With prolonged obstruction, PT can become elevated because of vitamin K malabsorption.

Radiologic imaging is central to the diagnosis and treatment planning for patients with cholangiocarcinomas. Given the increased reliance on imaging studies, Miller, Schwartz, and D'Angelica (2007) reviewed the optimal use of the various imaging modalities. The initial radiographic evaluation consists of either abdominal ultrasonography or CT scan. Intrahepatic cholangiocarcinomas are easily viewed on standard CT scans, but identifying extrahepatic cholangiocarcinomas with standard CT scans often is difficult.

Ultrasound is usually performed first because it is noninvasive, is readily available, and provides important diagnostic information if the patient is jaundiced. Ultrasonography may show intrahepatic biliary dilation without evidence of extrahepatic bile duct abnormality and without evidence of stones. Ultrasound with Doppler can delineate the biliary extent of disease, vascular encasement or thrombosis, presence of lymph node metastases in the porta hepatis, and presence of liver metastases. However, small lesions and extrahepatic cholangiocarcinomas are difficult to identify with ultrasound.

CT resembles ultrasonography in that it may demonstrate ductal dilation and large mass lesions. CT using delayed contrast can also be used to evaluate intra-abdominal lymph node involvement and distant metastases. These images are useful in determining tumor resectability by depicting the tumor's relationship to nearby major vessels and the biliary tree. If IV contrast is to be used, patient allergy to contrast should be determined and premedication given as needed.

MRI has been useful for examining the abdomen for disease extension into other tissues or for metastatic disease in the liver. It can provide details of the vasculature for preoperative planning via MRA and bile duct passages via MRCP. Because MRCP is noninvasive and considered a safer alternative to direct cholangiopancreatography, it is preferred over ERCP unless a therapeutic intervention is planned. Cholangiography, via a percutaneous route, or ERCP can be used to evaluate for hepatic and biliary invasion of tumor (Miller et al., 2007). Percutaneous cholangiography most reliably defines the proximal extent of tumor, especially when both right and left hepatic ducts are obstructed (Pitt et al., 1995).

Endoscopic ultrasound is performed by using high-frequency ultrasound probes placed on the endoscope. EUS has the advantage of interrogating tissues and organs in direct proximity to the stomach and duodenum, increasing the ability to detect abnormalities that would not be easily identified by percutaneous approach. This technique can also yield aspirate for cytologic studies. EUS-guided fine-needle aspiration (FNA) results may be positive when other diagnostic tests are inconclusive. However, a negative FNA does not necessarily exclude a cancer diagnosis (Aljiffry et al., 2009).

A routine chest radiograph should be obtained to assess for pulmonary metastases. PET scanning has not been established in the evaluation of patient with cholangiocarcinoma, but some evidence indicates that it is useful for detecting lymph node involvement and distant metastatic disease in patients with otherwise potentially resectable disease (Corvera et al., 2008; Kim et al., 2008; Petrowsky et al., 2006; Seo et al., 2008).

Staging

Cholangiocarcinoma can arise anywhere within the biliary tree. Approximately 10% of cholangiocarcinomas arise within the intrahepatic bile ducts; however, the extrahepatic varieties are far more common. More than 90% of cholangiocarcinomas are adenocarcinomas, well differentiated, and mucin-producing (Lim, 2003).

Intrahepatic cholangiocarcinoma is staged according to the TNM staging system (see Figure 4-4). Intrahepatic cholangiocarcinomas usually metastasize to other intrahepatic locations and the peritoneum, and subsequently to the lungs and pleura. The stage classification depends on the number of tumors, vascular invasion, perforation of the visceral peritoneum, and regional lymph node involvement. A separate TNM staging system is used for extrahepatic cholangiocarcinoma. As a result of differences in anatomy of the bile duct and consideration of local factors that relate to resectability, extrahepatic cholangiocarcinomas have been divided into perihilar and distal bile duct cancers (see Figures 4-5 and 4-6).

Treatment Options

Surgery

Complete surgical resection is the only effective therapy that is potentially curative. Unfortunately, only 10% of patients present with early-stage disease and are considered for curative resection. Surgical exploration should be undertaken in low-risk patients—those without radiologic evidence of metastatic or locally unresectable disease. Even in these selected patients, more than half are found intraoperatively to have either peritoneal or hepatic metastases or, more likely, locally unresectable disease (Pitt et al., 1995).

The operative approach depends on the site and extent of tumor. Intrahepatic tumors are treated with hepatic resection. Distal extrahepatic tumors are treated with pancreaticoduodenectomy. The perihilar tumors make up the largest group and are managed with resection of the bile duct with or without hepatic resection (Fong et al., 2001).

Debate exists about whether preoperative stenting to relieve biliary obstruction is warranted, but most surgeons believe that preoperative biliary decompression does not alter the outcome of surgery. Patients who have unresectable cancers at the time of laparotomy may undergo palliation for biliary obstruction with a surgical enteric bypass. Relief of jaundice will be achieved if at least one-third of the functioning hepatic parenchyma is adequately drained (Fong et al., 2001).

Figure 4-4. American Joint Committee on Cancer Turnor, Node, Metastasis (TNM) Staging System for Intrahepatic Bile Duct Cancer

Primary Tumor (T)

TX	Primary tumor cannot be assessed
T0	No evidence of primary tumor
Tis	Carcinoma in situ (intraductal)
T1	Solitary tumor without vascular invasion
T2a	Solitary tumor with vascular invasion
T2b	Multiple tumors, with or without vascular invasion
T3	Tumor perforating the visceral peritoneum or involving the local extrahepatic structures by direct invasion
T4	Tumor with periductal invasion

Regional Lymph Nodes (N)

NX	Regional lymph nodes cannot be assessed
N0	No regional lymph node metastasis
N1	Regional lymph node metastasis

Distant Metastasis (M)

M0	No distant metastasis
M1	Distant metastasis

Stage Grouping

Stage I	T1 N0 M0
Stage II	T2 N0 M0
Stage IIIA	T3 N0 M0
Stage IIIB	T4 N0 M0
Stage IIIC	Any T N1 M0
Stage IV	Any T Any N M1

Histologic Grade (G)

G1	Well differentiated
G2	Moderately differentiated
G3	Poorly differentiated
G4	Undifferentiated

Figure 4-5. American Joint Committee on Cancer Tumor, Node, Metastasis (TNM) Staging System for Perihilar Bile Duct Cancer

Primary Tumor (T)

TX	Primary tumor cannot be assessed
T0	No evidence of primary tumor
Tis	Carcinoma in situ
T1	Tumor confined to the bile duct, with extension up to the muscle layer or fibrous tissue
T2a	Tumor invades beyond the wall of the bile duct to surrounding adipose tissue
T2b	Tumor invades adjacent hepatic parenchyma
T3	Tumor invades unilateral branches of the portal vein or hepatic artery
T4	Tumor invades main portal vein or its branches bilaterally; or the common hepatic artery; or the second-order biliary radicals bilaterally; or unilateral second-order biliary radicals with contralateral portal vein or hepatic artery involvement

Regional Lymph Nodes (N)

NX	Regional lymph nodes cannot be assessed
N0	No regional lymph node metastasis
N1	Regional lymph node metastasis (including nodes along the cystic duct, common bile duct, hepatic artery, and portal vein)
N2	Metastasis to periaortic, pericaval, superior mesenteric artery, and/or celiac artery lymph nodes

Distant Metastasis (M)

M0	No distant metastasis
M1	Distant metastasis

Stage Grouping

Stage 0	Tis N0 M0
Stage I	T1 N0 M0
Stage II	T2a–b N0 M0
Stage IIIA	T3 N0 M0
Stage IIIB	T1–3 N1 M0
Stage IVA	T4 N0–1 M0
Stage IVB	Any T N2 M0
	Any T Any N M1

Hepatic transplantation is considered for some patients with proximal tumors who are not candidates for resection because of the extent of tumor spread in the liver. A multicenter study that treated these patients with neoadjuvant therapy followed by liver transplantation had a 65% rate of recurrence-free survival after five years, showing this therapy to be highly effective (Murad et al., 2012).

Figure 4-6. American Joint Committee on Cancer Tumor, Node, Metastasis (TNM) Staging System for Distal Bile Duct Cancer

Primary Tumor (T)

TX	Primary tumor cannot be assessed
T0	No evidence of primary tumor
Tis	Carcinoma in situ
T1	Tumor confined to the bile duct histologically
T2	Tumor invades beyond the wall of the bile duct
T3	Tumor invades the gallbladder, pancreas, duodenum, or other adjacent organs without involvement of the celiac axis, or the superior mesenteric artery
T4	Tumor involves the celiac axis, or the superior mesenteric artery

Regional Lymph Nodes (N)

NX	Regional lymph nodes cannot be assessed
N0	No regional lymph node metastasis
N1	Regional lymph node metastasis

Distant Metastasis (M)

M0	No distant metastasis
M1	Distant metastasis

Stage Grouping

Stage 0	Tis N0 M0
Stage IA	T1 N0 M0
Stage IB	T2 N0 M0
Stage IIA	T3 N0 M0
Stage IIB	T1–3 N1 M0

Note. From *AJCC Cancer Staging Manual* (7th ed., p. 229), by S.B. Edge, D.R. Byrd, C.C. Compton, A.G. Fritz, F.L. Greene, and A. Trotti III (Eds.), 2010, New York, NY: Springer, www.springer.com. Copyright 2010 by American Joint Committee on Cancer. Adapted with permission.

Palliative Therapy

Patients with unequivocal evidence of unresectable cholangiocarcinoma at initial evaluation should receive nonsurgical palliative care. Nonsurgical palliation to relieve biliary obstruction can be achieved with endoscopic and percutaneous stents. Percutaneous biliary drainage may be required if endoscopic drainage is unsuccessful. Metallic stents have been used to provide biliary drainage but are more expensive than plastic stents. Metal stents expand to a larger diameter and tend to stay patent and require fewer subsequent manipulations (Ahrendt & Pitt, 2001). Plastic stents usually occlude within three months and require replacement. Adequate biliary drainage can be achieved in a high percentage of cases.

Because patients with unresectable tumors will likely develop back pain, celiac-plexus block via regional injection of alcohol or another sclerosing agent can relieve pain in the mid-back. A meta-analysis showed that 89% of patients with can-cer (regardless of type of intra-abdominal malignancy) who underwent a celiac-plexus block reported to have good to excellent pain relief two weeks following the procedure. Additionally, partial to complete pain relief continued in approximately 90% of patients alive at three months and in 79%–90% of patients until death (Eisenberg, Carr, & Chalmers, 1995). Implementing celiac-plexus block prior to the onset of severe pain has been shown to maintain an improved overall quality of life (Lillemoe et al., 1993).

Radiation Therapy

Radiation therapy for treating resected extrahepatic bile duct cancer is controversial given the lack of randomized trials and small size of the studies in the literature. A few published studies have investigated the use of external beam radiation with boost doses administered using intraluminal brachytherapy (Golfieri et al., 2006; Ishii et al., 2004; Kuvshinoff et al., 1995; Takamura et al., 2003). This technique uses a wire or string of radioactive seeds introduced into the bile duct to deliver high-dose radiation to the duct itself, with minimal damage to the surrounding liver (Aljiffry et al., 2009). The previously described palliative radiotherapy is associated with increased incidence of complications, such as cholangitis and gastroduodenitis, in comparison to best supportive care and therefore is not routinely used in many centers (Bowling, Galbraith, Hatfield, Solano, & Spittle, 1996).

Photodynamic therapy is an emerging palliative strategy that is a two-step process: the first step is IV administration of a photosensitizing drug that preferentially accumulates in malignant cells; the second step is activation of the photosensitizer by light illumination at a specific wavelength to cause tumor cell necrosis (Ortner, 2004). The combination of photodynamic therapy with biliary stenting has been shown to significantly improve the overall survival of patients with unresectable cholangiocarcinoma in two small randomized clinical trials (Ortner, 2004; Zoepf, Jakobs, Arnold, Apel, & Riemann, 2005).

Chemotherapy

There is no established standard chemotherapy regimen for patients with locally advanced or metastatic biliary duct cancer because no single randomized study has ever been sufficiently robust to draw definitive conclusions. However, a phase III trial provided evidence that cisplatin plus gemcitabine is an effective treatment option for locally advanced or metastatic biliary duct cancer. Patients treated with cisplatin plus gemcitabine lived an average of 3.6 months longer than those treated with gemcitabine alone (Valle et al., 2010). Other drugs—including hormones, antiestrogens, cholecystokinin, somatostatin, and antibiotics used as cytotoxic agents—have been tried as novel approaches.

Chemoradiation in patients with advanced biliary duct cancer can provide control of symptoms caused by local tumor effects and may prolong overall survival (Czito, Anscher, &

Willett, 2006; Macdonald & Crane, 2002). The National Comprehensive Cancer Network recommends that chemotherapy administered concurrently with radiation should be limited to either IV 5-FU or oral capecitabine and that such treatment be restricted to patients without evidence of metastatic disease (Benson et al., 2009). Concurrent chemoradiation with gemcitabine is not recommended because of limited clinical data and the toxicity associated with this treatment.

Prognosis and Surveillance

Long-term survival in patients with cholangiocarcinoma depends largely on the stage of disease at presentation and whether such patients are treated by a palliative procedure or by complete tumor resection. The median survival in patients who undergo resection and postoperative chemoradiation may be as high as 17–27.5 months. An intermediate prognosis (median survival duration of 7–17 months) is achieved for patients who cannot undergo resection but can tolerate adjuvant chemoradiation or possibly photodynamic therapy. The poorest prognosis is for patients with unresectable disease, with or without overt metastatic disease, who can tolerate only palliative stent placement (median survival duration of five to eight months) (Ahrendt, Cameron, & Pitt, 1996).

For patients with resectable intrahepatic cholangiocarcinoma, overall five-year survival is 30%–40%. In comparison, overall five-year survival for patients with resectable extrahepatic (perihilar) tumors has been only 10%–20%, although it may be as high as 33%–46% in patients with negative margins on microscopy (Ahrendt et al., 1996; Sugiura et al., 1994). In patients with extrahepatic cholangiocarcinoma (distal bile duct), overall survival is 32–38 months, and five-year survival ranges 28%–45% (Nakeeb et al., 1996). Patterns of treatment failure after curative surgery show disappointingly high rates of recurrence in the tumor bed and regional nodes. These patterns may be due in part to the narrow pathologic margins; however, the regional node failure rate is approximately 50%, and the distal metastases rate is 30%–40%.

Currently, no data support aggressive surveillance in patients who have had surgical resection of bile duct cancer. The patient and healthcare provider should have a careful discussion regarding follow-up care. Imaging studies maybe considered every six months for two years, and periodic laboratory work every two to three months.

Nursing Implications and Future Directions

Similar to nursing care for patients with early-stage gallbladder cancer, nursing care for patients with early-stage cholangiocarcinoma focuses on support during treatment decision-making, attentive pre- and postoperative care, and symptom management. Nursing care of patients with advanced disease concentrates on palliation of symptoms and end-of-life care. Symptom management, patient and family education, and the current state of research are the same as were indicated for gallbladder cancer. As was true for gallbladder cancer, oncology nurses who provide care for patients with cholangiocarcinoma are in a unique position to advocate for both patients and caregivers.

Summary

The sudden onset, limited treatment options, and overall poor prognosis are challenges when caring for patients with gallbladder or bile duct cancer. Both cancers have limited success in achieving cure, and surgery is the most effective therapy. Advances in our understanding of genetic alterations in these cancers will ultimately lead to targeted therapies that can improve the outlook for these patients.

References

Ahrendt, S.A., Cameron, J.L., & Pitt, H.A. (1996). Current management of patients with perihilar cholangiocarcinoma. *Advances in Surgery, 30,* 427–452.

Ahrendt, S.A., & Pitt, H.A. (2001). Malignant diseases of the biliary tract. In P.J. Morris & W.C. Wood (Eds.), *Oxford textbook of surgery* (2nd ed., pp. 1699–1713). New York, NY: Oxford University Press.

Albores-Saavedra, J., & Henson, D.E. (1986). *Tumors of the gallbladder and extrahepatic bile ducts: Atlas of tumor pathology* (2nd series, fascicle 22). Washington, DC: Armed Forces Institute of Pathology.

Aljiffry, M., Walsh, M.J., & Molinari, M. (2009). Advances in diagnosis, treatment and palliation of cholangiocarcinoma: 1990–2009. *World Journal of Gastroenterology, 15,* 4240–4262. doi:10.3748/wjg.15.4240

American Cancer Society. (2012a, June 28). Bile duct (cholangiocarcinoma) cancer. Retrieved from http://www.cancer.org/Cancer/BileDuctCancer/DetailedGuide/bile-duct-cancer-what-is-bile-duct-cancer

American Cancer Society. (2012b). Cancer facts and figures 2012. Retrieved from http://www.cancer.org/acs/groups/content/@epidemiologysurveilance/documents/document/acspc-031941.pdf

Ames, B.N., & Gold, L.S. (1998). The causes and prevention of cancer: The role of environment. *Biotherapy (Dordrecht, Netherlands), 11*(2–3), 205–220. doi:10.1023/A:1007971204469

Barreto, S.G., Haga, H., & Shukla, P.J. (2009). Hormones and gallbladder cancer in women. *Indian Journal of Gastroenterology, 28,* 126–130. doi:10.1007/s12664-009-0046-8

Bartlett, D.L., Ramanthan, R.K., & Ben-Josef, E. (2008). Cancers of the biliary tree. In V.T. DeVita Jr., T.S. Lawrence, & S.A. Rosenberg (Eds.), *Cancer: Principles and practice of oncology* (8th ed., pp. 1156–1186). Philadelphia, PA: Lippincott Williams & Wilkins.

Benjamin, I.S. (2003). Biliary cystic disease: The risk of cancer. *Journal of Hepato-Biliary-Pancreatic Surgery, 10,* 335–339. doi:10.1007/s00534-002-0696-8

Ben-Menachem, T. (2007). Risk factors for cholangiocarcinoma. *European Journal of Gastroenterology and Hepatology, 19,* 615–617. doi:10.1097/MEG.0b013e328224b935

Benson, A.B., III, Abrams, T.A., Ben-Josef, E., Bloomston, P.M., Botha, J.F., Clary, B.M., … Zhu, A.X. (2009). NCCN clinical practice guidelines in oncology: Hepatobiliary cancers. *Journal of the National Comprehensive Cancer Network, 7,* 350–391. Retrieved from http://www.jnccn.org/content/7/4/350.long

Bowling, T.E., Galbraith, S.M., Hatfield, A.R., Solano, J., & Spittle, M.F. (1996). A retrospective comparison of endoscopic stenting alone with stenting and radiotherapy in non-resectable cholangiocarcinoma. *Gut, 39,* 852–855. doi:10.1136/gut.39.6.852

Carriaga, M.T., & Henson, D.E. (1995). Liver, gallbladder, extrahepatic bile ducts, and pancreas. *Cancer, 75*(Suppl. 1), 171–190. doi:10.1002/1097-0142(19950101)75:1+<171::AID-CNCR 2820751306>3.0.CO;2-2

Corvera, C.U., Blumgart, L.H., Akhurst, T., DeMatteo, R.P., D'Angelica, M., Fong, Y., & Jarnagin, W.R. (2008). 18F-fluorodeoxyglucose positron emission tomography influences management decisions in patients with biliary cancer. *Journal of the American College of Surgeons, 206,* 57–65. doi:10.1016/j.jamcollsurg.2007.07.002

Csendes, A., Becerra, M., Rojas, J., & Medina, E. (2000). Number and size of stones in patients with asymptomatic and symptomatic gallstones and gallbladder carcinoma: A prospective study of 592 cases. *Journal of Gastrointestinal Surgery, 4,* 481–485. doi:10.1016/S1091 -255X(00)80090-6

Czito, B.G., Anscher, M.S., & Willett, C.G. (2006). Radiation therapy in the treatment of cholangiocarcinoma. *Oncology, 20,* 873–884.

Darwin, P.E., Kennedy, A.S., & Bonheur, J.L. (2012, February 23). Cholangiocarcinoma. Retrieved from http://emedicine.medscape.com/ article/277393-overview

Department of Health, Education, and Welfare. (1973, November 16). Protection of human subjects policies and procedures. Federal Register, 38(221), Part II. Retrieved from http://www.hhs.gov/ohrp/archive/ documents/19731116.pdf

Diehl, A.K. (1983). Gallstone size and the risk of gallbladder cancer. *JAMA, 250,* 2323–2326. doi:10.1001/jama.1983.03340170049027

Donohue, J.H., Stewart, A.K., & Menck, H.R. (1998). The national cancer data base report on carcinoma of the gallbladder, 1989–1995. *Cancer, 83,* 2618–2628. doi:10.1002/(SICI)1097 -0142(19981215)83:12<2618::AID-CNCR29>3.0.CO;2-H

Duffy, A., Capanu, M., Abou-Alfa, G.K., Huitzil, D., Jarnagin, W., Fong, Y., ... O'Reilly, E.M. (2008). Gallbladder cancer (GBC): 10-year experience at Memorial Sloan-Kettering Cancer Center (MSKCC). *Journal of Surgical Oncology, 98,* 485–489. doi:10.1002/jso.21141

Edge, S.B., Byrd, D.R., Compton, C.C., Fritz, A., Greene, F.L., & Trotti, A., III. (Eds.). (2010). *AJCC cancer staging handbook from the AJCC cancer staging manual* (7th ed.). New York, NY: American Joint Committee on Cancer.

Eisenberg, E., Carr, D.B., & Chalmers, T.C. (1995). Neurolytic celiac plexus block for treatment of cancer pain: A meta-analysis. *Anesthesia and Analgesia, 80,* 290–295. Retrieved from http://www.anesthesia -analgesia.org/content/80/2/290.long

Fenster, L.F., Lonborg, R., Thirlby, R.C., & Traverso, L.W. (1995). What symptoms does cholecystectomy cure? Insights from an outcomes measurement project and review of the literature. *American Journal of Surgery, 169,* 533–538. doi:10.1016/S0002-9610(99)80212-8

Fong, Y., Brennan, M.F., Turnbull, A., Colt, D.G., & Blumgart, L.H. (1993). Gallbladder cancer discovered during laparoscopic surgery. Potential for iatrogenic tumor dissemination. *Archives of Surgery, 128,* 1054–1056. doi:10.1001/archsurg.1993.01420210118016

Fong, Y., Kemeny, N., & Lawrence, T.S. (2001). Cancer of the liver and biliary tree. In V.T. DeVita Jr., S. Hellman, & S.A. Rosenberg (Eds.), *Cancer: Principles and practice of oncology* (6th ed., pp. 1162–1216). Philadelphia, PA: Lippincott Williams & Wilkins.

Gebbia, V., Giuliani, F., Maiello, E., Colucci, G., Verderame, F., Borsellino, N., ... Valdesi, M. (2001). Treatment of inoperable and/or metastatic biliary tree carcinomas with single-agent gemcitabine or in combination with levofolinic acid and infusional fluorouracil: Results of a multicenter phase II study. *Journal of Clinical Oncology, 19,* 4089–4091.

Glajchen, M. (2004). The emerging role and needs of family caregivers in cancer care. *Journal of Supportive Oncology, 2,* 145–155.

Golfieri, R., Giampalma, E., Renzulli, M., Galuppi, A., Vicenzi, L., Galaverni, M.C., & Cappelli, A. (2006). Unresectable hilar cholangiocarcinoma: Multimodality approach with percutaneous treatment associated with radiotherapy and chemotherapy. *In Vivo, 20,* 757–760. Retrieved from http://iv.iiarjournals.org/content/20/6A/757.long

Halpert, D., & Erdek, M.A. (2008). Pain management for hepatobiliary cancer. *Current Treatment Options in Oncology, 9,* 234–241. doi:10.1007/s11864-008-0069-x

Hanks, G.W., Conno, F., Cherny, N., Hanna, M., Kalso, E., McQuay, H.J., ... Expert Working Group of the Research Network of the European Association for Palliative Care. (2001). Morphine and alternative opioids in cancer pain: The EAPC recommendations. *British Journal of Cancer, 84,* 587–593. doi:10.1054/bjoc.2001.1680

Hodgin, M.B. (2011). Gallbladder and bile duct cancer. In C.H. Yarbro, D. Wujcik, & B.H. Gobel (Eds.), *Cancer nursing: Principles and practice* (7th ed., pp. 1316–1333). Burlington, MA: Jones and Bartlett.

Hsing, A.W., Rashid, A., Devesa, S.D., & Fraumeni, J.F. (2006). Biliary tract cancer. In D. Schottenfeld & J.F. Fraumeni (Eds.), *Cancer epidemiology and prevention* (3rd ed., pp. 787–800). New York, NY: Oxford University Press.

Hu, B., Gong, B., & Zhou, D.Y. (2003). Association of anomalous pancreaticobiliary ductal junction with gallbladder carcinoma in Chinese patients: An ERCP study. *Gastrointestinal Endoscopy, 57,* 541–545. doi:10.1067/mge.2003.136

Huether, S.E. (2009). Structure and function of the digestive system. In K.L. McCance & S.E. Huether (Eds.), *Pathophysiology: The biologic basis for disease in adults and children* (6th ed., pp. 1420–1541). Maryland Heights, MO: Mosby.

Ishii, H., Furuse, J., Nagase, M., Kawashima, M., Ikeda, H., & Yoshino, M. (2004). Relief of jaundice by external beam radiotherapy and intraluminal brachytherapy in patients with extrahepatic cholangiocarcinoma: Results without stenting. *Hepato-Gastroenterology, 51,* 954–957.

Jacox, A., Carr, D.B., & Payne, R.E.A. (1994). *Management of cancer pain: Clinical practice guideline number 9* (AHCPR No. 94-0592). Rockville, MD: U.S. Department of Health and Human Services.

Kaza, R.K., Gulati, M., Wig, J.D., & Chawla, Y.K. (2006). Evaluation of gall bladder carcinoma with dynamic magnetic resonance imaging and magnetic resonance cholangiopancreatography. *Australasian Radiology, 50,* 212–217. doi:10.1111/j.1440-1673.2006.01564.x

Kim, J.H., Kim, T.K., Eun, H.W., Kim, B.S., Lee, M.G., Kim, P.N., & Ha, H.K. (2002). Preoperative evaluation of gallbladder carcinoma: Efficacy of combined use of MR imaging, MR cholangiography, and contrast-enhanced dual-phase three-dimensional MR angiography. *Journal of Magnetic Resonance Imaging, 16,* 676–684. doi:10.1002/jmri.10212

Kim, J.Y., Kim, M.H., Lee, T.Y., Hwang, C.Y., Kim, J.S., Yun, S.C., ... Lee, S.K. (2008). Clinical role of 18F-FDG PET-CT in suspected and potentially operable cholangiocarcinoma: A prospective study compared with conventional imaging. *American Journal of Gastroenterology, 103,* 1145–1151. doi:10.1111/j.1572-0241.2007.01710.x

Kuvshinoff, B.W., Armstrong, J.G., Fong, Y., Schupak, K., Getradjman, G., Heffernan, N., & Blumgart, L.H. (1995). Palliation of irresectable hilar cholangiocarcinoma with biliary drainage and radiotherapy. *British Journal of Surgery, 82,* 1522–1525. doi:10.1002/bjs.1800821122

Kwon, A.H., Inui, H., Matsui, Y., Uchida, Y., Hukui, J., & Kamiyama, Y. (2004). Laparoscopic cholecystectomy in patients with porcelain gallbladder based on the preoperative ultrasound findings. *Hepato-Gastroenterology, 51,* 950–953.

Lai, C.H., & Lau, W.Y. (2008). Gallbladder cancer—A comprehensive review. *The Surgeon: Journal of the Royal Colleges of Surgeons of Edinburgh and Ireland, 6,* 101–110. doi:10.1016/S1479-666X(08)80073-X

Lake, J.R. (1993). Benign and malignant neoplasms of the gallbladder, bile ducts and ampulla. In M.H. Sleisinger & J.S. Fordtran (Eds.), *Gastrointestinal disease: Pathophysiology, diagnosis, management* (5th ed., pp. 1891–1902). Philadelphia, PA: Saunders.

Levin, B. (1999). Gallbladder carcinoma. *Annals of Oncology, 10*(Suppl. 4), 129–130.

Levy, A.D., Murakata, L.A., & Rohrmann, C.A., Jr. (2001). Gallbladder carcinoma: Radiologic-pathologic correlation. *Radiographics, 21,* 295–314.

Lillemoe, K.D., Cameron, J.L., Kaufman, H.S., Yeo, C.J., Pitt, H.A., & Sauter, P.K. (1993). Chemical splanchnicectomy in patients with unresectable pancreatic cancer. A prospective randomized trial. *Annals of Surgery, 217,* 447–455. doi:10.1097/00000658-199305010-00004

Lim, J.H. (2003). Cholangiocarcinoma: Morphologic classification according to growth pattern and imaging findings. *American Journal of Roentgenology, 181,* 819–827.

Lindell, G., Holmin, T., Ewers, S.B., Tranberg, K.G., Stenram, U., & Ihse, I. (2003). Extended operation with or without intraoperative (IORT) and external (EBRT) radiotherapy for gallbladder carcinoma. *Hepato-Gastroenterology, 50,* 310–314.

Lipshutz, G.S., Brennan, T.V., & Warren, R.S. (2002). Thorotrast-induced liver neoplasia: A collective review. *Journal of the American College of Surgeons, 195,* 713–718. doi:10.1016/S1072-7515(02)01287-5

Macdonald, O.K., & Crane, C.H. (2002). Palliative and postoperative radiotherapy in biliary tract cancer. *Surgical Oncology Clinics of North America, 11,* 941–954. doi:10.1016/S1055-3207(02)00038-8

Mancuso, T.F., & Brennan, M.J. (1970). Epidemiological considerations of cancer of the gallbladder, bile ducts and salivary glands in the rubber industry. *Journal of Occupational Medicine, 12,* 333–341.

Merz, B.J., Dodge, G.G., Abellera, R.M., & Kisken, W.A. (1993). Implant metastasis of gallbladder carcinoma in situ in a cholecystectomy scar: A case report. *Surgery, 114,* 120–124.

Miller, G., & Jarnagin, W.R. (2008). Gallbladder carcinoma. *European Journal of Surgical, 34,* 306–312. doi:10.1016/j.ejso.2007.07.206

Miller, G., Schwartz, L.H., & D'Angelica, M. (2007). The use of imaging in the diagnosis and staging of hepatobiliary malignancies. *Surgical Oncology Clinics of North America, 16,* 343–368. doi:10.1016/j.soc.2007.04.001

Mizutani, M., Nawata, S., Hirai, I., Murakami, G., & Kimura, W. (2005). Anatomy and histology of Virchow's node. *Anatomical Science International, 80,* 193–198.

Molmenti, E.P., Marsh, J.W., Dvorchik, I., Oliver, J.H., III., Madariaga, J., & Iwatsuki, S. (1999). Hepatobiliary malignancies: Primary hepatic malignant neoplasms. *Surgical Clinics of North America, 79,* 43–57, viii. doi:10.1016/S0039-6109(05)70006-2

Muguruma, N., Okamura, S., Ichikawa, S., Tsujigami, K., Suzuki, M., Tadatsu, M., ... Ito, S. (2001). Endoscopic sonography in the diagnosis of gallbladder wall lesions in patients with gallstones. *Journal of Clinical Ultrasound, 29,* 395–400. doi:10.1002/jcu.1055

Murad, S.D., Kim, W.R., Harnois, D.M., Douglas, D.D., Burton, J., Kulik, L.M., ... Heimbach, J.K. (2012). Efficacy of neoadjuvant chemoradiation, followed by liver transplantation, for perihilar cholangiocarcinoma at 12 U.S. centers. *Gastroenterology, 143,* 88–98. doi:10.1053/j.gastro.2012.04.008

Musser, J.H. (1889). Primary cancer of the gallbladder and bile ducts. *Boston Medical Surgical Journal, 121,* 581. doi:10.1056/NEJM188912121212404

Nakeeb, A., Pitt, H.A., Sohn, T.A., Coleman, J., Abrams, R.A., Piantadosi, S., ... Cameron, J.L. (1996). Cholangiocarcinoma: A spectrum of intrahepatic, perihilar, and distal tumors. *Annals of Surgery, 224,* 463–473. doi:10.1097/00000658-199610000-00005

Namasivayam, S., Kalra, M.K., Torres, W.E., & Small, W.C. (2006). Adverse reactions to intravenous iodinated contrast media: An update. *Current Problems in Diagnostic Radiology, 35,* 164–169. doi:10.1067/j.cpradiol.2006.04.001

Ortner, M.A. (2004). Photodynamic therapy in cholangiocarcinomas. *Best Practice and Research: Clinical Gastroenterology, 18,* 147–154. doi:10.1016/S1521-6918(03)00100-8

Pack, D.A., O'Connor, K., & O'Hagan, K. (2001). Cholangiocarcinoma: A nursing perspective. *Clinical Journal of Oncology Nursing, 5,* 141–146.

Pagana, K.D., & Pagana, T.J. (1997). *Diagnostic and laboratory test reference* (3rd ed.). St. Louis, MO: Mosby.

Patel, T. (2006). Cholangiocarcinoma. *Nature Clinical Practice: Gastroenterology and Hepatology, 3,* 33–42. doi:10.1038/ncpgasthep0389

Petrowsky, H., Wildbrett, P., Husarik, D.B., Hany, T.F., Tam, S., Jochum, W., & Clavien, P.A. (2006). Impact of integrated positron emission tomography and computed tomography on staging and management of gallbladder cancer and cholangiocarcinoma. *Journal of Hepatology, 45,* 43–50. doi:10.1016/j.jhep.2006.03.009

Pitt, H.A., Dooley, W.C., Yeo, C.J., & Cameron, J.L. (1995). Malignancies of the biliary tree. *Current Problems in Surgery, 32,* 1–90. doi:10.1016/S0011-3840(05)80011-5

Rajagopalan, V., Daines, W.P., Grossbard, M.L., & Kozuch, P. (2004). Gallbladder and biliary tract carcinoma: A comprehensive update, part 1. *Oncology, 18,* 889–896.

Randi, G., Franceschi, S., & La Vecchia, C. (2006). Gallbladder cancer worldwide: Geographical distribution and risk factors. *International Journal of Cancer, 118,* 1591–1602. doi:10.1002/ijc.21683

Sauerland, C., Engelking, C., Wickham, R., & Pearlstone, D.B. (2009). Cancers of the pancreas and hepatobiliary system. *Seminars in Oncology Nursing, 25,* 76–92. doi:10.1016/j.soncn.2008.10.006

Seo, S., Hatano, E., Higashi, T., Nakajima, A., Nakamoto, Y., Tada, M., ... Uemoto, S. (2008). Fluorine-18 fluorodeoxyglucose positron emission tomography predicts lymph node metastasis, P-glycoprotein expression, and recurrence after resection in mass-forming intrahepatic cholangiocarcinoma. *Surgery, 143,* 769–777. doi:10.1016/j.surg.2008.01.010

Serra, I., Calvo, A., Baez, S., Yamamoto, M., Endoh, K., & Aranda, W. (1996). Risk factors for gallbladder cancer: An international collaborative case-control study. *Cancer, 78,* 1515–1517. doi:10.1002/(SICI)1097-0142(19961001)78:7<1515::AID-CNCR21>3.0.CO;2-1

Singh, S., Ansari, M.A., & Narayan, G. (2012). Pathobiology of gallbladder cancer. *Journal of Scientific Research, 56,* 35–35.

Stephen, A.E., & Berger, D.L. (2001). Carcinoma in the porcelain gallbladder: A relationship revisited. *Surgery, 129,* 699–703. doi:10.1067/msy.2001.113888

Stern, N., & Sturgess, R. (2008). Endoscopic therapy in the management of malignant biliary obstruction. *European Journal of Surgical Oncology, 34,* 313–317. doi:10.1016/j.ejso.2007.07.210

Stutes, M., Tran, S., & DeMorrow, S. (2007). Genetic and epigenetic changes associated with cholangiocarcinoma: From DNA methylation to microRNAs. *World Journal of Gastroenterology, 13,* 6465–6469. doi:10.3748/wjg.13.6465

Sugiura, Y., Nakamura, S., Iida, S., Hosoda, Y., Ikeuchi, S., Mori, S., ... Tsuzuki, T. (1994). Extensive resection of the bile ducts combined with liver resection for cancer of the main hepatic duct junction: A cooperative study of the Keio Bile Duct Cancer Study Group. *Surgery, 115,* 445–451.

Sun, V., Ferrell, B., Juarez, G., Wagman, L.D., Yen, Y., & Chung, V. (2008). Symptom concerns and quality of life in hepatobiliary cancers. *Oncology Nursing Forum, 35,* E45–E52. doi:10.1188/08.ONF.E45-E52

Takamura, A., Saito, H., Kamada, T., Hiramatsu, K., Takeuchi, S., Hasegawa, M., & Miyamoto, N. (2003). Intraluminal low-dose-rate ^{192}Ir brachytherapy combined with external beam radiotherapy and biliary stenting for unresectable extrahepatic bile duct carcinoma. *International Journal of Radiation Oncology, Biology, Physics, 57,* 1357–1365. doi:10.1016/S0360-3016(03)00770-3

Valle, J., Wasan, H., Palmer, D.H., Cunningham, D., Anthoney, A., Maraveyas, A., ... ABC-02 Trial Investigators. (2010). Cisplatin plus gemcitabine versus gemcitabine for biliary tract cancer. *New England Journal of Medicine, 362,* 1273–1281. doi:10.1056/NEJMoa0908721

Vogt, D.P. (1988). Current management of cholangiocarcinoma. *Oncology, 2,* 37–44, 54.

White, K., Kraybill, W.G., & Lopez, M.J. (1988). Primary carcinoma of the gallbladder: TNM staging and prognosis. *Journal of Surgical Oncology, 39,* 251–255. doi:10.1002/jso.2930390407

Yamamoto, S., Kubo, S., Hai, S., Uenishi, T., Yamamoto, T., Shuto, T., ... Tanaka, T. (2004). Hepatitis C virus infection as a likely etiology of intrahepatic cholangiocarcinoma. *Cancer Science, 95,* 592–595. doi:10.1111/j.1349-7006.2004.tb02492.x

Yasuhito, Y. (2006). Genetic alterations in gallbladder carcinoma. *Kantansui, 53,* 257.

Yee, K., Sheppard, B.C., Domreis, J., & Blanke, C.D. (2002). Cancers of the gallbladder and biliary ducts. *Oncology, 16,* 939–946, 949.

Zoepf, T., Jakobs, R., Arnold, J.C., Apel, D., & Riemann, J.F. (2005). Palliation of nonresectable bile duct cancer: Improved survival after photodynamic therapy. *American Journal of Gastroenterology, 100,* 2426–2430. doi:10.1111/j.1572-0241.2005.00318.x

CHAPTER 5

Primary Hepatocellular Carcinoma

Gail W. Davidson, RN, BSN, OCN®, and Lyn Wooten, RN, MSN

Introduction

Hepatocellular carcinoma (HCC) is the most common form of primary liver cancer, accounting for 75% of the reported cases. This tumor originates in the hepatocytes, which are the cells responsible for the primary functions of the liver (Gish, Marrero, & Benson, 2010). The major risk factors for developing HCC are a history of hepatitis B or hepatitis C viral infection, cirrhosis, and nonalcoholic fatty liver disease. A steady increase in the number of cases has been reported in part because of the screening guidelines now in place for patients with hepatitis B and C or cirrhosis and improved techniques for imaging the liver. The American Cancer Society estimated that in 2012, HCC would be the fifth most common cause of cancer death in men and the eighth most common cause of cancer death among women in the United States (Siegel, Naishadham, & Jemal, 2012). Great developments have occurred in curative therapies for patients diagnosed with early-stage disease, but the challenge of treating patients in the presence of chronic liver disease remains (Silva & Wigg, 2010).

Incidence

HCC is the fifth most common cancer in the world (International Agency for Research on Cancer [IARC], 2008). Because of its high fatality rate (HCC has a mortality-to-incidence ratio of 0.93), liver cancer is the third leading cause of cancer deaths worldwide, accounting for about 694,000 deaths in 2008 (IARC, 2008). Age-standardized incidence rates vary from 4/100,000 in North America to 36/100,000 in China, and 94/100,000 in Mongolia (IARC, 2008; World Cancer Research Fund International, 2008). Although HCC is relatively uncommon in the United States, the incidence has risen because of the spread of the hepatitis C virus (National Cancer Institute [NCI], 2012b). An increased incidence of as much as 75% has been attributed to both hepatitis C virus spread and the diagnosis of nonalcoholic fatty liver disease (Abou-Alfa & DeMatteo, 2009).

In the United States, 28,720 new cases of liver and intrahepatic bile duct cancers were expected to be diagnosed and 20,550 deaths attributable to the disease were expected in 2012 (Siegel et al., 2012). The disease is typically diagnosed in the fifth and sixth decades of life, and 80% of people are diagnosed in the advanced stages (Dugdale & Chen, 2011; Sun & Sarna, 2008). Due to diagnosis in the advanced stages, the five-year survival for HCC is less than 5% if the disease is unresectable at diagnosis (Sun & Sarna, 2008). Surgery is the only curative treatment for HCC, yet only 10%–20% of patients diagnosed are able to undergo complete resection (Dugdale & Chen, 2011). The prognosis for any patient with primary liver cancer who is treated for progressing, recurring, or relapsing disease is poor. Treatment of recurrence depends on prior treatment, the site of recurrence, presence of cirrhosis, hepatic function, and the patient's functional status. A re-resection should be considered if at all feasible as the best chance for a cure. If the patient's condition or location of disease precludes this, embolization or clinical trials should be considered (NCI, 2012b).

Risk Factors

Several risk factors are related to HCC, and exposure to many of these risks is avoidable. HCC is associated with cirrhosis in 50%–80% of patients, with 5% of patients with cirrhosis developing HCC (Abou-Alfa & DeMatteo, 2009). Cirrhosis can be caused by numerous factors, including alcohol abuse (alcoholic cirrhosis), obesity (nonalcoholic fatty liver disease), and an autoimmune disease causing biliary cirrhosis. Hepatitis B and hepatitis C bear the most significant risk worldwide, especially in those with chronic active hepatitis. Men with both hepatitis B and C are at the highest risk, and those consuming more than 80 g of alcohol daily even further increase their risk compared to those who do not drink (NCI, 2012b). In the United States, 2.7 million people have chronic hepatitis C. Chronic hepatitis B and C account for 30%–40% of all HCC diagnoses in the United States (NCI, 2012a).

Cirrhosis, regardless of the etiology, increases the risk of developing HCC. The risk of developing HCC once diagnosed with cirrhosis increases by 1%–6% annually (NCI, 2012a).

Inherited metabolic disorders such as hemochromatosis and Wilson disease are responsible for a higher risk of developing HCC. Hemochromatosis is a malabsorption disease that causes increased iron deposits in the liver. Wilson disease causes impaired copper absorption, creating stress on the liver (Abou-Alfa & DeMatteo, 2009). Other risk factors include alpha-1-antitrypsin deficiency, glycogen storage disease, pophyria cutanea tarda, tyrosinemia, and nonalcoholic steatohepatitis associated with obesity, type 2 diabetes, dyslipidemia, or insulin resistance (NCI, 2012a). Environmental factors can also contribute to HCC development through exposure to aflatoxins and vinyl chloride. Aflatoxins or mycotoxins are formed by specific *Aspergillus* species, which are a frequent contaminant of improperly stored grains and nuts, particularly in Africa and Asia (NCI, 2012a) (see Table 5-1). Workers exposed to polyvinyl chloride (PVC) or PVC dust prior to stringent industry controls are also at risk for developing HCC and liver angiosarcoma (NCI, 2012a).

Prevention of HCC can be facilitated through childhood vaccination against hepatitis B or treatment with antivirals if exposure occurs. Avoiding exposure to aflatoxins and vinyl chloride dust would also be prudent when possible, as well as avoiding alcohol abuse.

Familial Association

Associations based on genetic or familial factors continue to be studied. It has been proved that having a first-degree relative with hepatitis B and HCC is associated with an increased risk of developing HCC for family members who are also hepatitis B carriers (NCI, 2012b). In a study conducted at the University of Texas MD Anderson Cancer Center, a fourfold increase in HCC risk was found when first-degree family members reported having liver cancer (Hassan et al., 2009). However, no association was found if the family history included cancer other than liver cancer (Hassan et al., 2009). Familial polyposis coli is associated with childhood hepatoblastoma (Hassan et al., 2009). HCC and fibrolamellar HCC have been associated with Gardner syndrome, a variant of familial adenomatous polyposis (FAP). FAP is an autosomal-dominant inherited disease. Germline mutations in the adenomatous polyposis coli (APC) gene have been found in many patients diagnosed with FAP. This APC gene mutation has been seen in HCC; however, more research is needed in this area (Hassan et al., 2009).

Other genetic-related research includes the study of micro RNAs (miRNAs). miRNAs regulate the activity of multiple cancer-related genes and pathways and are prime candidates for coordinating the events that lead to metastasis (NCI, 2008). Research has found a unique pattern of miRNAs that can predict whether cancer will spread early in the disease.

Table 5-1. Likely Etiology of Hepatocellular Carcinoma

Causative Agents	Dominant Geographical Area
Hepatitis B virus	Asia and Africa
Hepatitis C virus	Europe, United States, and Japan
Alcohol	Europe and United States
Aflatoxins	East Asia and Africa

Note. From "Liver (Hepatocellular) Cancer Screening (PDQ®)" [Health Professional Version], by the National Cancer Institute, January 25, 2012. Retrieved from http://www.cancer.gov/cancertopics/pdq/screening/hepatocellular/HealthProfessional/page2.

They have also been found to predict whether patients with liver cancer will have a longer or shorter disease course or survival (NCI, 2008).

In other research, the RASSF1A tumor suppressor gene has been studied. The loss of RASSF1A expression is one of the most common occurrences in human cancers (Dallol et al., 2004). Although the mechanism of action is not yet understood, RASSF1A protein expression and hypermethylation have been found to play a role in the carcinogenesis of HCC (Hu, Chen, Yu, & Qui, 2010). Reduced RASSF1A levels demonstrate a relationship with both the development and aggressiveness of HCC and could be used in clinical prognostics as well as screening for HCC in the future (Hu et al., 2010). Other chromosome research indicates the region *TP53* is connected to hepatocarcinogenesis regardless of the etiology of the disease, yet the *TP53* mutation varies dependent on geographic area (Teufel et al., 2007). An example of this is that the location of the mutation within *TP53* (third position of codon 249) is often seen when HCC is found in those exposed to aflatoxins—typically in sub-Saharan Africa or China (Teufel et al., 2007). When hepatitis B and C virus are present prior to HCC, the *TP53* region demonstrates a different variation. In general, *TP53* mutations demonstrate an unfavorable prognosis (Teufel et al., 2007). Teufel et al. (2007) also speak to the Wnt signaling pathway with b-catenin having a role in the development of HCC, although correlated to a less aggressive form of the disease, and transforming growth factor (TGF), which is important in many cellular processes. An overexpression of TGF-beta is demonstrated in HCC. The field of genomics is rapidly evolving, and ongoing research will yield more answers, which should lead to earlier diagnosis and improved prognosis.

Clinical Presentation

A triad of symptoms—right upper quadrant pain, palpable mass, and weight loss—are present in 90%–95% of patients with HCC (Sun & Sarna, 2008). Other typical findings include hepatic bruits (25%), ascites, splenomegaly, jaundice, wasting, and fever. Patient complaints include fatigue, weakness, epigastric fullness, anorexia, weight loss, constipation or diarrhea, increasing abdominal girth, and pain in the abdomen or right shoulder (Volker, 2004). Easy bruising or bleeding are also often reported (Dugdale & Chen, 2011). Patients with a diagnosis of liver cancer report the third highest level of psychological distress when compared to eight other cancers (Sun & Sarna, 2008).

When a diagnosis and history of cirrhosis is known, screening alpha-fetoprotein (AFP) testing is often completed on a routine basis. An increase in AFP, an increase in alkaline phosphatase, and diminished liver function tests (LFTs) are present in 50%–70% of patients with liver cancer, both patients with cirrhosis and the general population (NCI, 2012b). Prognostically, if AFP is within normal limits when hepatocellular cancer is diagnosed, patients have a longer median survival than patients with an elevated AFP. Other blood testing may reveal polycythemia, hypoglycemia, hypercalcemia, or dysfibrinogenemia (NCI, 2012b). In later or terminal stages of the disease, decompensated cirrhosis symptoms occur, as demonstrated by ascites, variceal bleeding, peripheral edema, portal hypertension, and hepatic encephalopathy (Sun & Sarna, 2008). If laboratory work identifies a possible liver abnormality, further diagnostic testing should be completed.

Diagnosis and Staging

Patients with a history of hepatitis B or C or cirrhosis may receive their HCC diagnosis through a surveillance program. In 2004, the American Association for the Study of Liver Diseases stated that these programs, in which patients would have a liver panel and AFP level drawn, as well as a physical examination and abdominal ultrasound, must become the standard of care, as they would increase survival rates for patients diagnosed with HCC (Runyon, 2004). Surveillance visits occur every 6–12 months according to the risk and independent findings for each patient. These programs have become the standard of care in large academic medical centers (Gish et al., 2010).

Once a lesion has been found in the liver, a full assessment of the lesion, status of liver function/portal hypertension, and patient's overall performance status must be completed. Magnetic resonance imaging (MRI) has become the imaging modality of choice for HCC, as studies have shown it to have better specificity and sensitivity for HCC lesions than abdominal computed tomography (CT) scan or ultrasound. The new contrast agent, gadoxetate disodium, has better liver organ specificity and an increased rate of biliary excretion, deeming it safer for patients with renal insufficiency. HCC lesions will be hypervascular in the arterial phase and wash out in the venous phase. The MRI will demonstrate the number and size of the lesions, specific information on liver segments involved, vascular proximity, and vascular inva-

sion. This information is necessary to begin the formulation of a treatment plan for the patient (Gish et al., 2010). Fewer than 5% of patients need biopsies to confirm the diagnosis of HCC because the improvement of imaging techniques and the introduction of National Comprehensive Cancer Network (NCCN) guidelines for standard criteria: a lesion greater than 2 cm that is hypervascular in the arterial phase and washes out in the venous phase on any imaging modality (CT, ultrasound, or MRI) with an AFP greater than 200 ng/ml (Bruix & Sherman, 2011; NCCN, 2011). Although biopsies are not always mandated at the present time, they may become more important in the future for therapies that are tumor targeted.

Assessment of liver function and portal hypertension begins with the liver panel, chemistry panel, coagulation studies, and complete blood count. The liver panel will measure serum levels of bilirubin, aspartate transaminase (AST), alanine transaminase, alkaline phosphatase, lactate dehydrogenase (LDH), albumin, and protein. Other important tests are blood urea nitrogen to creatinine ratio, prothrombin time, and international normalized ratio (INR). If the etiology of the patient's liver disease is not known at the time of diagnosis, a hepatitis panel must be drawn for hepatitis B and/or C viral infection. All of these results can be entered into schemata that differentiate the patients into levels that determine overall liver function and hepatic reserve.

The Child-Pugh Score is the most common assessment tool used to share information about liver function. It puts patients into three classes (A–C) according to likelihood of survival (NCCN, 2011). It provides a rough estimate of those patients with cirrhosis who have compensated (class A) or decompensated (class B–C) liver function. An estimated 60%–80% of patients with HCC have underlying cirrhosis (NCCN, 2011; Volk & Marrero, 2008). The Child-Pugh Score is easy to calculate but does not evaluate signs and symptoms of portal hypertension.

The Model for End-Stage Liver Disease (MELD) Score is another score that is used to share assessment of liver function. It is a numeric scale ranging from 6 (less ill) to 40 (gravely ill) for patients older than 12 years old. It is an equation using three laboratory values (serum bilirubin, INR, and creatinine). It also does not evaluate the presence of portal hypertension. This score has recently been adopted by the United Network for Organ Sharing (UNOS) to stratify patients on the liver transplantation list according to risk of death in three months. It is becoming more popular than the Child-Pugh Score for measuring liver compensation in some centers because it includes a measure for renal function and is easier to calculate (NCCN, 2011; Volk & Marrero, 2008).

Performance status of the patient obviously contributes greatly to the decisions made in regard to treatment. A CT scan must be done upon diagnosis to assess the presence of metastatic disease. Eastern Cooperative Oncology Group, or ECOG, scores are also used to determine the patient's ability to tolerate certain treatment regimens.

HCC is not "staged" as other solid tumors are but rather stratified into groups according to treatment categories: potentially resectable or transplantable, operable by performance status or comorbidity, unresectable, inoperable because of performance status or comorbidity with local disease only, and metastatic disease (NCCN, 2011).

After all the data have been collected, the multidisciplinary team of a gastroenterologist, medical oncologist, surgical oncologist, interventional radiologist, and oncology nurse can discuss the treatment options available to the patient. This disease is very complex and requires a team approach to care. The underlying liver disease, if present, must remain controlled for optimization of outcomes. Surgery and interventional radiology may work together for an operative procedure. Chemotherapy may be needed with metastatic or recurrent disease. Patient education, financial resources evaluation, and emotional support will be needed throughout the trajectory of care.

Treatment Options

Surgical Intervention

The most effective treatment for HCC is the removal of the tumor(s). Two options are available: (a) remove the part of the liver where the lesion resides (liver resection or partial hepatectomy) or (b) remove the entire liver and replace it with a healthy one (liver transplantation) (Vullierme et al., 2010).

Liver resection or partial hepatectomy is appropriate for those patients with a localized tumor, in a noncirrhotic liver or with a Child-Pugh A score without major vascular invasion. The goal would be tumor removal with 2 cm margins to prevent local recurrence. Three-year survival rates are 54% in this population (Jelic & Sotiropoulos, 2010). Prior to surgery, assessment of the future liver remnant must also be made. The noncirrhotic patient must be left with at least 30% of a healthy remnant for the liver to regenerate. Those with cirrhosis should be left with 40%, as their livers take longer to regenerate and their liver function may not recover as quickly postoperatively. To increase the volume of the future liver remnant, the surgeon may request portal vein embolization (PVE) preoperatively to induce growth in the "healthy" side of the liver. By embolizing the blood supply to the side of the liver with the lesion, the other side should hypertrophy. Recalculation of the future remnant should occur 6–10 weeks later to determine the effectiveness of the PVE procedure. To prevent tumor progression during this period, chemoembolization can be used at the same time as the PVE. Once the remnant is 30%–40%, liver resection can be scheduled for the patient. If the liver does not hypertrophy to the needed percentage, this procedure was a good "stress test" indicating the patient was not a reasonable resection candidate (Manizate, Hiotis, Labow, Roayaie, & Schwartz, 2010). Figure 5-1 illustrates liver segmentectomy.

Liver transplantation is the treatment of choice for patients with advanced cirrhosis (Child-Pugh B or C) and HCC. It allows the removal of detectable and undetectable lesions and treats the underlying liver disease. Before 1996, liver transplant results were poor in this population with high recurrence rates and short survival. A 1996 Milan study found that by restricting selection criteria for transplantation, outcomes for this HCC population could mirror those receiving liver transplants for other diseases. This "Milan criteria" is now the standard: single tumor up to 5 cm or up to 3 tumors, each no larger than 3 cm, without macrovascular invasion or extrahepatic spread (Silva & Wigg, 2010). Overall four-year survival rates are 85%, and recurrence-free survival rates are 92% using these criteria (Mazzaferro et al., 2008). Patients must also meet the UNOS criteria for liver transplantation so they cannot be eligible for liver resection, thereby preserving transplantation for those patients with more severe liver disease. The MELD score is used to predict mortality risk for HCC patients on the donor waiting list. The score is updated regularly.

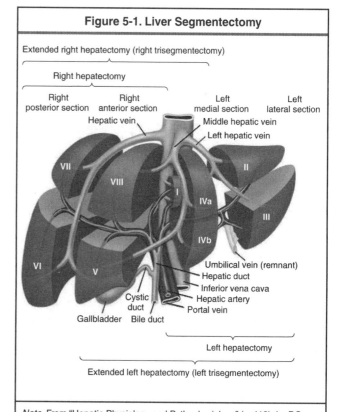

Figure 5-1. Liver Segmentectomy

Extended right hepatectomy (right trisegmentectomy)

Right hepatectomy

Right posterior section | Right anterior section | Left medial section | Left lateral section

Hepatic vein
Middle hepatic vein
Left hepatic vein

VII
VIII
I
IVa
II
III
IVb
VI
V

Umbilical vein (remnant)
Hepatic duct
Inferior vena cava
Cystic duct
Hepatic artery
Portal vein
Gallbladder
Bile duct

Left hepatectomy

Extended left hepatectomy (left trisegmentectomy)

Note. From "Hepatic Physiology and Pathophysiology" (p. 413), by P.S. Mushlin and S. Gelman in R.D. Miller, L.I. Eriksson, L.A. Fleisher, J.P. Wiener-Kronish, and W.L. Young (Eds.), *Miller's Anesthesia* (7th ed.), 2010, Philadelphia, PA: Churchill Livingstone. Copyright 2010 by Churchill Livingstone. Reprinted with permission.

Approximately 15%–33% patients are removed from the transplant list while waiting for an organ because of tumor progression (Vullierme et al., 2010). Shortage of cadaveric organs has increased the time patients spend on the list, so patients progress while waiting. Discussion has begun regarding use of living related donor transplants (LRDT) for patients who qualify to help offset this shortage. No clinical studies have been done to look at outcomes for LRDT versus cadaveric donors. Some evidence suggests that underestimation of tumor staging by radiology, as well as the broadening of tumor criteria suggested by the University of California, San Francisco, may affect the estimation of tumor progression for patients on the wait list. Many physicians opt for "bridging" therapy for patients while on the list to avoid this progression and subsequent dropoff. Therapies include radiofrequency ablation and transarterial chemoembolization (NCCN, 2011; Silva & Wigg, 2010).

Chemotherapy

For patients who do not qualify for liver surgery or transplantation, systemic therapy becomes their treatment option. Chemotherapeutic agents utilized in the past (doxorubicin, 5-fluorouracil) had limited response rates and offered marginal survival benefit. New therapies have begun to focus more on the molecular pathogenesis of HCC—an extremely vascular tumor with overexpression of vascular endothelial growth factor (VEGF). Underlying cirrhosis also inhibits the effects of chemotherapy on some level (Gish et al., 2010). A new class of chemotherapy agents has offered great hope for this population: the multitargeted kinase inhibitors. In November 2007, sorafenib was the first agent to gain U.S. Food and Drug Administration approval for treatment of unresectable HCC. Sorafenib targets not only tumor cell proliferation but also angiogenesis pathways. For this reason, it was thought to be ideal for the treatment of HCC. The Sorafenib Hepatocellular Carcinoma Assessment Randomized Protocol (SHARP) trial compared 400 mg sorafenib (oral, twice daily) versus placebo in 602 randomized patients with measurable, unresectable, advanced HCC (Llovet et al., 2008). Patients in the sorafenib group had a longer overall survival than placebo (10.7 months versus 7.9 months). In a second clinical trial in the Asia-Pacific, the overall survival was 6.5 months with sorafenib and 4.2 months with placebo (Cheng et al., 2009). Based on the results of the trials, NCCN guidelines recommend sorafenib as treatment for patients with Child-Pugh A or B liver function with disease not resectable, not suitable for liver transplant, or that has metastasized (NCCN, 2011).

The interference of cirrhosis in the treatment of HCC is an ongoing issue with the HCC population and one of continued debate. Hepatocyte necrosis and inflammation may contribute not only to problems with chemotherapy but also to early multifocal recurrences. Some clinicians feel that the reinstitution of antiviral therapies, including interferon, after sur-

gery, interventional radiology, or with chemotherapy will improve patient outcomes. The rationale is that these therapies help to prevent recurrence by "cleaning the carcinogenic soil and eliminating possibilities of novel tumorigenesis through their viral suppression and anti-inflammation action" (Miao et al., 2010, p. 2939).

Regional Chemotherapy

When disease is confined to the liver, regional infusion of the liver with chemotherapy may be an option. The hepatic artery supplies most liver tumors with their blood supply, providing a direct route to infuse chemotherapeutic agents (Paschos & Bird, 2008). Infusion may be done through a right upper abdominal subcutaneous port, a subcutaneously implanted pump, or other catheter placed directly into the hepatic artery (NCI, 2012b). The implantable pump has the advantage of providing both a bolus injection port for use and a small chamber that can be filled with high-dose chemotherapy for continuous infusion over the course of several weeks without interruption, and without the inconvenience of an external pump. Hepatic artery access devices require surgical insertion, which involves ligation and division of all accessory vessels distal to the site of the catheter to prevent misperfusion of the upper gastrointestinal tract. If not protected, a significant chemical gastritis or duodenitis could result. Catheter placement is evaluated by injection of fluorescein dye and adjusted as necessary. During the surgery, the gallbladder is typically removed to prevent chemotherapy-induced cholecystitis (Kemeny & Fata, 2001).

The preferred chemotherapy agent for hepatic arterial infusion has been floxuridine (FUDR) because of its high hepatic extraction rate. This allows a very high dose of the drug to be administered, as 94%–99% of the drug will be extracted by the liver during its first pass, meaning it will not recirculate through the bloodstream (Kemeny & Fata, 2001). By avoiding systemic infusion of the chemotherapy, not only can a very high dose of drug be given, but no systemic chemotherapy toxicities result. The use of hepatic arterial infusions has been limited because of the extremely technical nature of the surgical procedure as well as the commitment to implantable pump maintenance. Complications associated with hepatic arterial chemotherapy infusions include chemical hepatitis, biliary sclerosis, peptic ulceration, hepatic artery thrombus, and catheter displacement (Paschos & Bird, 2008).

Ablation Therapies

Ablation is a treatment option for HCC patients who have localized or locally advanced, unresectable disease confined to the liver (NCI, 2012b). Lesions must be accessible to the ablative probes or antennae. Multiple lesions (five to six) can be treated at one time, but lesions should be less than 5 cm in dimension (Abou-Alfa & DeMatteo, 2009). Ablation survival data equivalent to liver resection has been reported, but no overall survival improvement has been noted (NCI, 2012b). Ablation can be done percutaneously, laparoscopically, or during an open abdominal procedure. The first ablations used a chemical approach (ethanol), which was injected directly into the tumor, often called PEI (percutaneous ethanol injection) (Abou-Alfa & DeMatteo, 2009). The liver tumors absorbed the ethanol, which ablated (killed) the tumor cells. Lesions treated that were less than 3 cm demonstrated an 80% complete response (Lin & Lin, 2006). Many other types of ablations are more commonly performed today, including cryosurgery (the use of freezing technology), radiofrequency (the use of a heat-based technology), and microwave ablation (the use of microwave technology).

Cryosurgery involves the use of a liquid nitrogen-filled CryoProbe™ that is inserted into the tumor. Cycles of freezing and thawing are induced through the probe until cellular water is turned into a ball of ice, destroying the tumor (Paschos & Bird, 2008). Cryosurgery cannot be used if the tumor is close to a major blood vessel or a main bile duct. This procedure can be done through a laparoscopic or open procedure approach. Post-procedure care includes pain control and the monitoring of LFTs. Possible complications related to cryosurgery include myoglobinemia, acute tubular necrosis, thrombocytopenia, biliary leak or biliary stenosis, liver capsule cracking, and hemorrhage. Pleural effusions are common and can occur in 70% of patients. Typically, these resolve without intervention (Arciero & Sigurdson, 2008).

Radiofrequency ablation (RFA) employs a multiple array probe that is placed into the center of the tumor. Extreme heat (100°C) is directed into the tumor where tissue friction causes coagulative necrosis. RFA may be used when there is a concern that surgical resection may result in inadequate margins or inadequate postoperative liver reserve, or when comorbidities contraindicate a lengthy surgical procedure. RFA can be done percutaneously, laparoscopically, or in conjunction with an open procedure. Diligence in probe placement, particularly with the percutaneous approach, is required to avoid thermal injury of adjacent structures such as the colon and regional vasculature (Arciero & Sigurdson, 2008). Other possible complications include pleural effusions, fever, pain, liver hematomas, and liver abscesses (Paschos & Bird, 2008). Uncommonly, injuries to the biliary tree, hepatic artery, or diaphragm may occur, as well as hepatic artery pseudoaneurysms with bleeding, which may require hepatic artery embolization (Arciero & Sigurdson, 2008). Low morbidity and mortality rates, 7.2% and 0.3% respectively, have been reported (Paschos & Bird, 2008).

Microwave ablation uses magnetic energy that agitates water molecules. This thermal energy creates molecular friction, causing coagulative necrosis (Iannitti et al., 2007). The antenna and generators used are similar to those used in RFA, but a different part of the electromagnetic spectrum is employed.

A larger treatment diameter (larger lesion) can be addressed through the use of multiple antennas placed into the tumor (Iannitti et al., 2007). Microwave ablation is superior in comparison to RFA for the following reasons: (a) improved convection profile, (b) consistently higher intratumoral temperatures, (c) larger ablation volumes, (d) faster ablation times, and (e) the option to use multiple antennas simultaneously (Iannitti et al., 2007). Complications from microwave ablation are reported to be similar to those of RFA, with a similar caution related to skin burns with probe removal. A low morbidity of 16% and mortality of 1.4% are reported (Iannitti et al., 2007).

Postoperative or post-procedure care after ablation includes the management of right upper quadrant and right shoulder (referred) pain, as well as symptom management for fevers, flu-like symptoms, and tumor lysis symptoms (Gish et al., 2010). As with any procedure involving the liver, monitoring LFTs and for signs and symptoms of bleeding is critical.

Embolization Therapies

Embolization can be described as obstructing a blood vessel or an organ with an embolic agent to disrupt the circulation to specific blood vessels. When treating liver tumors, which tend to be quite vascular, the technique of manually introducing substances to block the nutrient-supplying tumor vessel can be very effective. Embolization therapies are typically used when liver tumors are unresectable, localized or locally advanced, but confined to the liver. However, chemoembolization may be indicated in the case of advanced-stage liver cancer—present in both lobes of the liver (NCI, 2012b). Embolization is contraindicated in patients with biliary obstruction, jaundice, or hepatic encephalopathy; when tumor replaces more than 50% of the liver; when the LDH is greater than 425 IU/L; AST is greater than 100 IU/L; or when the total bilirubin is greater than 32 mg/dl (Soulen, 2000).

Prior to the embolization procedure, cross-section imaging of the liver is completed, and laboratory work including a complete blood count, prothrombin time, partial thromboplastin time, creatinine, LFTs, and tumor markers are evaluated. A diagnostic arteriogram is completed to confirm portal vein patency and to determine the arterial blood supply within the liver as it feeds the tumor. Vessels that supply the gastrointestinal tract are also identified to ensure the embolization does not affect the stomach or small bowel vasculature. To perform the embolization, a catheter is advanced through the right or left hepatic artery, depending on the location of the tumor. Once the circulation to the tumor is reidentified and cannulated, embolic or blocking agents are injected into the vessel (Soulen, 2000). Although the physical obstruction of embolic material will obstruct the blood supply, and therefore the nutrients and oxygen that facilitate tumor growth, other agents may be used in combination to further affect the tumor. Types of embolization and agents include the following.

- Transarterial embolization (also known as bland embolization)—degradable starch microspheres, Lipiodol®, Gelfoam® (embolic agent only)
- Transarterial chemoembolization—cisplatin with or without doxorubicin, or mitomycin-coated spheres
- Selective internal radioactive therapy—yttrium-90-impregnated microspheres or coils
- Chemical embolization—ethanol or polyvinyl alcohol injection

When an agent is added to the embolic material, blood flow is impaired and chemotherapy or radioactive concentration and dwell time within the tumor tissue may be significant, but systemic toxicity is minimal (Soulen, 2000).

Patients should be instructed to fast prior to the procedure. Postembolization nausea and vomiting is reported by 80%–90% of patients (Soulen, 2000). Interventions to support hydration (IV support) and symptom management with antiemetics provide comfort. Other side effects from this treatment are often dependent on how much tumor is destroyed. Tumor necrosis releases toxins causing abdominal/liver pain, fevers, and nausea. Antipyretics and pain medication provide relief. If tumor necrosis is significant, liver abscesses may form, requiring drainage and antibiotic interventions. Other complications can include hepatic insufficiency or infarction, tumor rupture, cholecystitis, or embolization of the gastrointestinal tract. Serious complications are reported in 3%–4% of procedures, with a 30-day mortality rate reported at 1%–4% (Soulen, 2000). The response rate, measured by decrease in tumor volume and decrease in alpha-fetoprotein count, ranges from 60% to 83% (Soulen, 2000).

PVE is a similar procedure that is done for a very different reason. When aggressive surgical treatment for a large-volume hepatocellular carcinoma is planned, such as an extended hepatectomy, PVE may be considered. The science behind a PVE is that by obstructing the portal venous flow to the side of the liver invaded by tumor, the opposite side—the healthy side—of the liver will hypertrophy (Hemming et al., 2003; Hu et al, 2010). This process will add healthy liver volume, which will aid in the success of a significant liver resection. PVE is typically done six weeks prior to the surgical (liver resection) procedure and can increase the functional liver mass by approximately 35% (Hemming et al., 2003).

Oncology Nursing Implications

Special Needs, Side Effects, and Monitoring

Although the prognosis for hepatocellular carcinoma is often poor, there continue to be new treatments and improved symptom management to help people living with this disease. Along the disease continuum, individuals will experience differing levels of complications related to both the disease and treatment modalities. The oncology nurse must be knowledgeable of the many facets of the disease and interventions to expertly manage the patient with HCC.

Care of Psychosocial Needs and Quality of Life

Psychosocial and emotional needs must be addressed as well as medical needs. Often depression and guilt, especially if a potentially preventable cause (hepatitis or cirrhosis) may have contributed to development of the disease, are seen in patients with HCC (Abou-Alfa & DeMatteo, 2009). Antianxiety and antidepressant medications may need to be considered. As with any disease, compliance with treatment is associated with the best outcomes, so developing an open, trusting relationship are key for treatment, as are identifying and addressing any psychosocial or emotional needs of the patient, family, and caregivers. Because of the limitations of effective, curative treatments for HCC, preserving the physical function and quality of life of patients with HCC is important. Oncology nurses can play a significant role in addressing symptom management and improving the quality of life. Poor prognosis, pain, fatigue, anorexia, ascites, and jaundice are just a few issues that affect functional status and quality of life (Sun & Sarna, 2008). When surveyed, patients with HCC reported that their quality of life was diminished by depression, decrease in sexual function, sleep disorders, and pain. These and other factors such as level of liver function, age, complications faced, and primary or recurrent disease status all have an impact on quality of life (Sun et al., 2008). Spirituality is the least defined domain related to quality of life, and its full impact is not known, but patients with HCC reported a statistically significant decline in spirituality (Sun et al., 2008).

Nursing Implications With Diagnostic Testing

Laboratory work and ultrasonography are typically the first diagnostic tests completed when liver cancer is suspected, and they present minimal risk. However, to confirm a diagnosis, a liver biopsy may be needed. Because the liver is a very vascular organ, a liver biopsy can be risky. A liver biopsy can be done percutaneously, under CT guidance, laparoscopically, or during an open abdominal procedure. A needle is placed into the tumor, or abnormal tissue, and a piece of tissue is removed for microscopic examination. Complications are reported in 0.06%–0.32% of patients and often occur in the first few hours after the procedure. Complications include hemorrhage, bile peritonitis, penetration of the viscera, and pneumothorax. The mortality rate is 0.0009%–0.12%. One-third of patients complain of significant pain at the biopsy site, in the right upper quadrant, or in the right shoulder. Pain should decrease or stabilize over time (NCI, 2012a). The nurse should expect to check vital signs frequently after a liver biopsy. Tachycardia or hypotension could be signs of bleeding. The biopsy site should be checked frequently, as well, for any indication of hematoma formation, worsening tenderness, or swelling near the biopsy site. Finally, monitoring for respiratory changes related to pneumothorax should also be done frequently. Shortness of breath, a change in oxygen saturations or oxygen use, or a change in bilateral breath sounds should be immediately reported.

Care of Postsurgical Patients

Because HCC is potentially curable with surgery, this treatment modality will be offered whenever it is felt to be a safe procedure. An understanding of the patient's preoperative functional capacity, general health status, and postdischarge goals may help to develop the postsurgical care plan. If the patient was living independently prior to surgery, aggressive postoperative care would be warranted to facilitate the patient's return to independence. If a patient required help with activities of daily living and was in poor nutritional status prior to surgery, the patient may not tolerate an aggressive postoperative plan. Nursing care for all patients should be aimed at preventing postoperative complications. The most significant postoperative complications from liver surgery include respiratory compromise/atelectasis, deep vein thrombosis/pulmonary embolus, fluid shifting, and wound infection. Postoperatively, pain is always a concern, and uncontrolled pain can result in poor effort related to incentive spirometry and ambulation. Care in pain management must be undertaken as the surgical assault on the liver may diminish liver function and affect medication metabolism. Pulmonary toilet and early ambulation will decrease the risk for respiratory compromise as well as for thrombus formation. Fluid management to ensure appropriate circulating volume without overload can be challenging because nutritional status is often less than desired and third-spacing of fluid and peripheral edema is common. Finally, ensuring the incision remains clean, dry, and uncontaminated is essential to healing. Ongoing monitoring of LFTs will also need to be done. If a liver transplant was performed, additional risks identified include bleeding, formation of hepatic arterial clot or thrombus, biliary leak, or rejection of the new organ (Abou-Alfa & DeMatteo, 2009). These patients will continue to be closely monitored.

Care of Post-Procedure Patients

Postablation and postembolization care require interventions related to the site through which the treatment was performed (percutaneous or laparoscopic). The nursing care will be similar to that of the patient after a liver biopsy: evaluat-

ing for pain, bleeding, or changes in respiratory status (NCI, 2012a).

Care After Chemotherapy

The impact of systemic chemotherapy will depend on the medications chosen and their particular side effect profiles. Blood work is frequently monitored to evaluate the red blood cell count, which will affect oxygenation and can impact fatigue; white blood cell count, which contributes to fighting infection; platelets and liver functions to monitor clotting abilities; and risk of bleeding. Blood products or growth-stimulating factors may be given to decrease symptoms and risk. Many chemotherapeutic regimens cause nausea and vomiting, stomatitis, and esophagitis. Modifications in diet and medication management can ease these side effects. The oncology nurse must teach the patient, family, or caregivers strategies to manage symptoms and aid in treatment compliance.

Patient Management and Evaluation

The complexity of patients with HCC requires a multidisciplinary approach for the management of multidimensional symptoms. Many of the patients who develop HCC have a previous diagnosis of hepatitis B or C or cirrhosis and have been followed by a medical professional for a period of time in the treatment of that chronic disease. Coping with the HCC diagnosis can be difficult whether the patient has been in treatment for a precursor disease or it is a completely new diagnosis, as well as if the disease can be aggressively treated (surgical cure) or if only supportive care will be offered. Sun and Sarna (2008) reported that 80% of patients are diagnosed with advanced-stage disease. For those who have curative liver cancer surgery, coping with the diagnosis may be limited to the postoperative recovery period, but for those undergoing palliative treatment, the psychosocial, emotional, and financial ramifications will likely be much more significant. Expert mental health clinicians and financial counselors should be available to to support the patient and family. Patients living with HCC will likely have multiple medical interventions related to the symptoms and treatment of the disease. Ongoing medical management and evaluation should be anticipated, and oncology nurses can play a significant role in supportive care.

Pain

Pain is a common complaint related to HCC because of the visceral involvement in the abdomen and pelvis. Pain is often referred to the right shoulder as well (Sun & Sarna, 2008). Treatment-related pain (surgery, embolization) must also be considered, and medication may need to be increased during this acute phase. As pain becomes less tolerable, opioid analgesics will be necessary. Caution with medications that can cause liver damage such as acetaminophen should be discussed. As the disease progresses and liver function diminishes, pain (and other) medication dosing may need to be adjusted because the metabolism of the medication will be delayed.

Fatigue

Fatigue, described as mental and physical exhaustion, can be related to HCC disease processes and treatment. A thorough evaluation of the factors that can contribute to fatigue is necessary to direct appropriate symptom relief. These factors include pain, emotional distress, sleep disturbances, anemia, nutritional deficiencies, deconditioning, and comorbidities (Sun & Sarna, 2008). Treatment of these factors may alleviate some of the fatigue. For example, chemotherapy-induced anemia could be improved with the use of erythropoietin, or antidepressants could aid depression and anxiety. A review of all home-administered medication may reveal aggravating sources as well. Nonpharmacologic interventions are also plentiful. The literature supports aerobic exercise, counseling on sleep hygiene, and discussing tips to conserve energy (Sun & Sarna, 2008). Nutrition counseling to encourage healthy, small, frequent meals and adequate hydration can also improve fatigue.

Anorexia and Cachexia

Anorexia is a loss of appetite. Cachexia has a primary (metabolic) result, caused by anorexia, and a secondary (starvation) result. The term *anorexia-cachexia syndrome* is used for cancer wasting (Sun & Sarna, 2008). Beyond the physical attribution seen in cancer wasting, measurement parameters include hypoalbuminemia, asthenia (weakness), chronic nausea, low calorie intake, and low muscle and fat mass. Weight loss in patients with HCC may be masked by ascites and edema (Sun & Sarna, 2008). Management begins with an assessment of contributing factors and how each of these can be addressed. Patients with HCC often complain of chronic nausea, constipation, early satiety, and taste alterations, which may be alleviated through nutrition counseling. Small, frequent, healthy meals and adequate hydration can improve intake, nutritional status, bowel function, and quality of life. Appetite stimulants may help some patients. Patients with edema and ascites should decrease sodium intake to avoid additional fluid retention. Underlying depression may also affect anorexia and should be addressed as well. Artificial nutrition, such as total parenteral nutrition, is initiated occasionally, but it has not been shown to increase lean body mass (Sun & Sarna, 2008).

Obstruction

Jaundice

Jaundice, or icterus, the yellowing of the skin and sclera, is caused when too much bile is in the blood. It is also char-acterized by severe itching, dark tea-colored urine, and light, chalky stools. Jaundice occurs when a bile duct is obstructed or compressed, thus not allowing the liver to absorb the bile as it normally would (Abou-Alfa & DeMatteo, 2009). In 1%–12% of patients, jaundice is the initial symptom at clinical presentation (Sun & Sarna, 2008). To develop a care plan, the cause of the obstruction must be determined. In the case of a blocked or compressed duct, bile duct stenting through an endoscope or percutaneously may relieve the obstruction (Abou-Alfa & DeMatteo, 2009). If the obstruction is the result of tumor invasion or intraductal growth, stenting is likely not an option. A presentation of jaundice will delay treatment. If jaundice cannot be resolved, liver function will continue to deteriorate, and treatment cannot be administered (Abou-Alfa & DeMatteo, 2009). For this reason, facilitating a resolution is critical when jaundice is identified. If an internal stent can be placed, no further care is needed beyond monitoring LFTs, signs and symptoms of infection, or for a return of jaundice should the stent become obstructed. If an external drain is needed to resolve the bile duct blockage, the patient and family will need to be educated regarding the aforementioned concerns and taught proper care and management of the drain. Depending on the amount of drainage removed, electrolyte and fluid status will need to be monitored to ensure balance and hydration. Cholestatic pruritus may be managed with cholestyramine to decrease enterohepatic circulation of bile salts (Sun & Sarna, 2008). Diphenhydramine or hydroxyzine (antihistamines) may alleviate itching but can cause drowsiness. Use of skin moisturizers and mild, fragrance-free soaps can also decrease pruritus (Abou-Alfa & DeMatteo, 2009) (see Table 5-2).

Ascites

Ascites, the accumulation of fluid in the abdomen, may arise from an imbalance in the influx/efflux of peritoneal cavity fluid or from a lymphatic obstruction caused by tumor invasion (Sun & Sarna, 2008). Ascites can also occur in patients with cirrhosis or portal hypertension. Symptoms of ascites include increasing abdominal girth, intra-abdominal pressure, abdominal wall discomfort, dyspnea, anorexia, early satiety, nausea, vomiting, esophageal reflux, pain, and peripheral edema (Saif, Siddiqui, & Sohail, 2009; Sun & Sarna, 2008).

Ascites management can be quite difficult for the medical team and frustrating for the patient. A sodium-restricted diet of less than 2 g per day as well as the use of potassium-sparing diuretics may be initiated (Saif et al., 2009). In severe cases, particularly if causing dyspnea, an abdominal paracentesis may be performed (Saif et al., 2009). A paracentesis is a sterile procedure in which a needle is placed into the abdominal cavity and up to 5 L of fluid can be removed (Saif et al., 2009). The patient should be cautioned that dizziness can occur, as well as a decrease in blood pressure. The patient's blood pressure (orthostatic) and pulse should be mon-

Table 5-2. Management of Common Symptoms in Hepatocellular Carcinoma

Symptom	Interventions
Abdominal pain	Opioid analgesics (moderate to severe), nonsteroidal anti-inflammatory drugs (mild)
Fatigue	Treatment of contributing factors, if indicated: anemia (erythropoietin), depression (antidepressants), sleep disturbance, nutritional deficiencies, deconditioning (exercise), and decreased energy level (psychostimulants)
Anorexia or cachexia	Treatment of contributing factors, if indicated: chronic nausea (antiemetics), constipation (laxatives), antidepressants (depression) Pharmacologic: megestrol acetate Others: artificial nutrition, dietary counseling
Ascites	Pharmacologic: diuretics (potassium-sparing + loop) Procedural: paracentesis
Jaundice secondary to biliary obstruction	Percutaneous drainage and biliary stent For cholestatic pruritus: cholestyramine, self-care measures (emollients, perfume-free soaps)

Note. Based on information from Del Fabbro et al., 2006; Greenway et al., 1982; Jones & Bergasa, 2000; National Comprehensive Cancer Center, 2006, 2007.

From "Symptom Management in Hepatocellular Carcinoma," by V.C.-Y. Sun and L. Sarna, 2008, *Clinical Journal of Oncology Nursing, 12*, p. 762. doi:10.1188/08.CJON.759-766. Copyright 2008 by the Oncology Nursing Society. Reprinted with permission.

itored until they are restored. The patient should report a fever (higher than 100°F [37.8°C]), severe or increased abdominal pain, blood in urine, bleeding, or drainage from the needle site. A temporary improvement of symptoms may occur, but ascites often returns. To avoid repeated paracentesis procedures, the placement of a peritoneovenous shunt (e.g., Denver® shunt, LeVeen shunt) may be discussed (Saif et al., 2009). The shunt can be placed under local anesthesia with sedation and involves a shunting device placed in the peritoneal cavity inserted into the jugular vein. The shunt returns peritoneal ascitic fluid to venous circulation, improving symptoms. Patients must learn to pump the shunt at least twice each day to limit the accumulation of fibrin and debris that could clog it. Besides clogging, other complications include infection, leakage of ascitic fluid, body edema, and coagulopathy (Encyclopedia of Surgery, 2003). Another procedure used to manage diuretic-resistant ascites is a transjugular intrahepatic portosystemic shunt, or TIPS. A TIPS decreases portal pressure by shunting fluid from the hepatic vein to the right jugular vein. The procedure can be performed by an interventional radiologist (Runyon, 2009). A palliative procedure, the placement of an indwelling drainage device (PleurX® catheter), may be utilized for intractable ascites (Reisfield & Wilson, 2003).

Portal Hypertension

Portal hypertension is abnormally high blood pressure in the branches of the portal vein. It can be responsible for the development of collateral blood vessels, or varices. Varices along the esophagus and stomach can bleed at any time, causing coffee-ground emesis or bloody stools (Abou-Alfa & DeMatteo, 2009). Immediate medical intervention is needed to stop the bleeding, which may include an ice-water nasogastric lavage or endoscopic banding of the bleeding area. Portal hypertension can also cause blood to back up into the spleen. The spleen will enlarge to accommodate this but will store additional platelets, decreasing the circulating platelet volume (Abou-Alfa & DeMatteo, 2009). Patients must be taught protective care and to avoid activities that may cause bruising or bleeding.

Hepatic Encephalopathy

Hepatic encephalopathy is a term used to describe worsening brain function that occurs as the liver deteriorates and is unable to process and excrete toxins. As the toxins accumulate in the blood, the patient becomes confused or very drowsy (Abou-Alfa & DeMatteo, 2009). Ammonia is one of the toxins that causes confusion, and administering lactulose can sometimes help to reduce the ammonia level in the blood. Lactulose works by binding with ammonia in the colon, and its laxative property causes frequent stools, decreasing the ammonia level. Monitoring the serum ammonia level and titrating the lactulose dose may diminish confusion. In the advanced stage of HCC as liver function further deteriorates and toxin levels rise, the patient may become comatose. Supportive, end-of-life, and comfort care measures should be in place at that time.

Nursing Research

Data and Implications

Nursing research regarding HCC has been sparse. Symptom management and the impact on quality of life have been addressed and are clearly areas where oncology nurses can have an impact on patients with HCC and their families and caregivers. Patient advocacy has also been studied related to the need to bridge communication with providers and experts (Sun & Sarna, 2008). In many cases, patients with HCC have been followed for several years for precursor diseases, and facilitating competent care is critical for successful treatment.

On the Horizon: Future Considerations

Research

Patients with HCC often suffer from multiple symptoms; therefore, studying symptom management interventions needs to continue for ongoing improvements in patient care. Sun and colleagues (2008) noted that study of distinct disease is also important to discern differences among hepatobiliary cancers. Beyond the physical symptoms, the psychosocial, emotional, and spiritual components of this disease warrant further research to improve the overall care of patients with HCC. Any contribution related to the study of genetics, genomics, and the use of biomarker technology will advance the care of patients with HCC and should improve the outcomes related to care and management of the disease.

Patient Education and Advocacy

For these patients and their loved ones, education throughout the course of the illness can be crucial in keeping them within the healthcare system, compliant with treatment regimens, and partners with the healthcare team. Their contact with the system can begin as early as a screening program in a digestive health center with a gastroenterologist. Patients need to receive information about hepatitis B and C viral infections and cirrhosis management (e.g., treatments, health risks to others, alcohol withdrawal and abstinence) and the risk for HCC development. If a patient develops HCC, referral to a cancer center can interrupt provider relationships and necessitate travel outside the patient's hometown. Patients need to be told that the connection with the gastroenterologist will continue throughout their care trajectory as the maintenance of compensated liver function is critical to the completion of treatment and may improve success of treatment with reduction of recurrence.

For patients who have had liver resections, postoperative morbidity can be drastically decreased if clinicians teach patients and their caregivers about pain control and deep vein thrombosis (DVT) and pneumonia prevention prior to surgery and reinforce this information after surgery. Clinicians should discuss the pain scale, use of epidurals (if applicable in a specific institution), and the transition to oral medications before the patient enters the hospital. With DVT prevention, clinicians should teach patients that they will begin getting out of bed the day after surgery and that they should move their arms and legs around while they are in the bed. For patients with high-risk indicators (e.g., DVT history, obesity), some surgeons may opt for postoperative anticoagulation therapy. Clinicians should ensure that the proper patient education is provided before the patient goes home. Pneumonia prevention will include early ambulation, use of the incentive spirometer, and cough and deep breathing. If possible, patients should receive an incentive spirometer and instructions on its use prior to surgery so they may start using it at home before surgery to practice optimizing alveoli while they can. Patients who have had a liver transplant will need the same postoperative education provided but will also have a very strict regimen of antirejection medications to which they must adhere in order to maintain their new liver. This will require frequent physician visits at first to check serum levels and adjust the medications. Patient who receive transplants require frequent education about all of the changes that will be made. A social worker and psychologist will work with the medical team to ensure that costs can be covered and emotional needs are being met.

Education required for patients receiving chemotherapy includes information about short-term and long-term effects. Short-term side effects for sorafenib may include hypertension, hand-foot syndrome, nausea, diarrhea, hemorrhage, or neutropenia. Patients also need information related to long-term effects that may occur, such as prolonged hypertension and hemorrage. This information would need to be individualized to each patient. As survivorship programs become more the norm around the country, care plans will need to be developed for individual patients depending on the treatment regimen that they experienced and the goals that they have for the future. It is important that this plan is developed in collaboration with patients and follows them throughout their cancer journey.

Summary

Cancer nurses must continue to advocate for the screening programs that are vital in the hepatitis and cirrhosis population to diagnose HCC as early as possible. Nurses also need to be aware of the growing number of cases of HCC being diagnosed in the metabolic syndrome population (NCI, 2012a) and advocate for screening programs for them, as well as ways to get the word out about their risk for the disease. We have not had tremendous success in treating this disease once it takes hold of the liver, but caught in the early stages, surgery or liver transplant offers hope. We must advocate for hepatitis B and C vaccines to prevent the viruses from developing to decrease a major risk factor for this disease. Funding for vaccinations and health clinics (especially those in rural areas) need our help and our voice. The shortage of organs continues to be a problem, especially those for African American patients. We must find a way to increase the number so that our patients do not die while waiting for a donor organ. HCC is a cancer for which many risk factors are known and are preventable. If the public was more educated, fewer people would suffer from this disease.

References

Abou-Alfa, G., & DeMatteo, R. (2009). *100 questions and answers about liver cancer* (2nd ed.). Burlington, MA: Jones and Bartlett.

Arciero, C., & Sigurdson, E. (2008). Diagnosis and treatment of metastatic disease to the liver. *Seminars in Oncology, 35,* 147–159. doi:10.1053/j.seminoncol.2007.12.004

Bruix, J., & Sherman, M. (2011). Management of hepatocellular carcinoma: An update. *Hepatology, 53,* 1020–1022. doi:10.1002/hep.24199

Cheng, A.L., Kang, Y.K., Chen, Z., Tsao, C.J., Quin, S., Kim, J.S., … Guan, Z. (2009). Efficacy and safety of sorafenib in patients in the Asia-Pacific region with advanced hepatocellular cancer: A phase III randomized, double-blind placebo controlled study. *Lancet, 10,* 25–34.

Dallol, A., Agathanggelou, A., Fenton, S., Ahmed-Choudhury, J., Hesson, L., Vos, M., Clark, G., … Latif, F. (2004). RASSF1A interacts with microtubule-associated proteins and modulates microtubule dynamics. *Cancer Research, 64,* 4112–4116. doi:10.1158/0008-5472.CAN-04-0267

Del Fabbro, E., Dalal, S., & Bruera, E. (2006). Symptom control in palliative care—Part II: Cachexia/anorexia and fatigue. *Journal of Palliative Medicine, 9,* 409–421. doi:10.1089/jpm.2006.9.409

Dugdale, D.C., III, & Chen, Y.-B. (2011, August 24). Hepatocellular carcinoma. Retrieved from http://www.nlm.nih.gov/medlineplus/ency/article/000280.htm

Encyclopedia of Surgery. (2003). Peritoneovenous shunt. Retrieved from http://www.surgeryencyclopedia.com/Pa-St/Peritoneovenous-Shunt.html

Gish, R.J., Marrero, J.A., & Benson, A.B. (2010). A multidisciplinary approach to the management of hepatocellular carcinoma. *Gastroenterology and Hepatology, 6*(3, Suppl. 7), 1–16. Retrieved from http://www.ncbi.nlm.nih.gov/pmc/articles/PMC2886473/?tool=pubmed

Greenway, B., Johnson, P.J., & Williams, R. (1982). Control of malignant ascites with spironolactone. *British Journal of Surgery, 69,* 441–442. doi:10.1002/bjs.1800690802

Hassan, M., Apitz, M., Thomas, M., Curley, S., Patt, Y., Vauthey, J., … Li, D. (2009). The association of family history of liver cancer with hepatocellular carcinoma: A case-control study in the United States. *Journal of Hepatology, 50,* 334–341. doi:10.1016/j.jhep.2008.08.016

Hemming, A., Reed, A., Howard, R., Fujita, S., Hochwald, S., Caridi, J., … Vauthey, J. (2003). Preoperative portal vein embolization for extended hepatectomy. *Annals of Surgery, 237,* 686–693. doi:10.1097/01.SLA.0000065265.16728.C0

Hu, L., Chen, G., Yu, H., & Qui, X. (2010). Clinicopathological significance of RASSF1A reduced expression and hypermethylation in hepatocellular carcinoma. *Hepatology International, 4,* 423–432. doi:10.1007/s12072-010-9164-8

Iannitti, D., Martin, R., Simon, C., Hope, W., Newcomb, W., McMasters, K., & Dupuy, D. (2007). Hepatic tumor ablation with clustered microwave antennae: The U.S. Phase II Trial. *HPB, 9,* 120–124. doi:10.1080/13651820701222677

International Agency for Research on Cancer. (2008). Liver cancer incidence, mortality and prevalence worldwide in 2008. Retrieved from http://globocan.iarc.fr/

Jelic, S., & Sotiropoulos, G.C. (2010). Hepatocellular carcinoma: ESMO Clinical Practice Guidelines for diagnosis, treatment, and follow-up. *Annals of Oncology, 21*(Suppl. 5), v59–v64. doi:10.1093/annonc/mdq166

Jones, E.A., & Bergasa, N.V. (2000). Evolving concepts of the pathogenesis and treatment of the pruritus of cholestasis. *Canadian Journal of Gastroenterology, 14,* 33–40. Retrieved from http://www.pulsus.com/journals/abstract.jsp?HCtype=Consumer&sCurrPg=journal&jnlKy=2&atlKy=5414&isuKy=193&isArt=t&

Kemeny, N., & Fata, F. (2001). Hepatic-arterial chemotherapy. *Lancet Oncology, 2,* 418–428. doi:10.1016/S1470-2045(00)00419-8

Lin, X.-D., & Lin, L.-W. (2006). Local injection therapy for hepatocellular carcinoma. *Hepatobiliary and Pancreas Diseases International, 5,* 16–21.

Llovet, J.M., Ricci, S., Mazzaferro, V., Hilgard, P., Gane, E., Blanc, J., … Bruix, J. (2008). Sorafenib in advanced hepatocellular carcinoma. *New England Journal of Medicine, 359,* 378–390. doi:10.1056/NEJMoa0708857

Manizate, F., Hiotis, S.P., Labow, D., Roayaie, S., & Schwartz, M. (2010). Liver functional reserve estimation: State of the art and relevance for local treatments—The Western perspective. *Journal of Hepato-Biliary-Pancreatic Sciences, 17,* 385–388. doi:10.1007/s00534-009-0228-x

Mazzaferro, V., Chun, Y.S., Poon, R.T., Schwartz, M.E., Yao, F.Y., Marsh, J.W., … Lee, S.G. (2008). Liver transplantation for hepatocellular carcinoma. *Annals of Surgical Oncology, 15,* 1001–1007. doi:10.1245/s10434-007-9559-5

Miao, R.-U., Zhao, H.-T., Yang, H.-Y., Mao, Y.-L., Lu, X., Zhao, Y., … Huang, J.-F. (2010). Postoperative adjuvant antiviral therapy for hepatitis B/C virus-related hepatocellular carcinoma: A meta-analysis. *World of Gastroenterology, 16,* 2931–2942. doi:10.3748/wjg.v16.i23.2931

National Cancer Institute. (2008, January 7). Researchers discover new biomarker for predicting liver cancer spread and survival. Retrieved from http://www.cancer.gov/newscenter/pressreleases/microRNAlivercancers

National Cancer Institute. (2012a, January 25). Liver (hepatocellular) cancer screening (PDQ®) [Health professional version]. Retrieved from http://www.cancer.gov/cancertopics/pdq/screening/hepatocellular/healthprofessional

National Cancer Institute. (2012b, February 23). Adult primary liver cancer treatment (PDQ®) [Health professional version]. Retrieved from http://www.cancer.gov/cancertopics/pdq/treatment/adult-primary-liver/healthprofessional

National Comprehensive Cancer Network. (2006). *NCCN Clinical Practice Guidelines in Oncology: Adult cancer pain* [v.1.2006]. Fort Washington, PA: Author.

National Comprehensive Cancer Network. (2007). *NCCN Clinical Practice Guidelines in Oncology: Cancer-related fatigue* [v.2.2007]. Fort Washington, PA: Author.

National Comprehensive Cancer Network. (2011). *NCCN Clinical Practice Guidelines in Oncology: Hepatobiliary cancers* [v.2.2012]. Fort Washington, PA: Author.

Paschos, K.A., & Bird, N. (2008). Current diagnostic and therapeutic approaches for colorectal cancer liver metastasis. *Hippokratia, 12,* 132–138.

Reisfield, G.M., & Wilson, G.R.(2003). Management of intractable, cirrhotic ascites with an indwelling drainage catheter. *Journal of Palliative Medicine, 6,* 787–791. doi:10.1089/109662103322515365

Runyon, B.A. (2004). Management of adult patients with ascites due to cirrhosis. *Hepatology, 39,* 841–856. doi:10.1002/hep.20066

Runyon, B.A. (2009). Management of adult patients with ascites due to cirrhosis: An update. *Hepatology, 49,* 2087–2107. doi:10.1002/hep.22853

Saif, M.W., Siddiqui, I.A., & Sohail, M.A. (2009). Management of ascites due to gastrointestinal malignancy. *Annals of Saudi Medicine, 29,* 369–377. doi:10.4103/0256-4947.55167

Siegel, R., Naishadham, D., & Jemal, A. (2012). Cancer statistics, 2012. *CA: A Cancer Journal for Clinicians, 62,* 10–29. doi:10.3322/caac.20138.

Silva, M.F., & Wigg, A.J. (2010). Current controversies surrounding liver transplantation for hepatocellular carcinoma. *Journal of Gastroenterology and Hepatology, 25,* 1217–1226. doi:10.1111/j.1440-1746.2010.06335.x

Soulen, M.C. (2000). Image-guided therapy of hepatic malignancies. *Applied Radiology, 29,* 21–29. doi:10.1016/S0160-9963(00)80214-9

Sun, V., Ferrell, B., Juarez, G., Wagman, L.D., Yen, Y., & Chung, V. (2008). Symptom concerns and quality of life in hepatobiliary cancers. *Oncology Nursing Forum, 35,* E45–E52. doi:10.1188/08.ONF.E45-E52

Sun, V.C.-Y., & Sarna, L. (2008). Symptom management in hepatocellular carcinoma. *Clinical Journal of Oncology Nursing, 12,* 759–766. doi:10.1188/08.CJON.759-766

Teufel, A., Staib, F., Kanzler, S., Weinmann, A., Schulze-Bergkamen, H., & Galle, P. (2007). Genetics of hepatocellular carcinoma. *World Journal of Gastroenterology, 13,* 2271–2282.

Volk, M.L., & Marrero, J.A. (2008). Early detection of liver cancer: Diagnosis and management. *Current Gastroenterology Reports, 10,* 60–66. doi:10.1007/s11894-008-0010-2

Volker, D.L. (2004). Other cancers. In C.G. Varricchio, T.B. Ades, P.S. Hinds, & M. Pierce (Eds.), *A cancer source book for nurses* (8th ed., pp. 309–326). Burlington, MA: Jones and Bartlett.

Vullierme, M.P., Paradis, V., Chirica, M., Castaing, D., Belghiti, J., Soubrane, O., … Farges, O. (2010). Hepatocellular carcinoma—What's new? *Journal of Visceral Surgery, 147,* e1–e12. doi:10.1016/j.jviscsurg.2010.02.003

World Cancer Research Fund International. (2008). Liver cancer statistics. Retrieved from http://www.wcrf.org/cancer_statistics/liver_cancer_statistics.php

CHAPTER 6

Liver Metastases

Nicoletta Campagna, DNP, APRN-BC, AOCNP®, and Jamie Cairo, DNP, APRN-BC, AOCNP®

Introduction

The liver provides a welcoming environment in which metastases may become established, not only because of its rich, dual blood supply but also because of humeral factors that promote cell growth. The blood supply of the liver is exceeded only by that of the lung in terms of blood flow per minute (Bartlett, 2000). The liver is the second most commonly involved organ by metastatic disease, after the lymph nodes. A focal liver lesion is more likely to represent a metastatic deposit than a primary malignancy. Most liver metastases are multiple (Adam, 2002). Several factors influence the incidence and pattern of liver metastases. These include the patient's age, sex, primary site, histologic type, and duration of the tumor.

Pathophysiology

The liver has a rich blood supply from both the hepatic artery and the portal vein. Metastases can reach the liver from any organ, but the direct passage of blood from the gastrointestinal (GI) tract to the liver from the portal circulation plays a critical role in explaining the high rate of liver metastases from these sites (Kemeny, Kemeny, & Dawson, 2008).

The dual blood supply and microvasculature of the liver considerably contribute to the establishment of liver metastases. Tumor emboli entering the sinusoids through the liver's blood supply appear to be physically obstructed by the Kupfer cells, but if tumor cells are large, they tend to become lodged in the portal venous branches. The presence of stasis, damaged endothelium, and normally fenestrated endothelium is favorable to the implantation of tumor emboli. By contrast, tumor emboli do not adhere to intact endothelium. Access to underlying collagen in the space of Disse, the space between the fenestrated endothelium and the hepatic cords, provides various attachment points for cancer emboli arriving at the sinusoid (Khan & Pankhania, 2011). Not all implanted cancer cells in the space of Disse develop into liver metastases. The fenestrations in the sinusoidal lining facilitate cancer implantation.

The destruction of liver tissue by cancer cells and their metastases is linked to the release of a variety of proteinases from the cancer cells. Tumor emboli leaving the sinusoid move instantly to a subendothelial position or between layers of liver cells. As a result, in the early stages of tissue implantation, the tumor cells lie in close proximity to the diffusible nutrients.

The pathologic anatomy of metastases resembles that of the primary tumor. Metastases frequently show the same degree of vascularity as that of the primary tumor. Most metastases are hypovascular, but some tumors typically have hypervascular metastases. These include metastases from carcinoids, leiomyosarcomas, neuroendocrine tumors, renal carcinomas, thyroid carcinomas, and choriocarcinomas. Occasionally, cancers of the ovary, pancreas, or breast produce hypervascular metastases (Khan & Pankhania, 2011).

Blood flow is said to increase relative to the normal parenchyma in all metastases. Large metastases tend to displace the surrounding vessels and may occlude or compress the portal venous branches. However, neovascularity, vascular encasement, and arteriovenous shunting are rare (Bartlett, 2000). Large metastases often outgrow their blood supply, causing hypoxia and necrosis at the center of the lesion.

Metastatic liver tumors may be expansive or infiltrative. They vary in size, shape, vascularity, and growth pattern. They vary because of differences in blood supply, hemorrhage, cellular differentiation, fibrosis, and necrosis. The patterns of blood supply of liver metastases are of considerable clinical importance because the various diagnostic and therapeutic approaches depend on the degree of neovascularity and the source and type of blood supply.

Patterns of Metastatic Spread

Khan and Pankhania (2011) have identified the following main factors that dictate the mode of liver invasion by tumor cells: (a) the propensity to retain a round shape, (b) the adhesiveness of different types of tumor cells and their adhesiveness to hepatocytes, (c) the inability of some tumor cells to survive and multiply in the bloodstream for long periods, (d) the pressure on the adjacent tissues, (e) the formation of tumor cell and hepatocyte junction, (f) tumor cell movement, and (g) host tissue destruction by enzymes elaborated by tumor cells.

Colorectal carcinoma is the third most common cause of cancer death in the United States, with 103,170 new cases and 51,690 deaths annually (Lewis & Martin, 2006; Siegel, Naishadham, & Jemal, 2012). Ultimately, two-thirds of all patients with colorectal cancer will develop metastasis to the liver and other organs in their life span. Lewis and Martin (2006) have identified the liver as the most common site of metastatic disease from the colon because of the dominant portal venous flow from the entire colon and a majority of the rectum.

In addition to being a primary site for spread of colon cancer, the liver is also the primary site of metastases for many other malignant neoplasms. GI malignancies are especially prone to spread to the liver because of its portal venous drainage. Extraabdominal tumors such as bronchogenic carcinoma, breast cancer, and malignant melanoma often spread through the bloodstream to the liver (Kemeny & D'Angelica, 2010).

Differences are seen in the natural history of the hepatic metastases for GI tumors. In some situations, hepatic metastases are a sign of disseminated disease. When gastric and pancreatic cancers metastasize to the liver, the mean survival is short, and widespread metastases often exist so that radical measures such as hepatic resection or hepatic infusion are rarely suitable (Kemeny et al., 2008). In contrast, the liver may be the sole site of metastatic disease for colorectal cancer, and a noteworthy fraction of these patients may even have isolated liver metastasis. In this setting, there has been significant progress in the areas of hepatic resection, regional chemotherapy, and radiation therapy.

For non-GI tumors, metastases to the liver are less common as the initial site of relapse. Although breast, lung, and melanoma are the main extra-GI cancers to metastasize to the liver, initial isolated metastases in the liver occur in 4%, 15%, and 24% of these patients, respectively (Bartlett, 2000).

Signs and Symptoms

Metastatic liver disease is often asymptomatic, especially in the early stages, and is frequently found incidentally. The patient may present with nonspecific symptoms of cancer including unintentional weight loss, anorexia, abdominal pain, malaise, or fever. As disease progresses, the abdominal pain may become more prominent in the right upper abdomen and radiate to the back and right shoulder.

On physical examination the liver may be enlarged, hard, or tender. The patient may have palpable nodules at the free edge of the liver because of advanced disease. Hepatic tumors are typically quite vascular; thus, increased amounts of blood feed into the hepatic artery and cause turbulent blood flow in the artery. The turbulence may result in a hepatic bruit, which, although uncommon, is characteristic. With large tumors or disease that is in close proximity to the bile duct, signs of obstructive jaundice (including dark urine, pale feces, and pruritus) may be present (Khan & Pankhania, 2011). Splenomegaly is occasionally present, without portal hypertension, especially when the primary cancer is pancreatic.

Hepatic metastasis can lead to malignancy-related ascites. Patients often complain of abdominal pain and distention, shortness of breath, or early satiety. On physical examination, presence of ascites is suggested by abdominal distention, tympany, fluid wave, and shifting dullness. The puddle sign, in which the examiner has the patient lie prone for five minutes and then uses a stethoscope to detect the presence of ascites, can detect an amount of fluid as small as 120 ml. The presence of bulging flanks may be noted when peritoneal fluid exceeds 500 ml (Rahil & Field, 2008). The presence of an umbilical nodule, also known as a Sister Mary Joseph node, in combination with ascites may be seen with colon or gastric metastases (Runyon, 2010). If the patient develops ascites and lower limb edema, invasion or occlusion of the inferior vena cava may be present (Khan & Pankhania, 2011).

Laboratory Diagnostics

Biochemical laboratory tests in patients with hepatic metastases are not very sensitive (Kemeny, Kemeny, & Lawrence, 2004). These patients may have abnormalities on blood testing, including anemia, leukocytosis, elevated transaminases (glutamic-oxaloacetic transaminase and glutamic-pyruvic transaminase), alkaline phosphatase, bilirubin, prothrombin time, and lactate dehydrogenase.

Some biochemical markers may be useful in determining the source of the liver metastases. Alpha-fetoprotein is a glycoprotein synthesized by the fetal liver and some cancers and may be elevated in testicular germ cell, pancreatic, gastric, and colon cancers. Cancer antigen (CA) 19-9 is an antigen that is often elevated in pancreatic cancer but can also be elevated in gastric or colon cancers. CA 125 is a very specific antigen that is associated with ovarian carcinoma. The most specific tumor marker for colon cancer is the glycoprotein carcinoembryonic antigen, but it can also be elevated in pancreatic, gastric, lung, and breast cancers.

Imaging

The evaluation of suspected metastases is one of the most important indications for imaging. Imaging plays the principal role in staging, as well as monitoring the effectiveness of treatment and surveillance following treatment.

Ultrasound (Sonogram)

Ultrasound is frequently used to evaluate the liver. It has the benefit of being widely available and is able to detect metastatic lesions greater than 0.5 cm in diameter. Although ultrasound imaging is nonspecific in the workup of liver metastases, the presence of multiple hepatic nodules of different sizes within the liver is nearly always the result of metastases. Most metastatic deposits are solid and often have a hypoechoic halo surrounding the mass (Liu & Francis, 2010) (see Figure 6-1).

Despite some of its current limitations, recent technologic advances that use IV contrast agents and contrast-specific scan techniques have yielded promising results. In addition, ultrasound remains important as a guiding technology for the sampling of percutaneous lesions and in therapeutic interventions such as thermal ablation (Lencioni, Della Pina, Crocetti, Bozzi, & Cioni, 2007).

Computed Tomography

Computed tomography (CT) using contrast enhancement is the imaging technique that is most frequently chosen for assessing hepatic metastases. The diagnostic performance of the multidetector CT with helical scan technique in this setting is high and has essentially replaced CT arterial portography for diagnosis of hepatic metastases (Liu & Francis, 2010). It provides fast acquisition of images, provides detailed, cross-sectional images, and can evaluate the liver in several contrast-enhanced phases. CT is highly sensitive for the detection of liver metastases (80%–90% sensitivity and 99% specificity for contrast-enhanced scans) (Khan & Pankhania, 2011). Multiphase spiral CT scan using oral and IV contrast material is

done in three phases in order to obtain different phases of tissue enhancement.

Noncontrast CT can be used for patients with a history of contrast allergy reactions or renal impairment and can help to identify hypervascular tumors, calcifications, and hemorrhoids. However, it fails to adequately distinguish hypovascular tumors from the liver parenchyma (Kemeny et al., 2004). IV contrast is used to highlight blood vessels and to enhance the structure of the organ; thus, the appearance of the metastasis will vary based on vascularity (see Figure 6-2). Most liver metastases are hypovascular (hypo-attenuating) in comparison with surrounding hepatic tissue. Metastases that tend to be hypovascular include those from the colon, lung, prostate, and gynecologic primaries (Khan & Pankhania, 2011) (see Figures 6-3 and 6-4).

Helical CT allows scanning of the liver during the different phases of contrast medium distribution: arterial phase

Figure 6-2. Vascularity of Hepatic Lesions

Hypovascular Liver Lesions	Hypervascular Liver Lesions

• Benign cystic lesions
• Hemangioma
• Lymphoma
• Metastases from carcinoma of
  – Lung
  – Colon
  – Breast
  – Stomach
  – Head and neck tumors
	• Primary liver tumors
	• Metastases from
	  – Carcinoid
	  – Islet cell tumors
	  – Pheochromocytoma
	  – Thyroid
	  – Melanoma
	  – Breast
	  – Renal cell
	  – Sarcoma
	  – Choriocarcinoma

Figure 6-3. Coronal Reformat of Axial Computed Tomography Scan Post–IV Contrast in a 75-Year-Old Female With Metastatic Colon Cancer

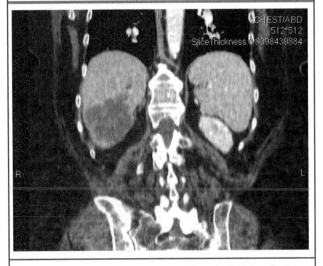

Note. Image courtesy of Dr. Cary Pallin and Kenosha Radiology Center. Used with permission.

Figure 6-1. Transverse Ultrasound of the Liver in a 72-Year-Old Female With Metastatic Endometrial Cancer

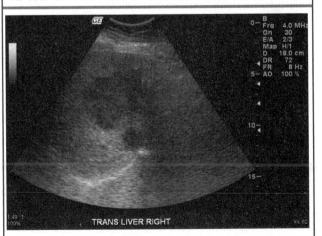

Note. Image courtesy of Dr. Cary Pallin and Kenosha Radiology Center. Used with permission.

Figure 6-4. Axial Computed Tomography Scan Post–IV
Contrast (140 cc Omnipaque® 300) in a 76-Year-Old
Male With Metastatic Colon Cancer

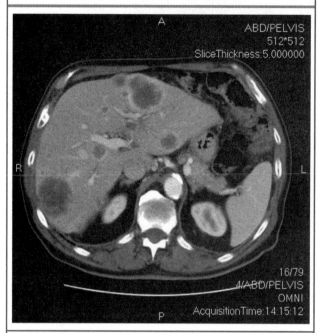

Note. Image courtesy of Dr. Cary Pallin and Kenosha Radiology Center. Used with permission.

acquisition (or early phase study), portal phase acquisition (or venous phase study), and delayed phase acquisition (or equilibrium phase study). Metastases with abundant arterial blood flow may enhance vividly during the arterial-predominant phase of enhancement, including metastases from neuroendocrine tumors, pheochromocytoma, carcinoid, breast, renal cell carcinoma, and thyroid (Paulson, 2001).

Magnetic Resonance Imaging

Magnetic resonance imaging (MRI) is a nonionizing, multiplanar technique that is highly effective for the evaluation of suspected hepatic metastases, with sensitivity ranging from 80%–100% and specificity up to 97% (Liu & Francis, 2010). MRI is frequently ordered prior to tumor resection to better characterize lesions of indeterminate appearance visualized on CT scan. MRI has better sensitivity in detection of small lesions compared to helical CT. Contrast enhancement is typically used. Metastatic lesions are usually of low signal intensity relative to the background liver tissue on T1-weighted scans and have high intensity signal on T2-weighted scans (Paulson, 2001) (see Figure 6-5).

MRI has advantages over CT scan in that it does not use radiation and has improved contrast sensitivity. In the case of diffuse metastases, CT scanning and ultrasound may underestimate the extent of disease. In addition, MRI can be used when

alternative imaging is contraindicated (Khan & Pankhania, 2011). MRI has some drawbacks in that it is prone to motion artifact, respiratory, and cardiac movements, which can negatively affect the images, and it is also expensive (Choi, 2006).

Intraoperative ultrasound is the most sensitive imaging technique for the detection of liver abnormalities, with 96% accuracy (Khan & Pankhania, 2011). This test involves the placement of the transducer directly on the surface of the liver. In patients who are undergoing hepatic resection, it can be helpful in delineating the extent of disease and vascular landmarks (Schwartz & Kruskal, 2009).

Positron-Emission Tomography

Positron-emission tomography (PET) can be used for the detection of metastatic lesions, and it is often used in com-

Figure 6-5. MRI Axial T1 Three Minutes Post–IV
Contrast (20 cc Omniscan®) in a 42-Year-Old Female
With Metastatic Leiomyosarcoma

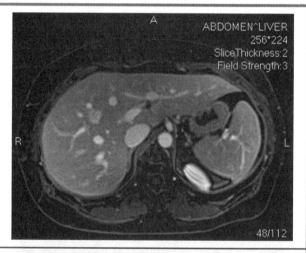

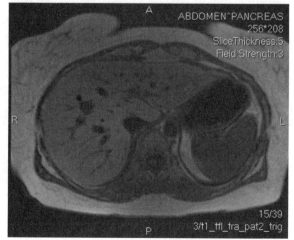

Note. Images courtesy of Dr. Cary Pallin and Kenosha Radiology Center. Used with permission.

bination with CT scanning. It is no more sensitive than MRI in detecting liver metastasis, and it does not provide the anatomic resolution of other imaging that gives cross-sectional views. However, it can be useful in the identification of extrahepatic disease. In particular, PET has been used successfully to identify GI carcinoid tumors and lymph node and organ metastases. In general, it should not be used in first-line imaging (Khan & Pankhania, 2011).

Diagnostic Liver Biopsy

Liver biopsy is a powerful tool that can be used to evaluate the etiology of liver abnormalities when radiologic imaging does not provide exact characterization of the lesion. Fine-needle aspiration biopsy under image guidance has gained increasing acceptance as the diagnostic procedure of choice for patients with focal hepatic lesions. It can be performed percutaneously or endoscopically. Fine-needle aspiration uses thin-walled needles of small diameter that can be directed into focal liver lesions. The aspirated specimen contains cells mixed with blood and tissue fluid that can be sent for cytologic and histologic examination. Fine-needle aspiration is not considered a true tissue biopsy because it only provides a small number of cells for cytologic examination (Bravo, Sheth, & Chopra, 2009). It is often used when a specific lesion needs to be sampled. Hemorrhage is a potential complication with liver biopsies, although the occurrence of complications after hepatic fine-needle aspiration is rare, about 0.5% (Chhieng, 2004). Potential seeding of neoplastic cells is also a potential concern (Schwartz & Kruskal, 2009). Laparoscopic liver biopsy has the highest diagnostic yield and is a good option for staging disease extent in patients with intra-abdominal malignancies, but it requires general anesthesia and is therefore associated with increased risk and cost (Bravo et al., 2009).

Treatment Modalities

Treatment of hepatic metastases often depends on the location of the primary cancer and histologic diagnosis. A number of systemic and regional treatment options are available for patients with isolated liver metastasis (see Figure 6-6). For many years, 5-fluorouracil (5-FU) was the primary chemotherapeutic agent used to treat metastatic colorectal cancer. Over the past decade, treatment options expanded with the approval of irinotecan and oxaliplatin, as well as the monoclonal antibodies bevacizumab, cetuximab, and panitumumab. A number of chemotherapy regimens including these agents, both alone and in combination, are used to treat metastatic disease (e.g., FOLFIRI, FOLFOX 6, XE-LOX, FOLFOXIRI) and are beyond the scope of this chapter. Despite the new agents introduced since 2000, the best way to combine and sequence these agents is still not established (Clark & Grothey, 2012).

Figure 6-6. Treatment Options for Patients With Isolated Liver Metastases

- Systemic treatment
- Regional therapy
  - Resection with or without adjuvant chemotherapy
  - Local ablative therapy
    * Cryotherapy
    * Radiofrequency ablation
    * Percutaneous ethanol injection
  - Infusion therapy
    * Hepatic artery infusion
    * Hepatic artery infusion with hemofiltration
    * Chemoembolization
    * Isolated hepatic perfusion
    * Selected internal radiation

Note. Based on information from Alexander, 2002.

The liver is a common metastasis site for ocular melanoma. It is quite refractory to systemic chemotherapy, and the prognosis is poor with a median overall survival of 11 months for patients receiving chemotherapy or best supportive care (Rivoire et al., 2005). Hepatic arterial chemoembolization can be used to treat ocular melanoma with hepatic metastasis. However, Gupta et al. (2010) found that the median overall survival was 6.7 months, and progression-free survival was 3.8 months. They also found that the extent of liver involvement, baseline lactate dehydrogenase levels, and response to therapy were significant predictors for overall and progression-free survival. Neuroendocrine tumors metastatic to the liver have a tendency to a somewhat indolent clinical course. Transarterial hepatic chemotherapy using mitomycin C and gemcitabine can be an effective therapeutic treatment for patients with neuroendocrine tumors. Vogl, Gruber, Naguib, and Nour-Eldin (2009) found that patients tolerated treatment with no major complications, and the median survival time from the initial diagnosis using this approach was 57.1 months. If surgical resection or interventional embolization cannot be performed, or if the disease has metastasized to places beyond the liver, systemic treatment can be used. Biotherapy using somatostatin analogs (e.g., octreotide) or interferon can be used (Fendrich, Michl, Habbe, & Bartsch, 2010). Chemotherapy is typically reserved for poorly differentiated metastatic tumors. Depending on the size and location of the tumor in the liver, first-line treatment chemotherapy using streptozotocin in combination with 5-FU and doxorubicin has been shown to achieve a response rate of 39% with an overall survival rate of 74% (Kouvaraki et al., 2004). In a subset of patients with highly proliferating tumors, cisplatin or carboplatin in combination with etoposide can be used with an overall survival of 20 months (Di Meglio et al., 2010).

Resection of metastatic disease confined to the liver has been associated with long-term disease-free survival in patients with colorectal cancer and other histologies. Unfortunately, only 10%–20% of individuals have metastatic deposits that are conducive to surgical resection based on size, number, and location (Alexander, 2002). Alexander noted that a number of studies have reported actuarial five-year survival rates of 25%–40% following hepatic resection for colorectal cancer and 10%–73% for individuals with other histologies, including neuroendocrine, breast, and genitourinary cancers.

Because of its unique vascular anatomy, the liver is a good site for delivery of various types of regional therapies for patients who have unresectable metastases. It is well known that established hepatic metastases derive the majority of their blood flow from the hepatic artery versus the portal venous system. Using chemotherapeutics with a high first pass extraction rate such as floxuridine for patients with colorectal cancer, there is selective accumulation of the drug in tumors versus normal hepatic parenchyma. In general, response rates are better with regional therapeutics delivered via the hepatic artery than with systemic therapy (Kemeny et al., 2008). Local ablative techniques are used with percutaneously or operatively positioned probes to deliver radiofrequency or cryotherapy sufficient to destroy established tumor deposits in the hepatic parenchyma with minimal injury to surrounding hepatic tissue. Vascular isolation and perfusion of the liver, also known as isolated hepatic perfusion or IHP, is a specialized surgical procedure designed to deliver high-dose biotherapy or chemotherapy to the liver (Bartlett, 2000).

Hepatic Resection

There is general agreement that surgical resection is the treatment of choice for patients with one to three metastases from colorectal cancer, producing a five-year survival of about 30%. A number of factors have resulted in decreased morbidity and mortality for patients undergoing hepatic resection (see Figure 6-7). Improved patient selection based on state-of-the-art imaging modalities and technical advances in performing hepatic resection are the factors having the highest impact.

Major hepatic resection should be based on an understanding of the segmental anatomy of the liver. The liver is composed of eight segments each fed by discrete pedicles of the portal triad (see Figure 5-1 in Chapter 5). Anatomically, the liver is divided into the left and right lobes by the principal plane, which lies between the gallbladder and the vena cava. Segments 2, 3, 4A, and 4B comprise the left lobe, and segments 5, 6, 7, and 8 comprise the right lobe. The caudate lobe is considered segment 1 and has a unique orientation behind the portal vein, deriving portal inflow from multiple main and left portal vein branches. The caudate lobe's venous drainage is largely by direct tributaries into the retrohepatic vena cava. The left branch of the portal triad divides in the umbilical fissure to feed segments 2 and 3 laterally and 4 medially. The main right branch of the portal triad branches posteriorly to segments 6 and 7 and anteriorly to segments 5 and 8. Focusing on segmental anatomy has provided the ability

---

Figure 6-7. Technical Advances in Hepatic Surgery Resulting in Improved Outcome and Decreased Morbidity and Mortality

Improved Patient Selection
- Accurate staging with high-resolution preoperative imaging studies
- Intraoperative ultrasound
  - Screens for occult metastases
  - Defines internal anatomy to guide resection

Improved Operative Technique
- Segmental approach to resection
- Avoidance of coagulopathy
  - Correction of preoperative coagulation abnormalities
  - Minimize blood loss
  - Routine use of warming devices
- Minimal blood loss during parenchymal dissection
  - Extrahepatic ligation of hepatic vein prior to dissection
  - Low central venous pressure
- No drains

Note. Based on information from Alexander, 2002.

---

to perform metastasectomies rather than formal lobectomies and total vascular exclusion.

During laparotomy when the abdominal cavity has been cautiously evaluated to exclude the presence of extrahepatic disease, intraoperative ultrasound is used to evaluate for the presence of occult metastases. When possible, resection should be based on segmental anatomic considerations to preserve normal hepatic parenchyma and minimize blood loss during the resection. In performing a standard right or left hepatectomy, the direct small venous branches between the liver and the vena cava are systemically ligated and divided. No drains are typically employed for uncomplicated hepatic resections, and Alexander (2002) has referred to mortality associated with major hepatic resection as being less than 4%.

A number of series have reported results of hepatic resection for patients with colorectal liver metastases with overall five-year survival ranging between 25% and 45% (Alexander, 2002). Resection of colorectal metastases to the liver can be curative in at least one-fourth of patients with certain requirements (Lim et al., 2007). The curability by resection of liver metastases from other primary cancers is not quite as clear. Resection of metastases from other GI malignancies, such as stomach and pancreas, has been disappointing because of the aggressive nature of these tumors by the time they become metastatic (Pocard, Pouillart, Asselain, & Salmon, 2000).

Occasionally, a single hepatic metastasis from a breast carcinoma is found and resected with good results, but this is generally not advisable because breast cancer is a systemic disease. Liver metastases from GI tumors can be considered regional spread, but for the metastases to go from the breast to the liver requires release of tumor cells into the systemic circulation. As a result, the concept that the liver could be the only site of spread is harder to prove, and as a result, curative intent is more difficult to achieve.

GI neuroendocrine tumors that have metastasized to the liver are frequently resected. According to Kemeny and D'Angelica (2010), these tumors present a special challenge to surgeons in that they are frequently indolent and are often associated with hormonal changes that can cause symptoms such as diarrhea, flushing, abdominal cramps, asthma, and edema. Five-year survival in patients who undergo hepatic resection range from 50% to 75%, and symptom control occurred in more than 90% of patients who underwent this procedure. The authors point out that these data are retrospective and prone to selection bias because these patients had indolent disease and a lesser degree of tumor burden.

Sarcomas also metastasize to the liver. A group from Memorial Sloan-Kettering reviewed retrospective data on hepatic resections for sarcoma. The review included 331 patients with liver metastases from a variety of primary sarcomas, 56 who underwent hepatectomy. Thirty-four of the 56 patients had a GI stromal tumor (GIST). Ten of the 56 patients actually survived for five years, but nearly all of these patients had recurrence. The disease-specific survival rate for three and five years was 50% and 30%, respectively. Patients with GIST had the same survival as those with other types of sarcoma (DeMatteo et al., 2001). These data were collected before imatinib was approved for the treatment of GIST. The time interval (less than or greater than two years) between the appearance of the primary sarcoma and that of the liver metastases had a significant influence on survival and was the only independent prognostic variable in a multivariate analysis (Kemeny & D'Angelica, 2010).

In the United States, the data on resection of colorectal metastases to the liver have changed over the past 30 years. According to Kemeny et al. (2008), more than 50,000 patients each year develop liver metastases from colorectal cancer. The resection of these metastases has been increasing over the years because patient eligibility data has expanded (Kemeny et al., 2008). Data interpretation guidance for hepatic resection can be found in Figure 6-8. Noncolorectal non-neuroendocrine metastases to the liver are labeled "NCCN metastases." Studies of resection on NCCN metastases are limited, mostly because of small numbers. However long-term survival is possible with more than one-third of patients. Of these, testicular, adrenal, and gynecologic cancers had the best outcomes (Kemeny & D'Angelica, 2010).

Several studies have addressed the matter of extrahepatic intra-abdominal metastases at the time of hepatic resection. In most instances, surgeons do not proceed with liver resection in the presence of extrahepatic metastases. In general, prognostic variables that influence survival after hepatic resection include the presence of extrahepatic disease, the stage of the primary colon cancer, the time interval between primary and the development of hepatic metastases, and the number of metastases as well as positive margins.

Figure 6-8. Guidelines for Data Interpretation in Hepatic Resection

- In colorectal primary, hepatic resection is the only available treatment that will result in a 25% five-year survival in one to three metastases.
- In four or more metastases from a colorectal primary, hepatic resection cannot be universally recommended at this time and should be limited to centers doing studies on these treatment modalities.
- Patients with hepatic metastases that developed 12 months after primary colon cancer resection have better survival after hepatic resection than patients with synchronous hepatic metastases with their primary colorectal lesions.
- Duke's stage C of primary colorectal resection is a poor prognostic sign for patients undergoing resection of hepatic metastases but should not exclude patients from hepatic resection.
- Patients with extrahepatic abdominal metastases should not be considered for hepatic resection unless the extrahepatic disease is part of a local recurrence in the colorectal area that can be completely excised.
- Bilobar hepatic disease and previous response to chemotherapy are not indicators that influence success with hepatic resection.

Note. Based on information from Kemeny et al., 2008.

Ablative Techniques

An alternative to surgical resection of metastatic tumors is local ablation techniques such as cryotherapy, local injection of toxic agents, or hyperthermic coagulative necrosis (see Table 6-1). In general, lesions conducive to surgical resection are also conducive to local ablation techniques. Lesions not conducive to resection because vessels involved are too large or lesions are too numerous are not conducive to local ablation.

Local ablation techniques can be beneficial in treating deep parenchymal hepatic metastases as a means of preserving hepatic parenchyma, compared to what may be necessary if a resection were done. This is vital in cirrhosis, in which minimal hepatic reserve is a limiting factor. Also, avoiding a lobectomy may preserve the vascular anatomy so that a lobectomy on either side could be performed for recurrence if necessary (Adam, 2002).

Consideration regarding local ablation as a procedure for hepatic metastases must involve thinking about limitations of each approach. In general, one has to consider the ability to access the lesion percutaneously, the capability to adequately ablate all regions of the tumor with special attention to the leading edge, and the potential side effects to normal surrounding tissues. Any bowel lying adjacent to the tumor must be taken into consideration. It is frequently difficult to interpret clinical studies on local ablation because of inconsistent end points. Predictably, the treated regions demonstrate low density on CT scans that can be difficult to distinguish from tumor and which should be larger than the initial tumor. The

			Table 6-1. Local Ablation Advantages and Disadvantages		
Mechanism	**Technique**	**Zone of Necrosis**	**Advantages**	**Disadvantages**
Freezing	Cryotherapy	3–5 cm	Large zone of necrosis Easily followed by ultrasound	Requires laparotomy Large probe size
Hyperthermic coagulative necrosis	Radiofrequency ablation	2 cm	Percutaneous technique	Small zone of necrosis
Local injection therapy	Ethanol Acetic acid Chemotherapy Hot saline	3 cm	Simple Inexpensive	Inhomogeneous distribution

Note. Based on information from Bartlett, 2000.

appearance of low density is at times considered a response but is in no way objective. As a result, response data are typically unable to be evaluated. Survival is also a problematic end point because the treated lesion frequently has no influence on survival. Therefore, success of treatment is not reflected in longer survival. The most important factor to consider in interpreting response data for these therapies is the time to progression in the treated lesions. Unfortunately, this end point is frequently not described.

Different hepatic tumors respond to local injection of toxic agents, such as ethanol. It is a simple and inexpensive technique with guaranteed efficacy of the agent against cancer cells. Limitations of ethanol injection include the inability to evenly distribute the toxic agent throughout a tumor and the potential toxicity of ethanol leaking outside of the tumor into normal cells. One potential limiting factor is that each lesion usually requires about four treatments. Cancers ideal for alcohol injection are the small hepatocellular cancers in a cirrhotic liver because these tumors are relatively soft compared to surrounding liver.

Cryosurgery uses subzero temperatures for in situ destruction of tissues. Cellular destruction and death is a result of rapid freeze and thaw of tissues. One big advantage of cryosurgery is the ability to use this local treatment without damaging normal tissue. Difficulties with this technique include defining the full extent of the tumor and inability to monitor the amount of freezing. As a result, the possibility of overtreatment of surrounding susceptible normal tissues exists. Technical developments that have improved the use of cryotherapy include cryoprobes cooled by liquid nitrogen allowing more precise freezing, even within the liver, along with intraoperative ultrasound allowing precise placement of the cryoprobe and more accurate monitoring of the freezing process (Kemeny et al., 2008). Cryotherapy can be used intraoperatively or percutaneously.

However, cryotherapy involves some technical issues, including that adequate hydration is needed before surgery to avoid myoglobinuria and tumor lysis; attention must be paid to bile ducts to avoid biliary fistula formation; two freeze/thaw cycles are preferred, and vigorous pulling or twisting of the probe could cause cracking (Khan & Pankhania, 2011).

Potential complications include hepatic cracking secondary to the thermal stresses that occur with rapid freezing. These are usually associated with hemorrhage, which could require packing. Other potential complications include biliary fistula, which then requires percutaneous drainage, and myoglobinuria resulting in acute tubular necrosis.

Just as tumors can be destroyed by cold, they can also be destroyed by heat. Techniques such as radiofrequency and microwave have been used to destroy tumors. Radiofrequency ablation involves placing a small electrode within the tumor, which is then used to deliver energy to the tumor tissue. Radiofrequency current produces ionic agitation, which is transformed into frictional heat and results in breakdown of proteins and cellular membranes. Larger tumors have the potential of being destroyed by cryoablation. Candidates for radiofrequency ablation must have one to three lesions located in the periphery of the liver that are not adjacent to the bowel, kidney, gallbladder, or diaphragm. Lesions should optimally be smaller than 3 cm, although current research is investigating the use of ablation in lesions as large as 7 cm (Kemeny & D'Angelica, 2010). During ablation, a hyperechoic area is formed around the tip of the needle, which matches the area treated.

Cancer cells have the ability to be more sensitive than normal cells to heat because of the decreased vasodilation capacity of the neurovascular bed (Kemeny et al., 2008). Microwave coagulation is useful in very small tumors (less than 3 cm). Microwave coagulation and percutaneous ethanol injection therapy may be more useful if combined with embolization. Lesions near hilar structures are not good candidates for microwave coagulation, but lesions next to hepatic veins are good candidates (Lewis & Martin, 2006).

There is no doubt that these techniques successfully ablate tumor tissue. However, these techniques have a limited ability to accurately address all regions of a spherical tumor, including a margin beyond the leading edge in three dimensions, when the lesion is larger than the achievable zone of necrosis and the real-time imaging is in two dimensions. Numerous overlapping zones of necrosis may be necessary. This is difficult to achieve without leaving regions of the tumor untreated. Also, because tissue injury is in no way specific for tumor cells, surrounding bile ducts, vessels, bowel, diaphragm, and other structures can be injured during the ablation. Large vessels near the tumor can act to prevent adequate heating or cooling of adjacent tissue, resulting in escape of viable tumor cells in this region. Although killing 99% of cells within a tumor using regional ablation may be a satisfactory result when palliating patients at high risk for recurrence in new sites, it may not compare favorably to surgical resection in patients with curative potential in which a negative margin can frequently be guaranteed with surgery, and the risk of local recurrence at the site of resection is minimal (Bartlett, 2000). For tumors not conducive to surgical resection or local ablation, regional hepatic treatment approaches can be considered. These include chemoembolization, hepatic artery infusion (HAI) therapy, and isolated hepatic perfusion techniques.

Hepatic Artery Infusion

The use of HAI chemotherapy was intended to take advantage of increased concentration of chemotherapy delivered to the tumor vasculature while minimizing systemic side effects by utilizing drugs that are rapidly metabolized by the liver in their first pass through the liver (Kemeny et al., 2008). FUDR® (floxuridine) is the regimen most widely studied for use as HAI. The treatment is done as typically a monthly two-week infusion delivered by a surgically implanted pump with its catheter placed in the gastroduodenal artery directed into the hepatic artery. According to Kemeny and D'Angelica (2010), the response rate is higher with HAI (41%) than with systemic therapy (14%). The regimen is generally well tolerated and does not cause myelosuppression, nausea, vomiting, or diarrhea. The most common problems associated with HAI are hepatic toxicity and ulceration of the stomach and duodenum. Biliary sclerosis may also occur leading to obstructive jaundice, which can be difficult to manage.

The rationale for hepatic arterial chemotherapy has an anatomic and pharmacologic basis (see Figure 6-9). Regional HAI can be done using either a hepatic arterial port, a percutaneously placed catheter connected to an external pump, or a totally implanted pump.

Although FUDR is the optimal drug for HAI, other drugs can be used in the event of toxicity side effects or intolerance and can be found in Table 6-2 with their half-lives and exposure. More recent studies have focused on the use of irinotecan and oxaliplatin (Venook, 2012).

It is important to closely monitor liver function. Biliary toxicity typically manifests as elevations of serum glutamic-oxaloacetic transaminase, alkaline phosphatase, and bilirubin. Early manifestation of toxicity is shown with elevation of aspartate transferase. If the bilirubin rises above 3 mg/dl, no further treatment should be given until it normalizes, and then treatment can be resumed at a 75% reduction in order to prevent sclerosing cholangitis (Kemeny et al., 2008). Endoscopic retrograde cholangiopancreatography (ERCP) can be performed in patients who develop jaundice and may demonstrate lesions resembling idiopathic sclerosing cholangitis in 5%–29% (Kemeny & D'Angelica, 2010). In some patients, these strictures may be more focal and worse at the hepatic

---

Figure 6-9. Hepatic Arterial Chemotherapy Rationale

- Almost exclusively, the hepatic artery perfuses liver metastases while the normal liver is primarily perfused by the portal vein and minimally from the hepatic artery.
- Certain drugs have high hepatic extractions during the first pass through the arterial circulation. This results in high local concentrations of the drug while minimizing systemic toxicity. This is what makes floxuridine an optimal drug for hepatic arterial infusion.
- Many drugs have a steep dose response curve, and these will be the most useful when given by an intrahepatic route because a large dose can be given regionally.
- Drugs with a high total body clearance are more effective because if the drug is not cleared rapidly, recirculation through the systemic circulation diminishes the advantage of hepatic arterial delivery.
- Frequently the liver is the first and only site of metastatic disease. The theory of stepwise pattern of metastatic progression dictates that hematogenous spread occurs first via the portal vein to the liver, then from the liver to the lungs, and then to other organs. As a result, aggressive treatment of metastases confined to the liver could lead to prolonged survival for some patients.

Note. Based on information from Kemeny et al., 2008; Stratmann, 2002.

Table 6-2. Hepatic Artery Infusion Drugs

Drug	Estimated Half-Life (Minutes)	Increased Exposure by Hepatic Artery Infusion
Fluorouracil (5-FU)	10	5–10-fold
5-FU, 2-deoxyuridine, floxuridine	< 10	100–400-fold
Carmustine (also known as bischloroethyl nitrosourea or BCNU)	< 5	6–7-fold
Mitomycin C	< 10	6–8-fold
Cisplatin	20–30	4–7-fold
Doxorubicin	60	2-fold

Note. Based on information from Bartlett, 2000; Kemeny et al., 2008.

duct bifurcation. In these cases, drainage procedures either by ERCP or by transhepatic cholangiogram can be helpful. However, one should first exclude duct obstruction from metastases before any invasive interventions.

Inadvertent perfusion of the stomach and duodenum with drug via small collateral branches from the hepatic artery can cause severe ulcer disease. According to Kemeny et al. (2008), this complication can be prevented with careful dissection of the collaterals at the time of pump placement. However, even without radiologically visible perfusion of the stomach, mild gastritis and duodenitis still can occur.

Hepatic Arterial Embolization and Chemoembolization

Regional hepatic treatment approaches such as hepatic arterial embolization (HAE) and hepatic arterial chemoembolization (HACE) are frequently used for the management of patients with primary and secondary malignant liver tumors not conducive to surgical resection or local ablation. Hepatic tumor types that typically respond to HAE and HACE include hepatocellular carcinoma, intrahepatic cholangiocarcinoma, and metastases from neuroendocrine tumors, melanomas, colorectal carcinoma, and sarcomas (Kamat et al., 2008). Although typically relatively safe, HAE and HACE can be connected with serious complications, such as hepatic failure, hepatic infarction, tumor lysis syndrome, renal failure, sepsis, and even death. Replacement of more than 75% of the normal liver has been regarded as a relative contraindication to HAE and HACE because of the high risk of postembolization hepatic failure in these patients (Patel et al., 2005).

As a treatment, HACE has been used since the mid-1970s. Although typically the prognosis in metastatic liver disease is poor, the use of more aggressive treatment procedures in patients with neuroendocrine tumors and colorectal metastases may result in favorable outcome.

Chemoembolization is a technique that combines intra-arterial chemotherapy with obstruction of the arterial inflow to tumors via embolization of small particles (e.g., iodized oil, gel foam, polyvinyl alcohol, starch microspheres) into the tumor vasculature (Bartlett, 2000). This is based on the concept that blocking the arterial system will produce ischemic necrosis of the tumor. Because tumors receive 100% of their blood supply from the arterial system compared to the normal liver, which receives 25% of its supply from here, the normal liver should recover from embolization, whereas the tumor should not. Also, obstructed arterial inflow should prevent washout of chemotherapy delivered to the tumors. Using embolization compared to intra-arterial alone allows 20 times higher chemotherapy concentrations being achieved in tumors and lasts up to 30 days (Kress et al., 2003). Although chemotherapy response varies by histology, response to embolization is applicable to all histologies.

Khan and Pankhania (2011) have specified three circumstances in which effective chemoembolization of the liver is possible.
- The liver has a unique blood supply: 75% of the hepatic blood supply is derived from the portal vein, whereas 25% of the blood supply is derived from the hepatic artery.
- The hepatic artery supplies approximately 95% of the blood in both primary and metastatic hepatic tumors.
- Development of catheter technology has allowed extremely selective placement of catheters for safe and effective delivery of therapeutic agents to hepatic tumors.

The development of microcatheters has afforded safe placement, even with aberrant vessels or collateral blood supply. It was discovered in the early 1980s that when iodized poppy-seed oil is injected into the hepatic artery, it actually remains in the neovascularity of the hepatic cellular carcinoma, acting as a vehicle for delivering cytotoxic agents to tumor sites within the liver.

Side effects of chemoembolization are generally tolerable in patients with sufficient hepatic reserve. Common but transient side effects include fever, pain, and nausea. Liver failure occurs in patients with minimal hepatic reserve. As with local ablation techniques, evaluation of response is especially difficult after chemoembolization because of the change in density of the tumors and surrounding tissues because of ischemia. This frequently leads to a perceptible increase in the size of the tumor mass on CT scans. In general, chemoembolization has the ability to provide rapid palliation for large tumors or neuroendocrine tumors with syndromes of hormone excess. The duration of palliation is usually three to six months. However, multiple repeat embolizations can be performed until normal hepatic reserve is depleted. Improvements in the embolic materials and chemotherapy compounds have the potential to improve these overall results in the future.

Khan and Pankhania (2011) have listed the following contraindications for embolization: (a) biliary obstruction, (b) hepatic encephalopathy, (c) tumor load more than 50%, (d) bilirubin level greater than 2 mg/dl, (e) lactate dehydrogenase level greater than 425 U/L, and (f) aspartate aminotransferase level greater than 100 U/L.

Systemic Chemotherapy

The response of hepatic metastases to systemic chemotherapy is variable and typically reflects the response of the primary tumor. Some tumor types are more responsive to chemotherapy than others. In metastatic breast cancer, liver tumors have been found to have fewer estrogen-positive receptors. In patients who receive systemic chemotherapy, liver metastasis is a poor prognostic indicator, and these patients have a median survival time of about 10 months (Kemeny et al., 2008). A number of new agents are used in the treatment of metastatic colorectal cancer. Combination regimens using irinotecan, 5-FU, and leucovorin or oxaliplatin, 5-FU, and leucovorin (FOLFOX) have increased response rates over 5-FU and leucovorin alone. In addition, the use of the anti–vascular endothelial growth factor monoclonal antibody bevacizumab with these regimens has improved survival in select patient groups (Kemeny & D'Angelica, 2010).

Metastases from gastric cancer are more responsive to chemotherapy than any other GI cancers. Approximately 70% of patients with colorectal cancer develop liver metastasis (Kemeny & D'Angelica, 2010). One may question when to start systemic chemotherapy for patients with liver metastases from breast, gastric, or colon cancer. For patients with gastric or colon cancer who are asymptomatic and have a volume of disease less than 20%, if the liver is involved with tumor and not resectable, earlier treatment increases survival and increases time with good performance status. If the patient has rapidly progressive disease or is symptomatic, chemotherapy should be started as soon as possible. Before starting treatment, a baseline CT scan and laboratory values should be obtained. Scans should be repeated at two- to three-month intervals to assess whether the tumor is responding. Because hepatic metastases from a primary breast cancer typically progress rapidly and response rates to chemotherapy are high, patients are usually started on chemotherapy early.

The potential benefits of neoadjuvant chemotherapy with resectable disease include the opportunity to test for chemoresponsiveness, the potential elimination of micrometastatic disease, and the possibility of shrinkage with a higher likelihood of complete resection and reduced extent of resection. In addition, response to neoadjuvant treatment has been highlighted as a prognostic indicator for survival, which may help to select suitable candidates for surgery. Potential disadvantages of neoadjuvant treatment include the possibility of hepatic damage and inducing a complete response that renders previously resectable patients unsuitable for surgery. The ability to visualize the metastases at the time of surgery, either on a preoperative scan or through direct visualization in the operating room, permits a higher likelihood of a complete resection. A complete radiologic response may necessitate that a large resection be performed in order to ensure that all microscopic disease is resected and may also result in an incomplete resection through the lack of ability to visualize the metastases (Alberts & Wagman, 2008).

The term *conversion therapy* is frequently used when the intent of treatment is to render unresectable disease resectable with preoperative chemotherapy. Neoadjuvant chemotherapy is reserved for the treatment administered to patients with liver metastases that are resectable. Thus the intent of conversion therapy is obviously different from the intent of neoadjuvant therapy although both treatments are given before planned hepatic resection (Halfdanarson, Kendrick, & Grothey, 2010).

Radiotherapy

Improvements with systemic therapy in controlling occult metastatic liver disease have raised renewed interest in local therapies that can treat isolated sites of metastatic disease within the liver. Radiotherapy (RT) is a treatment option that can be offered to patients inappropriate for surgery or other ablative therapies.

Improvements in RT planning and delivery have made it possible for RT to be delivered more evenly with sharp falloff in dose surrounding the target volume. Strategies that have improved the conformity of RT delivery include reducing breathing motion, reproducible immobilization, diagnostic quality imaging for RT planning, and imaging and repositioning at the time of its delivery (Swaminath & Dawson, 2010). All of these strategies improve accuracy and precision of RT delivery that improves the similarity of planned doses with delivered doses, minimizing the risk of long-term normal tissue toxicity and improving the odds of long-term tumor control.

Stereotactic body RT (SBRT) refers to the delivery of large and potent doses of radiation in a small number of fractions (usually less than 10), with high accuracy and precision to extracranial tumor sites (Chang & Timmerman, 2007). SBRT involves the use of highly ablative doses with sharp dose gradients around the target and has been used mostly in smaller target volumes (less than 6 cm), but larger tumors have also been treated with SBRT (Lee, Kim, et al., 2009).

An important potential toxicity to consider from liver toxicity is radiation-induced liver disease (RILD) that is pathologically characterized by marked congestion of the sinusoids in the central aspect of the liver lobule and hepatocyte atrophy in areas next to the congested veins (Lawrence et al., 1995). In modern clinical studies of focal liver RT, the RILD risk is low as a result of awareness of the partial liver tolerance to RT and the availability of advanced RT planning and delivery technologies. Other hepatic toxicities such as reactivation of hepatitis B can occur during liver RT, but in the setting of liver metastases without cirrhosis or viral hepatitis these are rare (Lee, Zia, Oluwadamilola, Michie, & White, 2009). Lee, Zia, et al. (2009) noted occasional toxicity after SBRT with grade 3 or higher elevated gamma glutamyl transferase enzymes, asthenia, thrombocytopenia (more common after previous extensive chemotherapy), and elevated liver enzymes. Transient skin erythema and intermittent chest wall pain may occur after high-dose SBRT (Rusthoven et al., 2009).

Nursing Diagnosis: Implications for Oncology Practice

Ascites-Related Respiratory Dysfunction

Patients with ascites may experience impaired gas exchange when fluid accumulation results in diaphragmatic displacement. Clinicians should observe for signs and symptoms of respiratory difficulty, including dyspnea, tachypnea, signs of hypoxia, changes in mental status, or skin color change.

Nurses should encourage positioning for comfort and enhanced chest expansion with elevation of the head of the bed and facilitate the use of oxygen therapy as needed. Medications that may be helpful include morphine sulfate, bronchodilators, corticosteroids, anxiolytics, diuretics, and anticholinergics. Diuretics (loop and aldosterone inhibiting) may be prescribed, but their effectiveness in the malignant ascites setting is less efficacious in comparison to other causes of ascites (Murphy, 2009).

Increased Fall Risk

Patients with ascites may experience weakness and therefore may become at increased risk for falls. Patient positioning and safe mobilization are important considerations. Fluid accumulation from ascites is often very heavy and causes abdominal distention that is very uncomfortable. It can also throw off the patients' center of balance and potentially shift it suddenly with movement, increasing the risk of falls. The cognitive function issues associated with hepatic encephalopathy can be associated with negative physiologic consequences, such as falls, personality changes, intellectual impairment, and a depressed level of consciousness. Sedation and confusion caused by opiates or other narcotics can also potentiate falls.

Anxiety

Patients may experience anxiety related to respiratory compromise, physical deterioration, becoming aware of a poor prognosis, and reaching end-stage disease. Comprehensive assessment is necessary to determine the cause of the anxiety and to then construct an appropriate plan of care and intervention. There are two types of intervention: nonpharmacologic and pharmacologic. Medications that can alleviate anxiety include benzodiazepines and antidepressants. Education, problem-focused cognitive-behavioral psychotherapy, and support services can help to reduce emotional and physical distress for both patients and their caregivers (Shell & Kirsch, 2001).

Increased Infection Risk

Patients with ascites need special care to prevent infections related to procedures, such as repeated paracentesis catheter insertion, which may cause leakage of ascetic fluid at the insertion site. These patients may require periodic paracentesis where the fluid is drained by aseptically puncturing the abdominal wall with a needle attached to a closed collection system. Because paracentesis involves penetration of the skin and abdominal wall, it presents a risk of peritonitis. Aseptic technique should be maintained both during the procedure and with dressing changes after the procedure. The procedure is typically performed with ultrasound guidance. If the patient requires repeated paracentesis procedures, fluid volume de-

pletion and protein loss can occur (Winkelman, 2004). After the procedure, the puncture site should be dressed with gauze and pressure dressing tape. Sometimes fluid may continue to ooze or drip from the puncture site and an ostomy collection bag may be appropriate for placement around the puncture site. Indwelling intraperitoneal catheters can be used for refractory malignant ascites management. Retrospective studies have shown that these catheters are a safe and effective palliative strategy (Fleming, Alvarez-Secord, Von Gruenigen, Miller, & Abernathy, 2009).

Pain Management

Patients may require frequent alterations in their pain management regimen because of hepatic tumor growth, procedures, or surgery. Hepatic metastases can occasionally enlarge and cause pain from liver capsule distention. Comprehensive pain assessments should be conducted frequently. Beneficial interventions include analgesics, regional nerve block, and whole liver radiation for symptom relief (Rubatt, Boardman, Segreti, & Wheelock, 2010). Nurses can educate patients and their caregivers about the risks of acetaminophen use in patients with liver disease. Frequent evaluation of the effectiveness of the pain management plan should be performed.

Pruritus and Impaired Skin Integrity

Patients with hepatic dysfunction may experience endogenous pruritus that may result in impaired skin integrity. Treatment should be directed at symptom relief and eliminating causative factors when possible. Pruritus can also be medication induced, and opioids can be a causative agent. If possible, medications that are causing pruritus should be stopped. Antipruritic medications may be required. Encourage patients to keep their fingernails short and clean and to wear mittens if necessary to prevent infection and excoriations from scratching (Bain, 1998). Skin emollients, lotion with menthol, soft clothing, air humidification, and tepid baths can also provide relief (Murphy-Ende, 2009).

Inadequate Nutrition

Nurses should assess patients' nutritional status. Patients with hepatic metastases may be receiving chemotherapy or radiation, which can lead to nausea and vomiting. Antiemetics can help with these symptoms. Ascites can cause impaired gastric emptying secondary to pressure on the diaphragm. Proper patient positioning with patients on their right side with the head of the bed raised may help because the stomach empties toward the right. Medications that promote upper GI motility, such as metoclopramide, may also be ordered (Bain, 1998).

Small, frequent meals that are high in protein should be encouraged. Patients with ascites may require a low-sodium, high-protein, fluid-restricted diet. However, excessive protein in the diet of patients with hepatic encephalopathy may precipitate symptoms by increasing nitrogen load in the GI tract (Murphy-Ende, 2009). Frequent patient reassessment is important. For more information about nutritional considerations, please refer to Chapter 8.

Alteration in Bowel Function

The weight of the fluid can impair bowel motility and contribute to constipation, and it can also be difficult to assess bowel sounds. Aggressive bowel care is required, especially if the patient is taking opioids. Proper positioning with the patient on his or her right side with the head of the bed raised can help because the stomach empties toward the right. Medications that promote upper GI motility, such as metoclopramide, may also be ordered (Bain, 1998).

Mental Status Changes

Extensive metastases to the liver are an underlying cause for hepatic encephalopathy. In suspected cases, monitor serum ammonia levels, vital signs, and neurologic status. Medication can be used to control the rapid release and progression of neuroactive toxins. Mannitol, an osmotic diuretic that draws fluid out of the brain tissue, is the main pharmacologic treatment used in cases of hepatic encephalopathy. Other agents that may be ordered include dexamethasone, thiopental, indomethacin, acetylcysteine, and lactulose (Wright, Chattree, & Jalan, 2011).

Bleeding Risk

Patients who undergo diagnostic liver biopsy also require special care and monitoring. Aspirin should be discontinued a week prior to the procedure, and nonsteroidal anti-inflammatory drugs should be stopped three days prior. Fasting is optional and at the discretion of the clinician performing the test. Eating allows for gallbladder contraction, which reduces the risk of gallbladder puncture (Pinelo & Presa, 2009). On the day of biopsy, review recent laboratory diagnostics including a prothrombin time and complete blood count. It is important to obtain informed consent. Complications are rare but can occur. Vasovagal response and pain are the most common. Post-procedure bleeding can also occur, with intraperitoneal hemorrhage being the most serious event. It typically happens within the first few hours, although late hemorrhage can occur up to 24 hours after the biopsy (Zaman, Ingram, & Flora, 2009).

Advocacy, Education, and Support

Although there are no support services specifically for patients with hepatic metastases, advocacy can be found from site-specific groups such as the National Breast Cancer Coalition (www.stopbreastcancer.org) and the Colon Cancer Alliance (http://ccalliance.org). Support groups and educational services, such as those provided by the American Cancer Society (www.cancer.org), National Cancer Institute (www.cancer.gov), and CancerCare (www.cancercare.org), can also offer emotional and educational information for patients, families, and caregivers.

Future Trends

Much research activity in regard to the diagnosis and treatment of liver metastases is currently under way. As in other areas of cancer research, the goals of treatment development are to develop and continue to refine technologies and techniques that avoid toxicity and are less invasive (Timmerman et al., 2009). Further refinement of chemotherapy and biotherapy, both alone and in combination with surgical technique, should reduce the number of patients with hepatic metastases that are considered unresectable (Mayo & Pawlik, 2009).

Another area of research centers on redirecting the body's own immune response to attack metastases through the adapted use of tumor antigens (Timmerman et al., 2009). In addition, advances in molecular tumor marker technology are being expanded in an effort to improve targeted therapies (Mayo & Pawlik, 2009).

Hepatic perfusion and percutaneous hepatic perfusion selectively deliver high-dose therapeutic agents directly into the hepatic arterial system. These procedures limit systemic toxicity and are currently under clinical evaluation for patients with liver metastases from various solid organ cancers (Alexander & Butler, 2010).

Therasphere® (MDS Nordion, 2010), which is currently indicated for use in patients with unresectable hepatocellular carcinoma, is being actively tested in the metastatic setting. Therasphere is a technology that delivers radiation directly to the area of hepatic metastasis. This technique uses yttrium-90 microspheres that are delivered through a catheter directly into the hepatic artery. In a phase II trial conducted with colorectal hepatic metastases, this radioembolization therapy was found to produce sustained stable disease in some patients and will likely have a future role in combination with systemic chemotherapy (Mulcahy et al., 2009).

Summary

The liver provides a particularly hospitable secondary environment for metastasis from other cancers, most notably for patients with breast, colorectal, esophageal, lung, pancreatic, stomach, and adrenal cancers and melanoma. A number of factors influence the pattern of cancer spread, including portal venous flow and hematogenous spread, the primary site and histology of the cancer. Metastatic liver disease is often asymptomatic in its early stages. However, as disease progresses, symptoms can be debilitating and difficult to manage.

Imaging plays a key role in the staging of liver metastasis, but in general the appearance of these lesions tends to be nonspecific. Biopsy specimens are required for histologic diagnosis. CT using contrast enhancement remains the imaging modality of choice at this time for evaluating liver metastases.

Unfortunately, many tumors that metastasize to the liver, such as breast and lung cancers, will spread to other sites in the body as well. Treatment is dependent upon the primary cancer site, the number of lesions that are present in the liver, their size and location within the liver, and whether the cancer has spread to other organs. The patient's general health and comorbidities also influence factors in treatment decision making.

When cancer has spread to other organs in the body, systemic chemotherapy is generally recommended. However, if the metastasis is isolated to the liver in one or a few areas, it may be amenable to surgical intervention. In select patients, the use of hepatic arterial infusion, cryoablation, radiofrequency ablation, embolization, or percutaneous ethanol injection may provide palliative benefit. The goals of treatment for hepatic metastasis are to delay progression of disease, prolong life, relieve cancer-related symptoms, and improve quality of life.

A diagnosis of metastatic cancer is devastating. It can leave patients feeling afraid and isolated. In addition to medical treatment, nursing assessment and intervention that address symptom management, spiritual, emotional, and social guidance are of vital importance. This care is beneficial to both patients and their caregivers. Fortunately, a number of national and regional cancer and disease-specific organizations and programs are dedicated to helping patients who are living with metastatic disease. These groups can help individuals cope with their cancer diagnosis as well as assist in the navigation of specific challenges via peer support, education, and counseling, both online and in person.

References

Adam, A. (2002). Interventional radiology in the treatment of hepatic metastases. *Cancer Treatment Reviews, 28,* 93–99. doi:10.1053/ctrv.2002.9258

Alberts, S.R., & Wagman, L.D. (2008). Chemotherapy for colorectal cancer liver metastases. *Oncologist, 13,* 1063–1073. doi:10.1634/theoncologist.2008-0142

Alexander, H.R., Jr. (2002). Surgical approaches to liver metastases. *Cancer Journal, 8*(Suppl. 1), s68–s81.

Alexander, H.R., Jr., & Butler, C. (2010). Development of isolated hepatic perfusion via the operative and percutaneous techniques for patients with isolated and unresectable liver metastases. *Cancer Journal, 16,* 132–141. doi:10.1097/PPO.0b013e3181db9c0a

Bain, V. (1998). Jaundice, ascites and hepatic encephalopathy. In D. Doyle, G. Hanks, & N. Macdonald (Eds.), *Oxford textbook of palliative medicine* (pp. 573–583). New York, NY: Oxford University Press.

Bartlett, D.L. (2000). Treatment of patients with hepatic metastases. *Cancer Journal, 6*(Suppl. 2), s169–s176.

Bravo, A., Sheth, S., & Chopra, S. (2009, August 13). Percutaneous liver biopsy. Retrieved from http://www.uptodate.com

Chang, B.K., & Timmerman, R.D. (2007). Stereotactic body radiation therapy: A comprehensive review. *American Journal of Clinical Oncology, 30,* 637–644. doi:10.1097/COC.0b013e3180ca7cb1

Chhieng, D. (2004). Fine needle aspiration biopsy of liver—An update. *World Journal of Surgical Oncology, 2,* 5. doi:10.1186/1477-7819-2-5

Choi, J. (2006). Imaging of hepatic metastases. *Cancer Control, 13,* 6–12. doi:10.1097/PPO.0b013e3181d823c8

Clark, J., & Grothey, A. (2012). Systemic chemotherapy for metastatic colorectal cancer: Completed clinical trials [UpToDate, current as of June 2012]. Retrieved from http://www.uptodate.com/contents/systemic-chemotherapy-for-metastatic-colorectal-cancer-completed-clinical-trials

DeMatteo, R., Shah, A., Fong, Y., Jarnagin, W., Blumgart, L.H., & Brennan, M.F. (2001). Results of hepatic resection for sarcoma metastatic to liver. *Annals of Surgery, 234,* 540–548. doi:10.1097/00000658-200110000-00013

Di Meglio, G., Massacesi, C., Radice, D., Boselli, S., Pelosi, G., Squadroni, M., … Fazio, N. (2010). Carboplatin with etoposide in patients with extrapulmonary "aggressive" neuroendocrine carcinoma. *Journal of Clinical Oncology, 28*(Suppl.), Abstract e13072.

Fendrich, V., Michl, P., Habbe, N., & Bartsch, D.K. (2010). Liver-specific therapies for metastases of neuroendocrine pancreatic tumors. *World Journal of Hepatology, 2,* 367–373. doi:10.4254/wjh.v2.i10.367

Fleming, N., Alvarez-Secord, A., Von Gruenigen, V., Miller, M.J., & Abernathy, A. (2010). Indwelling catheters for the management of refractory malignant ascites: A systematic literature overview and retrospective chart review. *Journal of Pain and Symptom Management, 38,* 341–349. doi:10.1016/j.jpainsymman.2008.09.008

Gupta, S., Bedikian, A.Y., Ahrar, J., Ensor, J., Ahrar, K., Madoff, D.C., … Hwu, P. (2010). Hepatic artery chemoembolization in patients with ocular melanoma metastatic to the liver: Response, survival, and prognostic factors. *American Journal of Clinical Oncology, 33,* 474–480. doi:10.1097/COC.0b013e3181b4b065

Halfdanarson, T.R., Kendrick, M.L., & Grothey, A. (2010). The role of chemotherapy in managing patients with resectable liver metastases. *Cancer Journal, 16,* 125–131. doi:10.1097/PPO.0b013e3181d823c8

Kamat, P.P., Gupta, S., Ensor, J.E., Murthy, R., Ahrar, K., Madoff, D.C., … Hicks, M.E. (2008). Hepatic arterial embolization and chemoembolization in the management of patients with large volume liver metastases. *Cardiovascular and Interventional Radiology, 31,* 299–307. doi:10.1007/s00270-007-9186-3

Kath, R., Hayungs, J., Bornfeld, N., Sauerwein, W., Hoftkein, K., & Seeber, S. (1993). Prognosis and treatment of disseminated uveal melanoma. *Cancer, 72,* 2219–2223. doi:10.1002/1097-0142(19931001)72:7<2219::AID-CNCR2820720725>3.0.CO;2-J

Kemeny, N., & D'Angelica, M. (2010). Treatment of liver metastasis. In W. Hong, R. Bast, W. Hait, D. Kufe, R. Pollock, R. Weichselbaum, … E. Frei (Eds.), *Holland-Frei cancer medicine* (8th ed., pp. 1109–1123). Shelton, CT: American Association for Cancer Research.

Kemeny, N., Kemeny, M., & Dawson, L. (2008). Liver metastases. In M. Abeloff, J. Armitage, J. Niederhuber, M. Kastan, & W. McKenna (Eds.), *Clinical oncology* (4th ed., pp. 885–923). Philadelphia, PA: Elsevier Churchill Livingstone.

Kemeny, N., Kemeny, M., & Lawrence, T. (2004). Liver metastases. In M. Abeloff, J. Armitage, J. Niederhuber, M. Kastan, & W. McKenna (Eds.), *Clinical oncology* (3rd ed., pp. 1141–1176). Philadelphia, PA: Elsevier Churchill Livingstone.

Khan, A.N., & Pankhania, A. (2011, August). Liver metastases imaging. Retrieved from http://emedicine.medscape.com/article/369936-overview#showall

Kouvaraki, M.A., Ajani, J.A., Hoff, P., Wolff, R., Evans, D.B., Lozano, R., & Yao, J.C. (2004). Fluorouracil, doxorubicin, and streptozocin in the treatment of patients with locally advanced and metastatic pancreatic endocrine carcinomas. *Journal of Clinical Oncology, 23,* 4762–4771. doi:10.1200/JCO.2004.04.024

Kress, O., Wagner, H.J., Wied, M., Klose, K.J., Arnold, R., & Alfke, H. (2003). Transarterial chemoembolization of neuroendocrine tumors—A retrospective single center analysis. *Digestion, 68,* 94–101. doi:10.1159/000074522

Lawrence, T.S., Robertson, J.M., Anscher, M.S., Jirtle, R.L., Ensminger, W.D., & Fajardo, L.F. (1995). Hepatic toxicity resulting from cancer treatment. *International Journal of Radiation Oncology, Biology, Physics, 31,* 1237–1248.

Lee, M.T., Kim, J.J., Dinniwell, R., Brierley, J., Lockwood, G., Wong, R., … Dawson, L.A. (2009). Phase I study of individualized stereotactic body radiotherapy of liver metastases. *Journal of Clinical Oncology, 27,* 1585–1591. doi:10.1200/JCO.2008.20.0600

Lee, C.L., Zia, F., Oluwadamilola, O., Michie, J., & White, J.D. (2009). Survey of complementary and alternative medicine practitioners regarding cancer management and research. *Journal of the Society for Integrative Oncology, 7,* 26–54.

Lencioni, R., Della Pina, C., Crocetti, L., Bozzi, E., & Cioni, D. (2007). Clinical management of focal liver lesions: The key role of real-time contrast-enhanced US. *European Radiology Supplements, 17*(Suppl. 6), 73–79. doi:10.1007/s10406-007-0231-8

Lewis, A.M., & Martin, R.C. (2006). The treatment of hepatic metastases in colorectal carcinoma. *American Surgeon, 72,* 466–473.

Lim, E., Thomson, B.N., Heinze, S., Chao, M., Gunawardana, D., & Gibbs, P. (2007). Optimizing the approach to patients with potentially resectable liver metastases from colorectal cancer. *ANZ Journal of Surgery, 77,* 941–947. doi:10.1111/j.1445-2197.2007.04287.x

Liu, P., & Francis, I. (2010). Hepatic imaging for metastatic disease. *Cancer Journal, 16,* 93–102. doi:10.1097/PPO.0b013e3181d7ea21

MDS Nordion. (2010). Therasphere: An innovative treatment for liver cancer. Retrieved from http://www.mdsnordion.com

Mayo, S., & Pawlik, T. (2009). Current management of colorectal hepatic metastasis. *Expert Reviews in Gastroenterology and Hepatology, 3,* 131–144. doi:10.1586/egh.09.8

Mulcahy, M., Lewandowski, R.J., Ibrahim, S., Sato, K.T., Ryu, R.K., Atassi, B., … Salem, R. (2009). Radioembolization of colorectal hepatic metastases using yttrium-90 microspheres. *Cancer, 115,* 1849–1858. doi:10.1002/cncr.24224

Murphy, D. (2009). Malignant ascites. In C. Chernecky & K. Murphy-Ende (Eds.), *Acute care oncology nursing* (2nd ed., pp. 26–34). Madison, WI: Elsevier Saunders.

Murphy-Ende, K. (2009). Malignant ascites. In C. Chernecky & K. Murphy-Ende (Eds.), *Acute care oncology nursing* (2nd ed., pp. 274–283). Madison, WI: Elsevier Saunders.

Patel, K., Sullivan, K., Berd, D., Mastrangelo, M.J., Shields, C., Shields, J., & Sato, T. (2005). Chemoembolization of the hepatic artery with BCNU for metastatic uveal melanoma: Results of a phase II study [Abstract]. *Melanoma Research, 12,* 297–304. doi:10.1097/00008390-200508000-00011

Paulson, E.K. (2001). Evaluation of the liver for metastatic disease. *Seminars in Liver Disease, 21,* 225–236. doi:10.1055/s-2001-15498

Pinelo, E., & Presa, J. (2009). Outpatient percutaneous liver biopsy: Still a good option. *European Journal of Internal Medicine, 20,* 487–489. doi:10.1016/j.ejim.2009.02.002

Pocard, M., Pouillart, P., Asselain, B., & Salmon, R. (2000). Hepatic resection in metastatic breast cancer: Results and prognostic factors. *European Journal of Surgical Oncology, 26,* 155–159. doi:10.1053/ejso.1999.0761

Rahil, S., & Field, J. (2012, January 4). Ascites. Retrieved from http://emedicine.medscape.com/article/170907

Rivoire, M., Kodjikian, L., Baldo, S., Kaemmerlen, P., Négrier, S., & Grange, J. (2005). Treatment of liver metastases from uveal melanoma. *Annals of Surgical Oncology, 12,* 422–428. doi:10.1245/ASO.2005.06.032

Rubatt, J.M., Boardman, C.H., Segreti, E.M., & Wheelock, J. (2011, March 29). Palliative care of the patient with advanced gynecologic cancer. Retrieved http://emedicine.medscape.com/article/270646-overview

Runyon, B. (2010). Malignancy-related ascites [UpToDate, current as of June 2012]. Retrieved from http://www.uptodate.com/contents/malignancy-related-ascites

Rusthoven, K.E., Kavanagh, B.D., Burri, S.H., Chen, C., Cardenes, H., Chidel, M.A., … Shefter, T.E. (2009). Multi-institutional phase I/II trial of stereotactic body radiation therapy for liver metastases. *Journal of Clinical Oncology, 27,* 1572–1578. doi:10.1200/JCO.2008.19.6329

Schwartz, J., & Kruskal, J. (2009, September 30). Approach to the patient with a focal liver lesion. Retrieved from http://www.uptodate.com

Siegel, R., Naishadham, D., & Jemal, A. (2012). Cancer statistics 2012. *CA: A Cancer Journal for Clinicians, 62,* 10–29. doi:10.3322/caac.20138

Shell, J., & Kirsch, S. (2001). Psychosocial issues, outcomes, and quality of life. In S.E. Otto (Ed.), *Oncology nursing* (4th ed., pp. 948–972). St. Louis, MO: Elsevier Mosby.

Stratmann, S. (2002). Hepatic artery chemotherapy in the management of colorectal metastases. *Baylor Medical Center Proceedings, 15,* 376–379. Retrieved from http://www.ncbi.nlm.nih.gov/pmc/articles/PMC1276641/pdf/bumc0015-0376.pdf

Swaminath, A., & Dawson, L.A. (2010). Emerging role of radiotherapy in the management of liver metastases. *Cancer Journal, 16,* 150–155. doi:10.1097/PPO.0b013e3181d7e8b3

Timmerman, R.D., Bizekis, C.S., Pass, H.I., Fong, Y., Dupuy, D., Dawson, L.A., … La, D. (2009). Local surgical, ablative, and radiation treatment of metastases. *CA: A Cancer Journal for Clinicians,* 145–170. doi:10.3322/caac.20013

Venook, AP. (2012). Nonsurgical local treatment strategies for colorectal cancer liver metastases [UpToDate, current as of June 2012]. Retrieved from http://www.uptodate.com/contents/nonsurgical-local-treatment-strategies-for-colorectal-cancer-liver-metastases?source=search_result&search=Venook%2C+AP.+%282012%29.+Nonsurgical+local+treatment+strategies+for+colorectal+cancer+liver+metastases.&selectedTitle=1%7E150

Vogl, T., Gruber, T., Naguib, N., & Nour-Eldin, N. (2009). Liver metastases of neuroendocrine tumors: Treatment with hepatic transarterial chemotherapy using two therapeutic protocols. *American Journal of Roentgenology, 193,* 941–947. doi:10.2214/AJR.08.1879

Winkelman, L. (2004). Malignant ascites. In C.H. Yarbro, M.H. Frogge, & M. Goodman (Eds.), *Cancer symptom management* (3rd ed., pp. 401–419). Burlington, MA: Jones and Bartlett.

Wright, G., Chattree, A., & Jalan, R. (2011). Management of hepatic encephalopathy. *International Journal of Hepatology, 2011,* Article 841407. doi:10.4061/2011/841407

Zaman, A., Ingram, K., & Flora, K. (2009, November 18). Diagnostic liver biopsy. Retrieved from http://emedicine.medscape.com

CHAPTER 7

Quality of Life and Symptom Management

Virginia Sun, RN, PhD, and Betty Ferrell, PhD, FAAN, MA, FPCN, CHPN

Introduction

Quality-of-life (QOL) assessment and optimal symptom management are important aspects of quality cancer care for patients with pancreatic and hepatobiliary cancers. These patients often suffer from multiple symptoms and existential concerns that negatively affect QOL, particularly in an advanced disease setting. The primary goals of palliative care include the alleviation of symptom distress and the enhancement of overall QOL. To achieve these goals of care, it is important to assess QOL and identify factors that contribute to diminished QOL. This chapter will discuss QOL and symptom management issues for patients with pancreatic and hepatobiliary cancers.

Quality of Life

QOL is defined as a multidimensional construct, and measurement of QOL involves assessing overall QOL and QOL domains (physical, psychological, social, and spiritual), as well as individual QOL items. This definition includes a focus on illness and is limited to the subjective assessment of the impact of disease and its treatment across the dimensions of functioning and well-being.

Research by Grant, Padilla, and Ferrell over the past 20 years has also emphasized the need for a multidimensional definition for QOL, including an existential dimension (Ferrell, Dow, Leigh, Ly, & Gulasekaram, 1995). These investigators defined QOL as consisting of four dimensions or domains: (a) physical well-being, (b) psychological well-being, (c) social well-being, and (d) spiritual well-being. Figure 7-1 presents a QOL model for patients with advanced cancer. Each dimension consists of generic items of concern to all cancer populations and may also include items specific to a type of cancer or treatment. Physical well-being issues are focused on common disease- or treatment-related symptoms such as pain, fatigue, and sleep disturbance. Psycho-

logical well-being issues include anxiety, depression, fear of recurrence, and coping. Social well-being domain issues include family distress, financial burden, sexual function, and employment. Finally, spiritual well-being concerns include hope, finding meaning, and religiosity (Hills, Paice, Cameron, & Shott, 2005). The model has been validated across studies in a number of cancer patient populations (Ferrell, 1995; Ferrell, Dow, & Grant, 1995; Ferrell, Dow, Leigh, et al., 1995; Ferrell, Grant, Funk, Otis-Green, & Garcia, 1998a, 1998b). The City of Hope Quality-of-Life Model acknowledges that QOL is subjective, based on the patient's self-report, which is always changing and dynamic and a multidimensional concept (Ferrell, Dow, Leigh, et al., 1995).

Quality of Life at the End of Life

A growing body of literature describes QOL issues at the end of life (EOL) for patients with cancer, including those with pancreatic and hepatobiliary cancers. Aspects of QOL that are important at the EOL include multiple symptoms (e.g., pain, dyspnea), anxiety, fear, meaning of the illness, spirituality, and relationships. In a systematic review of palliative cancer care literature, Jocham, Dassen, Widdershoven, and Halfens (2006) found that nurses, especially those in oncology and palliative care, have actively contributed to the development of the concept of overall QOL through instrument development and research. Hwang, Chang, Fairclough, Cogswell, and Kasimis (2003) documented QOL, symptom distress, and Karnofsky Performance Scale (KPS) over time in 67 patients with advanced cancer for purposes of defining a longitudinal model of QOL at the EOL. Results suggest that patterns of change in QOL as measured by the Functional Assessment of Cancer Therapy–General (FACT-G) scale up to six months before death were detected and revealed that different domains of symptom distress, functional status, and QOL change at different rates and at different selected time points (Hwang et al., 2003). The FACT-G is a cancer-specific QOL measure that contains a 27-item compilation of gen-

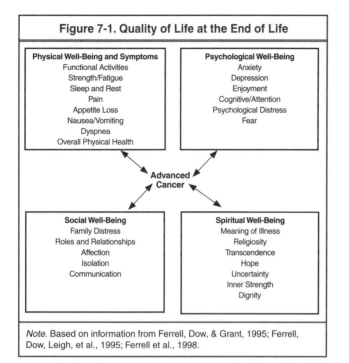

Figure 7-1. Quality of Life at the End of Life

Physical Well-Being and Symptoms
Functional Activities
Strength/Fatigue
Sleep and Rest
Pain
Appetite Loss
Nausea/Vomiting
Dyspnea
Overall Physical Health

Psychological Well-Being
Anxiety
Depression
Enjoyment
Cognitive/Attention
Psychological Distress
Fear

Advanced
Cancer

Social Well-Being
Family Distress
Roles and Relationships
Affection
Isolation
Communication

Spiritual Well-Being
Meaning of Illness
Religiosity
Transcendence
Hope
Uncertainty
Inner Strength
Dignity

Note. Based on information from Ferrell, Dow, & Grant, 1995; Ferrell, Dow, Leigh, et al., 1995; Ferrell et al., 1998.

eral questions divided into four QOL domains: physical, social/family, emotional, and functional well-being. A statistically significant decline in QOL, symptom distress, and functioning began two to three months before death, and these declines were often associated with clinical changes and hospitalizations (Hwang et al., 2003). Based on these observations, Hwang and colleagues (2003) proposed the Longitudinal Terminal Decline QOL Model. In the model, slow and steady changes in symptom distress, functional status, and QOL dimensions can occur six months prior to death. At three months before death, worsening symptom distress initiates changes in psychological well-being. Following increase in symptom distress, worsening KPS and QOL occur at two months prior to death. Finally, one month prior to death, dramatic increases in psychological distress and decreases in functional status occur (Hwang et al., 2003). This dramatic decrease in QOL has been observed in other studies and is referred to as the *terminal drop* (Diehr et al., 2007). Monitoring QOL changes at the EOL, particularly for patients with pancreatic and hepatobiliary cancers, can provide the clinician with valuable information on what symptoms are distressing and need to be addressed, physical support the patient needs in order to monitor safety as functional status decreases, and a focus on psychological/spiritual support as the distress associated with EOL increases.

Few studies in the literature have reported the impact of disease on overall QOL in patients with pancreatic and hepatobiliary cancers. Perception of QOL in these patients was found to be mediated not by symptom burden but rather by coping processes. Patients' perceived threat of symptoms and effectiveness of chosen coping strategies were important to

perceived QOL (Fitzsimmons, George, Payne, & Johnson, 1999). Global QOL and family functioning were significantly associated with survival in a cohort of patients with pancreatic cancer, even after controlling for stage at diagnosis (Lis, Gupta, & Grutsch, 2006). In pancreatic cancer, onset of symptoms at diagnosis such as jaundice was associated with better prognosis, whereas prognosis was significantly worse for patients presenting with back pain (Watanabe et al., 2004).

Symptoms in Pancreatic and Hepatobiliary Cancers

Physical Concerns

Patients with pancreatic cancers experience a significant number of symptoms as a direct or indirect result of disease, treatment, and comorbidities (see Figure 7-2). The symptoms that patients with cancer experience are often complex, multifactorial, and challenging to manage. Treatment modalities may lead to post-treatment morbidity and symptom burden, with modest or no improvements in survival (Fazal & Saif, 2007). Fatigue, loss of appetite, and impaired sense of overall well-being have been reported in pancreatic cancer (Labori, Hjermstad, Wester, Buanes, & Loge, 2006). Reyes-Gibby and colleagues (2007) explored symptom prevalence and interference with function in patients with locally advanced pancreatic cancer receiving chemoradiation. Findings suggested that 95% of patients reported at least one symptom. The most common moderate- to severe-intensity symptoms at presentation included lack of appetite, pain, fatigue, and sleep disturbance (Reyes-Gibby et al., 2007). Severe fatigue, nausea, and sleep disturbance increased during chemoradiation (Reyes-Gibby et al., 2007).

In advanced pancreatic and hepatobiliary cancers, it is common for multiple symptoms to occur simultaneously. Patients experiencing pain may also experience fatigue, depression, and anorexia, each with prevalence rates reported to be greater

Figure 7-2. Commons Symptoms of Pancreatic Cancer

- Abdominal pain
- Anorexia-cachexia
- Depression
- Dyspepsia
- Early satiety
- Fatigue
- Jaundice
- Nausea
- Sleep disturbance
- Steatorrhea

Note. Based on information from Krech & Walsh, 1991; Labori et al., 2006; Reyes-Gibby et al., 2007; Watanabe et al., 2004.

than 50% (Chang, Hwang, & Kasimis, 2002; Grosvenor, Bulcavage, & Cheblowski, 1989; McCorkle & Quint-Benoliel, 1983; Portenoy et al., 1994). Impaired physical functioning and diminishing daily activities as a result of multiple symptoms are additional concerns for patients. Evidence suggests that some symptoms, such as knee pain, have a particularly high prevalence. Kelsen and colleagues (1995) reported that patients with pancreatic cancer having moderate to severe pain had significantly impaired functional activity compared to patients with mild or no pain. Furthermore, a significant correlation between increased pain and depression were found, and this correlation resulted in impaired QOL and function (Kelsen, Portenoy, Thaler, Tao, & Brennan, 1997).

Pain-related distress has been reported to be the most substantial factor in the interference of patients' ability to perform daily activities (Wells, Murphy, Wujcik, & Johnson, 2003). Other physical symptoms that are found to cluster with pain include fatigue, nausea, insomnia, weight loss, immobility, and constipation (Chen & Tseng, 2006; Gift, Stommel, Jablonski, & Given, 2003; Walsh & Rybicki, 2006). Involuntary weight loss is common among patients with pancreatic cancer. Krech and Walsh (1991) found that gastrointestinal symptoms, such as anorexia (64%), early satiety (62%), and weight loss (51%), are common among patients with unresectable pancreatic cancer. Davidson, Ash, Capra, and Bauer (2004) explored whether stabilizing weight loss for patients with unresectable pancreatic cancer was associated with improved survival and QOL. Findings suggested that weight stabilization in unresectable pancreatic cancer was associated with improved survival duration and QOL. Survival was longer in patients who experienced weight stabilization compared to those who continued to lose weight with a difference in median survival of three months. Independent determinants of weight stabilization include the absence of nausea and vomiting at baseline and female gender (Davidson et al., 2004).

Figure 7-3 provides a detailed list of the common symptoms in hepatobiliary cancers. Patients may present with a variety of symptoms related to decompensated cirrhosis. These include ascites, variceal bleeding, peripheral edema, and hepatic encephalopathy (Lin et al., 2004). In a cohort of patients with hepatocellular carcinoma (HCC) in Taiwan, the most common symptom was abdominal pain (75.5%), which originated from enlarged tumor mass and was characterized as dull visceral pain (Lin et al., 2004). Other common complaints include fatigue or weakness, peripheral edema, cachexia, ascites, dyspnea, anorexia, and vomiting (Lin et al., 2004).

Pain is one of the most common and distressing symptoms for patients with hepatobiliary cancers. This is due primarily to visceral involvement that originates from a primary or metastatic lesion involving the abdominal or pelvic viscera (Mercadante, 2002). Treatment-related pain is also common. For example, 80%–90% of patients treated with transarterial chemoembolization (TACE) experience a postembolization syndrome. This syndrome often includes abdominal pain, ileus,

---

Figure 7-3. Common Symptoms of Hepatobiliary Cancers

- Ascites
- Asthenia
- Hepatic bruits
- Jaundice
- Nausea and vomiting
- Palpable liver mass
- Peripheral edema
- Pruritus
- Right upper quadrant pain
- Weight loss

Note. Based on information from Di Bisceglie, 2002; Watanabe et al., 2004.

---

fever, nausea, and vomiting, which can last from hours to days (Ramsey, Kernagis, Soulen, & Geschwind, 2002). Pain can occur during and after TACE, and patients who did not experience distressing levels of pain during the procedure are also vulnerable to post-procedural pain (Lee, Hahn, & Park, 2001).

Fatigue is part of the postembolization syndrome associated with TACE for patients with HCC. Patients usually experience mild to moderate levels of fatigue that peaks on the second day after TACE (Shun et al., 2005). Although fatigue gradually decreases two days post-treatment, level of fatigue is higher than pretreatment six days post-treatment (Shun et al., 2005). The incidence of weight loss is greater than 54% in most patients with hepatobiliary cancers, and incidence reaches 80% in the terminal stage (Strasser & Bruera, 2002). Cachexia can be separated into primary (metabolic) and secondary (starvation) cachexia (Strasser & Bruera, 2002). Anorexia is a symptom related to weight loss and a leading symptom of the primary metabolic cachexia syndrome. A common term for cancer wasting syndrome is *anorexia-cachexia syndrome* (Strasser & Bruera, 2002). The diagnosis of anorexia-cachexia syndrome is based on simple assessment of weight loss and anorexia, but currently no established tools or guidelines are available to distinguish primary and secondary cachexia. Other parameters, such as hypoalbuminemia, asthenia, chronic nausea, reduced caloric intake, or clinical judgment of reduced muscle and fat mass, can serve as additional criteria for assessment of the presence of cachexia (Strasser & Bruera, 2002). These criteria can be helpful in patients with relevant fluid retention (ascites, edema) where the extent of weight loss is masked by the accumulation of excess fluid (Strasser, 2000).

Jaundice is present in 19%–40% of patients at the time of HCC diagnosis and usually also occurs in later cancer stages (Qin & Tang, 2003). Obstructive jaundice occurs secondary to diffuse tumor invasion of the liver parenchyma or progressive liver failure. Intraductal tumor growth may occur in the common hepatic duct or common bile duct, causing obstructive jaundice (Qin & Tang, 2003). Ascites is a result of an imbalance in the normal state of influx and efflux of fluid from the peritoneal cavity. This decreased rate of efflux may occur as a result of lymphatic blockage from tumor invasion (Keen & Fallon, 2002). Symptoms related to ascites include increased intra-abdominal pressure, abdominal wall discomfort, dyspnea, anorexia, early satiety, nausea and vomiting, esophageal reflux, pain, and peripheral edema (Keen & Fallon, 2002).

Psychological Concerns

A cancer diagnosis is devastating for the person who hears those words "It's cancer" but often even more so when the specific cancer diagnosis carries a poor prognosis or is at late stage. Pancreatic and hepatobiliary cancers may also be associated with greater psychological distress because they are less common, and patients may feel isolated with fewer available resources (Brintzenhofe-Szoc, Levin, Li, Kissane, & Zabora, 2009; Zabora, Brintzenhofe-Szoc, Curbow, Hooker, & Piantadosi, 2001).

Literature regarding the psychological needs of patients with pancreatic and hepatobiliary cancers reinforces the common responses of anxiety, depression, and fear (Carney, Jones, Woolson, Noyes, & Doebbeling, 2003; Coleman et al., 2005; Fazal & Saif, 2007; Fitzsimmons & Johnson, 1998; Holland et al., 1986; Joffe & Adsett, 1985; Krishnan et al., 2006). With the wide access to information on the Internet, patients and families are often immediately confronted with survival statistics of these cancers, and at the time of diagnosis they may also be confronting the likelihood of death in the months ahead. With limited treatment options available, patients' emotional responses may be further challenged as they face difficult decisions about participation in clinical trials, treatment options that may impose extensive toxicities, and transition to hospice.

Careful assessment of psychological responses is essential for nurses. Patients may have a preexisting psychological diagnosis such as chronic depression or other life stresses (e.g., financial concerns, other concurrent illness, loss of employment) that are adding to the emotional response to the cancer diagnosis (National Comprehensive Cancer Network [NCCN], 2012). Use of the NCCN Distress Thermometer is widely recommended as an efficient clinical assessment tool. Additionally, an excellent resource for the assessment and management of distress is the *NCCN Clinical Practice Guidelines in Oncology: Distress Management*, which is updated frequently and available at www.nccn.org after free registration with the Web site.

Social Concerns

The social realm of QOL encompasses the person in relationship with others. A diagnosis of pancreatic or hepatobiliary cancer affects the patients' family, friends, and communi-

ty. Family members may become overwhelmed by the impact of the initial diagnosis, difficult treatment choices, and assisting the patient with recognition of the often poor prognosis of this diagnosis. Family members are challenged to maintain hope and support for the patient while also facing their own anticipatory grief (Coleman et al., 2005). Families may face financial burdens because of patients' immediate loss of ability to work and the anticipated costs of care and potential death. Patients who are diagnosed at an earlier stage may still experience a sense of uncertainty and fear of recurrence (Coleman et al., 2005).

Spiritual Concerns

Patients facing cancer may experience many spiritual concerns as they cope with life-threatening disease. Regardless of the ultimate outcome, patients face existential concerns as they question the meaning of illness, and often their religious beliefs are tested. Patients and families also seek to renew their lives and relationships as they search for a purpose in this altered life.

In 2009, a national consensus conference was conducted that included experts from the fields of palliative care and spiritual care to provide recommendations for improving the quality of spiritual care in palliative care (Puchalski et al., 2009). One outcome of that conference was the development of a consensus definition of spirituality that portrays the wide spectrum of spirituality and opportunities for care:

> *Spirituality* is the aspect of humanity that refers to the way individuals seek and express meaning and purpose and the way they experience their connectedness to the moment, to self, to others, to nature, and to the significant or sacred. (Puchalski et al., 2009, p. 887)

Case Example

Mr. Yuen Chang was a 58-year-old man employed as a high school math teacher. His wife of 20 years died of breast cancer five years ago, and Mr. Chang recently married Jennie, a teacher from the high school where he works. Mr. Chang was in excellent health but then developed weight loss, nausea, and then jaundice, which led to his diagnosis of liver cancer.

At the time of diagnosis, Mr. Chang and his wife opted for aggressive treatment, including surgery and chemotherapy. Although both were aware of his poor prognosis, they were adamant that they wanted as much time together as possible, especially because they were married for such a short time. Mr. Chang experienced numerous symptoms related to his disease and treatment, but the oncology clinic and palliative care service were successful in managing his nausea, pain, and depression. Jennie was directed to a support group for family caregivers. Mr. Chang was also seen by the oncology chaplain, who arranged for a visit from a

Buddhist priest based on his request to be reconnected with his faith community.

After completion of his chemotherapy, Mr. Chang's scans revealed that his tumor had not responded to the treatment, and new areas of metastasis were identified in the spine and lungs. Mr. and Mrs. Chang decided that he would forgo further treatment and admission to hospice was arranged.

Symptom Management in Pancreatic and Hepatobiliary Cancers

The treatment of pain begins with a comprehensive assessment of the clinical characteristic of visceral pain. For example, referred visceral pain in patients with hepatobiliary cancers is often found in the right shoulder (Mercadante, 2002). When pain is moderate or severe, opioid analgesics remain the gold standard. Several options for the delivery of opioids exist, such as oral, parenteral, transdermal, transmucosal/sublingual, rectal, and spinal. Indications for administration route must be based on the patient's ability to use the specific route, efficacy of the route in delivering adequate analgesia, ease of use for patient and family, associated complications, and cost (Mercadante, 2002). In the setting of visceral pain, nonsteroidal anti-inflammatory drugs (NSAIDs) have been found to produce a similar analgesic effect to those produced by opioids, although NSAIDs should be used with caution in patients with coagulopathies. They are particularly useful when pain is mild (Mercadante et al., 1999).

Fatigue management should begin with an in-depth assessment of the following contributing factors: pain, emotional distress, sleep disturbance, anemia, nutritional deficiencies, deconditioning, and comorbidities (Mock, 2004). Treating these factors as an initial approach may increase the tolerability of fatigue. Pharmacologic interventions are targeted toward the contributing factors associated with fatigue: erythropoietin for chemotherapy-induced anemia, antidepressants when depression is a cause of fatigue, and psychostimulants to increase energy level. Some evidence in the literature supports the use of methylphenidate in reducing fatigue in advanced cancer (Bruera et al., 2006). Considerable evidence in the current literature supports the efficacy of nonpharmacologic interventions, such as aerobic exercise, on fatigue reduction (Courneya et al., 2003; Dimeo, Stieglitz, Novelli-Fischer, Fetscher, & Keul, 1999; Mock, 2004; Schwartz, Mori, Gao, Nail, & King, 2001; Segal et al., 2003). Counseling on proper sleep hygiene and energy conservation tips are helpful self-care strategies that patients can use at home. A careful review of patients' medications may identify adverse effects that aggravate fatigue.

The management of anorexia-cachexia syndrome begins with a thorough assessment of potential contributors, such as chronic nausea, constipation, early satiety, taste alterations, and depression (Del Fabbro, Dalal, & Bruera, 2006). Phar-

macologically, at least 15 randomized controlled trials have demonstrated that megestrol acetate (doses ranging from 160 to 1,600 mg/day) significantly improves appetite when compared to placebo (Lopez et al., 2004). Artificial nutrition such as total parenteral nutrition is frequently used but has not been shown to increase lean body mass (Muscaritoli, Bossola, Aversa, Bellantone, & Fanelli, 2006). Individualized dietary counseling in recent randomized controlled trials in patients with cancer is effective in improving patients' food intake, nutritional status, and QOL (Ravasco, Monteiro-Grillo, Vidal, & Camilo, 2005).

The management of obstructive jaundice can be achieved using percutaneous drainage or the placement of a biliary stent. Cholestatic pruritus associated with obstructive jaundice can be managed using cholestyramine to decrease the enterohepatic circulation of bile acids (Jones & Bergasa, 2000). Other self-care measures include the use of emollients to maintain skin moisture and mild and fragrance-free soaps to prevent skin irritation that may further exacerbate pruritus (Cherny, 2002).

Diuretics remain the gold standard in management of ascites in patients with cancer. The rates of response to diuretics range from 38% to 86% (Gough & Balderson, 1993; Greenway, Johnson, & Williams, 1982). A potassium-sparing diuretic in combination with a loop diuretic is helpful in the treatment of ascites secondary to hepatic cirrhosis (Keen & Fallon, 2002). Abdominal paracentesis remains the most commonly used procedure for the management of ascites. This procedure affords quick symptomatic relief and is useful in HCC patients when diuretics are either ineffective or require a significant lag period prior to efficacy (Keen & Fallon, 2002).

The use of evidence-based interventions to manage cancer-related symptoms is crucial to quality patient care. The Oncology Nursing Society (ONS) Putting Evidence Into Practice (PEP) Resources provide comprehensive syntheses of the state of the science for the management of several common cancer-related symptoms, including pain, fatigue, anorexia, depression, and anxiety. Results from the PEP initiative are available online through the ONS Web site (www.ons.org/Research/PEP), as well as through journal articles (Adams et al., 2009; Aiello-Laws et al., 2009; Fulcher, Badger, Gunter, Marrs, & Reese, 2008; Mitchell, Beck, Hood, Moore, & Tanner, 2007; Sheldon, Swanson, Dolce, Marsh, & Summers, 2008) and books (Eaton & Tipton, 2009; Eaton, Tipton, & Irwin, 2011).

Nursing Implications

It is important for nurses caring for patients with pancreatic and hepatobiliary cancers in clinical settings to understand that the meaning of QOL varies across different disease trajectories. The QOL needs for patients at the EOL are unique, and nurses should be sensitive to these needs. The focus of QOL at the EOL may be different from the focus during the diagnosis or treatment phases. This focus involves not only the patient but also his or her family and healthcare providers (Egan & Labyak, 2006). For the patient, physical symptoms, meaning, spirituality, and relationships become particularly important (Glass, Cluxton, & Rancour, 2006). Because of the importance of physical symptoms in predicting QOL at the EOL, it is essential to provide aggressive symptom management to control common symptoms at the EOL, such as pain, fatigue, nausea, and dyspnea. Optimal pain management is essential for patients at the EOL (Deandrea, Montanari, Moja, & Apolone, 2008). Nurses should be vigilant in the routine assessment of pain and manage any uncontrolled pain with the appropriate medications. Routine assessment of side effects from pain medications, such as constipation, should be managed with a regular bowel regimen.

In the EOL setting, nurses should not only focus on the management and elimination of uncontrolled symptoms for patients but also foster the patient's search for meaning and spirituality. As patients move closer to death, confusion, restlessness, and agitation may occur. Such symptoms can challenge healthcare providers and impact the family members. Approaches include providing a soothing environment, speaking softly and touching the patient for reassurance, and providing medications to decrease the agitation (Kuebler, Heidrich, Vena, & English, 2006).

For family caregivers of patients with pancreatic and hepatobiliary cancers, the EOL phase can be particularly traumatic. Family caregivers need support in terms of what to expect physically for the patient at the EOL while simultaneously struggling with their needs (Bee, Barnes, & Luker, 2009). In this setting, nurses should support family caregivers in understanding the expected physical changes at the EOL as well as focus on the QOL needs of family caregivers. Functional declines should be expected in patients at the EOL, and nurses should address safety concerns at home with both patients and caregivers.

The task of supporting patients and their family caregivers at the EOL can be daunting. Therefore, it is important for nurses to assess QOL at the EOL using an interdisciplinary model. As available, nurses should coordinate EOL care for a variety of interdisciplinary colleagues (e.g., nurses, physicians, social workers, psychologists, chaplains, dietitians) who can help with supporting the QOL needs of patients and family caregivers at the EOL.

The early integration of palliative care is essential in maximizing QOL for patients with pancreatic and hepatobiliary cancers. The complex interplay of physical, psychological, social, spiritual, existential, medical, financial, and social burdens experienced by those facing pancreatic and hepatobiliary cancers make it imperative that an interdisciplinary team approach be used. Quality symptom management can best be delivered in a collaborative environment that integrates the skills of medicine, nursing, and supportive care professionals. The interdisciplinary care model encourages collaboration, and members of the team work to proactively care for the symptom needs of patients. Furthermore, an interdisciplinary care model provides an opportunity to administer tailored interventions of symptom management because the model is completely driven by the needs of patients individually rather than as a group.

The majority of symptom-related research has focused on a single symptom. However, symptom presentation in the patient with pancreatic or hepatobiliary cancer is not reduced to the experience of a single symptom alone. In fact, this experience includes multiple symptoms, and the relationship among these symptoms, their underlying mechanisms, and the impact on patient outcomes is still being explored. Furthermore, it is well-documented that unrelieved symptoms have a negative effect on patient outcomes, including functional status, mood states, and QOL (Kim, McGuire, Tulman, & Barsevick, 2005; Krech & Walsh, 1991; Labori et al., 2006; McMillan & Small, 2002; Miaskowski, Dodd, & Lee, 2004).

The concept of symptom clusters has gained incredible momentum in symptom-related research in the past few years. Although the occurrence of multiple symptoms has been studied in the past (Sarna, 1993), only recently this phenomenon was labeled *symptom clusters*. Currently, several working definitions for symptom clusters are used in nursing research. Dodd, Miaskowski, and Paul (2001) defined symptom clusters as three or more concurrent symptoms that are related to each other but may not share a common etiology. Kim and colleagues (2005) developed a more comprehensive definition of symptom clusters through a review of symptom clusters research. Symptom clusters consist of two or more symptoms that are related to each other and occur together (Kim et al., 2005). The clusters are composed of stable groups of symptoms, are relatively independent from other clusters, and may uncover specific underlying dimensions of symptoms. Symptoms within a cluster may or may not share a common etiology, and the relationship among symptoms within a cluster is associative rather than causal (Kim et al., 2005).

Few studies have described symptom clusters specifically in pancreatic and hepatobiliary cancers. Gupta, Rodeghier, Grutsch, and Lis (2010) described the role of symptom clusters in predicting survival in advanced pancreatic cancer. The cluster of fatigue and pain was found to be associated with survival independent of other symptoms and select patient characteristics, such as age, gender, stage of disease, and treatment history. In a sample of patients with hepatobiliary cancer, Steel and colleagues (2010) found that the symptom cluster of pain, fatigue, and depression was prevalent in patients. In this study, 25% of patients experienced high levels of pain, depression, and fatigue, and another 35% reported persistent fatigue (Steel et al., 2010). The three symptoms were reported in 62%–85% of patients at all follow-up time points of this six-month study (Steel et al., 2010).

The exploration of potential symptom clusters is critical to the development of effective symptom management strategies for patients with pancreatic and hepatobiliary cancers. This understanding is of particular importance in caring for patients with unresectable metastatic disease. The identification of clusters specific to therapies, such as surgery, chemotherapy, and organ-directed therapies, will also contribute to the specific symptom management needs of patients with pancreatic and hepatobiliary cancers based on treatment modalities.

Summary

QOL continues to be an important concept for patients with cancer at the EOL. Terminally ill patients with cancer are faced with challenges in all aspects of QOL, including physical, psychological, social, and spiritual well-being. In this setting, maximizing QOL is of the utmost importance. As the interest in QOL issues at the EOL continues to increase, nurses will continue to be actively involved locally, regionally, nationally, and internationally.

Considerable evidence points to the symptom burden that patients with pancreatic and hepatobiliary cancers experience. Symptom management and relief is a relevant and important topic in the discipline of nursing, and nurses are ideally positioned to positively impact patient outcomes through effective clinical assessment and management of cancer-related symptoms. It is imperative for nurses to foster collaborative, multidisciplinary methods of symptom management to optimize physical functioning and QOL in patients with pancreatic and hepatobiliary cancers.

References

Adams, L.A., Shepard, N., Caruso, R.A., Norling, M.J., Belansky, H., & Cunningham, R.S. (2009). Putting evidence into practice: Evidence-based interventions to prevent and manage anorexia. *Clinical Journal of Oncology Nursing, 13,* 95–102. doi:10.1188/09.CJON.95-102

Aiello-Laws, L., Reynolds, J., Deizer, N., Peterson, M., Ameringer, S., & Bakitas, M. (2009). Putting evidence into practice: What are the pharmacologic interventions for nociceptive and neuropathic cancer pain in adults? *Clinical Journal of Oncology Nursing, 13,* 649–655. doi:10.1188/09.CJON.649-655

Bee, P.E., Barnes, P., & Luker, K.A. (2009). A systematic review of informal caregivers' needs in providing home-based end-of-life care to people with cancer. *Journal of Clinical Nursing, 18,* 1379–1393. doi:10.1111/j.1365-2702.2008.02405.x

Brintzenhofe-Szoc, K.M., Levin, T.T., Li, Y., Kissane, D.W., & Zabora, J.R. (2009). Mixed anxiety/depression symptoms in a large cancer cohort: Prevalence by cancer type. *Psychosomatics, 50,* 383–391. doi:10.1176/appi.psy.50.4.383

Bruera, E., Valero, V., Driver, L., Shen, L., Willey, J., Zhang, T., & Palmer, J.L. (2006). Patient-controlled methylphenidate for cancer fatigue: A double-blind, randomized, placebo-controlled trial. *Journal of Clinical Oncology, 24,* 2073–2078. doi:10.1200/JCO.2005.02.8506

Carney, C.P., Jones, L., Woolson, R.F., Noyes, R., Jr., & Doebbeling, B.N. (2003). Relationship between depression and pancreatic cancer in the general population. *Psychosomatic Medicine, 65,* 884–888. doi:10.1097/01.PSY.0000088588.23348.D5

Chang, V.T., Hwang, S.S., & Kasimis, B. (2002). Longitudinal documentation of cancer pain management outcomes: A pilot study at a VA medical center. *Journal of Pain and Symptom Management, 24,* 494–505. doi:10.1016/S0885-3924(02)00516-X

Chen, M.L., & Tseng, H.C. (2006). Symptom clusters in cancer patients. *Supportive Care in Cancer, 14,* 825–830. doi:10.1007/s00520-006-0019-8

Cherny, N.I. (2002). Jaundice in gastrointestinal malignancy. In C. Ripamonti & E. Bruera (Eds.), *Gastrointestinal symptoms in advanced cancer patients* (pp. 291–298). New York, NY: Oxford University Press.

Coleman, J., Olsen, S.J., Sauter, P.K., Baker, D., Hodgin, M.B., Stanfield, C., ... Nolan, M.T. (2005). The effect of a Frequently Asked Questions module on a pancreatic cancer Web site patient/family chat room. *Cancer Nursing, 28,* 460–468. doi:10.1097/00002820-200511000-00009

Courneya, K.S., Mackey, J.R., Bell, G.J., Jones, L.W., Field, C.J., & Fairey, A.S. (2003). Randomized controlled trial of exercise training in postmenopausal breast cancer survivors: Cardiopulmonary and quality of life outcomes. *Journal of Clinical Oncology, 21,* 1660–1668. doi:10.1200/JCO.2003.04.093

Davidson, W., Ash, S., Capra, S., & Bauer, J. (2004). Weight stabilisation is associated with improved survival duration and quality of life in unresectable pancreatic cancer. *Clinical Nutrition, 23,* 239–247. doi:10.1016/j.clnu.2003.07.001

Deandrea, S., Montanari, M., Moja, L., & Apolone, G. (2008). Prevalence of undertreatment in cancer pain. A review of published literature. *Annals of Oncology, 19,* 1985–1991. doi:10.1093/annonc/mdn419

Del Fabbro, E., Dalal, S., & Bruera, E. (2006). Symptom control in palliative care—Part II: Cachexia/anorexia and fatigue. *Journal of Palliative Medicine, 9,* 409–421. doi:10.1089/jpm.2006.9.409

Di Bisceglie, A.M. (2002). Epidemiology and clinical presentation of hepatocellular carcinoma. *Journal of Vascular and Interventional Radiology, 13*(9, Pt. 2), S169–S171. doi:10.1016/S1051-0443(07)61783-7

Diehr, P., Lafferty, W.E., Patrick, D.L., Downey, L., Devlin, S.M., & Standish, L.J. (2007). Quality of life at the end of life. *Health and Quality of Life Outcomes, 5,* 51. doi:10.1186/1477-7525-5-51

Dimeo, F.C., Stieglitz, R.D., Novelli-Fischer, U., Fetscher, S., & Keul, J. (1999). Effects of physical activity on the fatigue and psychological status of cancer patients during chemotherapy. *Cancer, 85,* 2273–2277. doi:10.1002/(SICI)1097-0142(19990515)85:10<2273::AID-CNCR24>3.0.CO;2-B

Dodd, M.J., Miaskowski, C., & Paul, S.M. (2001). Symptom clusters and their effect on the functional status of patients with cancer. *Oncology Nursing Forum, 28,* 465–470.

Eaton, L.H., & Tipton, J.M. (Eds.). (2009). *Putting evidence into practice: Improving oncology patient outcomes.* Pittsburgh, PA: Oncology Nursing Society.

Eaton, L.H., Tipton, J.M., & Irwin, M. (Eds.). (2009). *Putting evidence into practice: Improving oncology patient outcomes, Volume 2.* Pittsburgh, PA: Oncology Nursing Society.

Egan, K.A., & Labyak, M. (2006). Hospice palliative care: A model for quality end-of-life care. In B. Ferrell & N. Coyle (Eds.), *Textbook of palliative nursing* (2nd ed., pp. 13–52). New York, NY: Oxford University Press.

Fazal, S., & Saif, M.W. (2007). Supportive and palliative care of pancreatic cancer. *JOP: Journal of the Pancreas, 8,* 240–253.

Ferrell, B.R. (1995). The impact of pain on quality of life. A decade of research. *Nursing Clinics of North America, 30,* 609–624.

Ferrell, B.R., Dow, K.H., & Grant, M. (1995). Measurement of the quality of life in cancer survivors. *Quality of Life Research, 4,* 523–531. doi:10.1007/BF00634747

Ferrell, B.R., Dow, K.H., Leigh, S., Ly, J., & Gulasekaram, P. (1995). Quality of life in long-term cancer survivors. *Oncology Nursing Forum, 22,* 915–922.

Ferrell, B.R., Grant, M.M., Funk, B.M., Otis-Green, S.A., & Garcia, N.J. (1998a). Quality of life in breast cancer survivors: Implications for developing support services. *Oncology Nursing Forum, 25,* 887–895.

Ferrell, B.R., Grant, M., Funk, B., Otis-Green, S., & Garcia, N. (1998b). Quality of life in breast cancer. Part II: Psychological and spiritual well-being. *Cancer Nursing, 21,* 1–9. doi:10.1097/00002820 -199802000-00001

Fitzsimmons, D., George, S., Payne, S., & Johnson, C.D. (1999). Differences in perception of quality of life issues between health professionals and patients with pancreatic cancer. *Psycho-Oncology, 8,* 135–143. doi:10.1002/(SICI)1099-1611(199903/04)8:2<135::AID -PON348>3.0.CO;2-Q

Fitzsimmons, D., & Johnson, C.D. (1998). Quality of life after treatment of pancreatic cancer. *Langenbeck's Archives of Surgery, 383,* 145–151. doi:10.1007/s004230050106

Fulcher, C.D., Badger, T., Gunter, A.K., Marrs, J.A., & Reese, J.M. (2008). Putting evidence into practice: Interventions for depression. *Clinical Journal of Oncology Nursing, 12,* 131–140. doi:10.1188/08. CJON.131-140

Gift, A.G., Stommel, M., Jablonski, A., & Given, W. (2003). A cluster of symptoms over time in patients with lung cancer. *Nursing Research, 52,* 393–400. doi:10.1097/00006199-200311000-00007

Glass, E., Cluxton, D., & Rancour, P. (2006). Principles of patient and family assessment. In B. Ferrell & N. Coyle (Eds.), *Textbook of palliative nursing* (2nd ed., pp. 87–106). New York, NY: Oxford University Press.

Gough, I.R., & Balderson, G.A. (1993). Malignant ascites. A comparison of peritoneovenous shunting and nonoperative management. *Cancer, 71,* 2377–2382. doi:10.1002/1097-0142(19930401)71:7<2377::AID -CNCR2820710732>3.0.CO;2-H

Greenway, B., Johnson, P.J., & Williams, R. (1982). Control of malignant ascites with spironolactone. *British Journal of Surgery, 69,* 441– 442. doi:10.1002/bjs.1800690802

Grosvenor, M., Bulcavage, L., & Cheblowski, R.T. (1989). Symptom potentially influencing weight loss in a cancer population: Correlations with primary site, nutritional status, and chemotherapy administration. *Cancer, 63,* 330–334. doi:10.1002/1097 -0142(19890115)63:2<330::AID-CNCR2820630221>3.0.CO;2-U

Gupta, D., Rodeghier, M., Grutsch, J.F., & Lis, C.G. (2010). Predicting survival in advanced pancreatic cancer: The role of symptom clusters [Abstract 265]. Abstract presented at the 2010 Gastrointestinal Cancers Symposium, January 22–24, 2010, Orlando, FL.

Hills, J., Paice, J.A., Cameron, J.R., & Shott, S. (2005). Spirituality and distress in palliative care consultation. *Journal of Palliative Medicine, 8,* 782–788. doi:10.1089/jpm.2005.8.782

Holland, J.C., Korzun, A.H., Tross, S., Silberfarb, P., Perry, M., Comis, R., & Oster, M. (1986). Comparative psychological disturbance in patients with pancreatic and gastric cancer. *American Journal of Psychiatry, 143,* 982–986.

Hwang, S.S., Chang, V.T., Fairclough, D.L., Cogswell, J., & Kasimis, B. (2003). Longitudinal quality of life in advanced cancer patients: Pilot study results from a VA medical cancer center. *Journal of Pain and Symptom Management, 25,* 225–235. doi:10.1111/j.1365-2702.2006.01274.x

Jocham, H.R., Dassen, T., Widdershoven, G., & Halfens, R. (2006). Quality of life in palliative care cancer patients: A literature review. *Journal of Clinical Nursing, 15,* 1188–1195. doi:10.1111/j.1365 -2702.2006.01274.x

Joffe, R.T., & Adsett, C.A. (1985). Depression and carcinoma of the pancreas. *Canadian Journal of Psychiatry, 30,* 117–118.

Jones, E.A., & Bergasa, N.V. (2000). Evolving concepts of the pathogenesis and treatment of the pruritus of cholestasis. *Canadian Journal of Gastroenterology, 14,* 33–39.

Keen, J., & Fallon, M. (2002). Malignant ascites. In C. Ripamonti & E. Bruera (Eds.), *Gastrointestinal symptoms in advanced cancer patients* (pp. 279–290). New York, NY: Oxford University Press.

Kelsen, D.P., Portenoy, R., Thaler, H., Tao, Y., & Brennan, M. (1997). Pain as a predictor of outcome in patients with operable pancreatic carcinoma. *Surgery, 122,* 53–59. doi:10.1016/S0039-6060(97)90264-6

Kelsen, D.P., Portenoy, R.K., Thaler, H.T., Niedzwiecki, D., Passik, S.D., Tao, Y., ... Foley, K.M. (1995). Pain and depression in patients with newly diagnosed pancreas cancer. *Journal of Clinical Oncology, 13,* 748–755.

Kim, H.J., McGuire, D.B., Tulman, L., & Barsevick, A.M. (2005). Symptom clusters: Concept analysis and clinical implications for cancer nursing. *Cancer Nursing, 28,* 270–282.

Krech, R.L., & Walsh, D. (1991). Symptoms of pancreatic cancer. *Journal of Pain and Symptom Management, 6,* 360–367. doi:10.1016/0885 -3924(91)90027-2

Krishnan, S., Rana, V., Janjan, N.A., Abbruzzese, J.L., Gould, M.S., Das, P., ... Crane, C.H. (2006). Prognostic factors in patients with unresectable locally advanced pancreatic adenocarcinoma treated with chemoradiation. *Cancer, 107,* 2589–2596. doi:10.1002/ cncr.22328

Kuebler, K., Heidrich, D., Vena, C., & English, N. (2006). Delirium, confusion, and agitation. In B. Ferrell & N. Coyle (Eds.), *Textbook of palliative nursing* (2nd ed., pp. 449–468). New York, NY: Oxford University Press.

Labori, K.J., Hjermstad, M.J., Wester, T., Buanes, T., & Loge, J.H. (2006). Symptom profiles and palliative care in advanced pancreatic cancer: A prospective study. *Supportive Care in Cancer, 14,* 1126–1133. doi:10.1007/s00520-006-0067-0

Lee, S.H., Hahn, S.T., & Park, S.H. (2001). Intra-arterial lidocaine administration for relief of pain resulting from transarterial chemoembolization of hepatocellular carcinoma: Its effectiveness and optimal timing of administration. *Cardiovascular and Interventional Radiology, 24,* 368–371. doi:10.1007/s00270-001-0073-z

Lin, M.H., Wu, P.Y., Tsai, S.T., Lin, C.L., Chen, T.W., & Hwang, S.J. (2004). Hospice palliative care for patients with hepatocellular carcinoma in Taiwan. *Palliative Medicine, 18,* 93–99. doi:10.1191/0269216304pm851oa

Lis, C.G., Gupta, D., & Grutsch, J.F. (2006). Patient satisfaction with quality of life as a predictor of survival in pancreatic cancer. *International Journal of Gastrointestinal Cancer, 37,* 35–44. doi:10.1385/ IJGC:37:1:35

Lopez, A., Figuls, M., Cuchi, G., Pasies, B., Alegre, M., & Herdman, M. (2004). Systematic review of megestrol acetate in the treatment of anorexia-cachexia syndrome. *Journal of Pain and Symptom Management, 27,* 360–369. doi:10.1016/j.jpainsymman.2003.09.007

McCorkle, R., & Quint-Benoliel, J. (1983). Symptom distress, current concerns and mood disturbance after diagnosis of life-threatening disease. *Social Science and Medicine, 17,* 431–438. doi:10.1016/0277 -9536(83)90348-9

McMillan, S.C., & Small, B.J. (2002). Symptom distress and quality of life in patients with cancer newly admitted to hospice home care. *Oncology Nursing Forum, 29,* 1421–1428. doi:10.1188/02 .ONF.1421-1428

Mercadante, S. (2002). Abdominal pain. In C. Ripamonti & E. Bruera (Eds.), *Gastrointestinal symptoms in advanced cancer patients* (pp. 223–234). New York, NY: Oxford University Press.

Mercadante, S., Casuccio, A., Agnello, A., Pumo, S., Kargar, J., & Garofalo, S. (1999). Analgesic effects of nonsteroidal anti-inflammatory drugs in cancer pain due to somatic or visceral mechanisms. *Journal of Pain and Symptom Management, 17,* 351–356. doi:10.1016/ S0885-3924(98)00141-9

Miaskowski, C., Dodd, M., & Lee, K. (2004). Symptom clusters: The new frontier in symptom management research. *Journal of the National Cancer Institute Monographs, 2004*(32), 17–21. doi:10.1093/ jncimonographs/lgh023

Mitchell, S.A., Beck, S.L., Hood, L.E., Moore, K., & Tanner, E.R. (2007). Putting evidence into practice: Evidence-based interventions for fatigue during and following cancer and its treatment. *Clinical Journal of Oncology Nursing, 11,* 99–113. doi:10.1188/07. CJON.99-113

Mock, V. (2004). Evidence-based treatment for cancer-related fatigue. *Journal of the National Cancer Institute Monographs, 2004*(32), 112– 118. doi:10.1093/jncimonographs/lgh025

Muscaritoli, M., Bossola, M., Aversa, Z., Bellantone, R., & Fanelli, F. (2006). Prevention and treatment of cancer cachexia: New insights into an old problem. *European Journal of Cancer, 42,* 31–41.

National Comprehensive Cancer Network. (2012). *NCCN Clinical Practice Guidelines in Oncology: Distress management* [v.2.2012]. Retrieved from http://www.nccn.org/professionals/physician_gls/pdf/distress.pdf

Portenoy, R.K., Thaler, H.T., Kornblith, A.B., Lepore, J.M., Friedlander-Klar, H., Coyle, N., ... Hoskins, W. (1994). Symptom prevalence, characteristics and distress in a cancer population. *Quality of Life Research, 3,* 183–189. doi:10.1007/BF00435383

Puchalski, C., Ferrell, B., Virani, R., Otis-Green, S., Baird, P., Bull, J., ... Sulmasy, D. (2009). Improving the quality of spiritual care as a dimension of palliative care: The report of the Consensus Conference. *Journal of Palliative Medicine, 12,* 885–904. doi:10.1089/jpm.2009.0142

Qin, L.X., & Tang, Z.Y. (2003). Hepatocellular carcinoma with obstructive jaundice: Diagnosis, treatment and prognosis. *World Journal of Gastroenterology, 9,* 385–391. Retrieved from http://www.wjgnet.com/1007-9327/full/v9/i3/385.htm

Ramsey, D.E., Kernagis, L.Y., Soulen, M.C., & Geschwind, J.F. (2002). Chemoembolization of hepatocellular carcinoma. *Journal of Vascular and Interventional Radiology, 13*(9, Pt. 2), S211–S221. doi:10.1016/S1051-0443(07)61789-8

Ravasco, P., Monteiro-Grillo, I., Vidal, P.M., & Camilo, M.E. (2005). Dietary counseling improves patient outcomes: A prospective, randomized, controlled trial in colorectal cancer patients undergoing radiotherapy. *Journal of Clinical Oncology, 23,* 1431–1438. doi:10.1200/JCO.2005.02.054

Reyes-Gibby, C.C., Chan, W., Abbruzzese, J.L., Xiong, H.Q., Ho, L., Evans, D.B., ... Crane, C. (2007). Patterns of self-reported symptoms in pancreatic cancer patients receiving chemoradiation. *Journal of Pain and Symptom Management, 34,* 244–252. doi:10.1016/j.jpainsymman.2006.11.007

Sarna, L. (1993). Correlates of symptom distress in women with lung cancer. *Cancer Practice, 1,* 21–28.

Schwartz, A.L., Mori, M., Gao, R., Nail, L.M., & King, M.E. (2001). Exercise reduces daily fatigue in women with breast cancer receiving chemotherapy. *Medicine and Science in Sports and Exercise, 33,* 718–723. doi:10.1097/00005768-200105000-00006

Segal, R.J., Reid, R.D., Courneya, K.S., Malone, S.C., Parliament, M.B., Scott, C.G., ... Wells, G.A. (2003). Resistance exercise in men re-ceiving androgen deprivation therapy for prostate cancer. *Journal of Clinical Oncology, 21,* 1653–1659. doi:10.1200/JCO.2003.09.534

Sheldon, L.K., Swanson, S., Dolce, A., Marsh, K., & Summers, J. (2008). Putting evidence into practice: Evidence-based interventions for anxiety. *Clinical Journal of Oncology Nursing, 12,* 789–797. doi:10.1188/08.CJON.789-797

Shun, S.-C., Lai, Y.-H., Jing, T.-T., Jeng, C., Lee, F.-Y., Hu, L.-S., & Cheng, S.-Y. (2005). Fatigue patterns and correlates in male liver cancer patients receiving transcatheter hepatic arterial chemoembolization. *Supportive Care in Cancer, 13,* 311–317. doi:10.1007/s00520-004-0740-0

Steel, J.L., Kim, K.H., Dew, M.A., Unruh, M.L., Antoni, M.H., Olek, M.C., ... Gamblin, T.C. (2010). Cancer-related symptom clusters, eosinophils, and survival in hepatobiliary cancer: An exploratory study. *Journal of Pain and Symptom Management, 39,* 859–871. doi:10.1016/j.jpainsymman.2009.09.019

Strasser, F. (2000). Impact of fluid retention on evaluation of cancer cachexia. *Supplement to Supportive Care in Cancer, 8,* 249.

Strasser, F., & Bruera, E. (2002). Cancer anorexia/cachexia syndrome: Epidemiology, pathogenesis, and assessment. In C. Ripamonti & E. Bruera (Eds.), *Gastrointestinal symptoms in advanced cancer patients* (pp. 39–80). New York, NY: Oxford University Press.

Walsh, D., & Rybicki, L. (2006). Symptom clustering in advanced cancer. *Supportive Care in Cancer, 14,* 831–836. doi:10.1007/s00520-005-0899-

Watanabe, I., Sasaki, S., Konishi, M., Nakagohri, T., Inoue, K., Oda, T., & Kinoshita, T. (2004). Onset symptoms and tumor locations as prognostic factors of pancreatic cancer. *Pancreas, 28,* 160–165.

Wells, N., Murphy, B., Wujcik, D., & Johnson, R. (2003). Pain-related distress and interference with daily life of ambulatory patients with cancer with pain. *Oncology Nursing Forum, 30,* 977–986. doi:10.1188/03.ONF.977-986

Zabora, J., Brintzenhofe-Szoc, K., Curbow, B., Hooker, C., & Piantadosi, S. (2001). The prevalence of psychological distress by cancer site. *Psycho-Oncology, 10,* 19–28. doi:10.1002/1099-1611(200101/02)10:1<19::AID-PON501>3.0.CO;2-6

CHAPTER 8

Nutritional Challenges

Maria Petzel, RD, CSO, LD, CNSC

Introduction

Nutritional status may be affected by both cancer and its treatments. Nutrient needs may be altered by the disease or treatment, and both can change patients' ability to ingest, digest, and absorb the appropriate nutrients to meet these needs (Hurst & Gallagher, 2006). Malnutrition is reported to occur in 40%–80% of patients with cancer (Bruera, 1997; National Cancer Institute [NCI], 2011).

Patients with pancreatic and hepatobiliary cancers are at an especially high risk for nutrition problems because of the anatomic location of the cancer and its potential effects on exocrine, endocrine, and biliary function, as well as treatment toxicity (Ottery, 1996b). Incidence of malnutrition in patients with pancreatic or hepatobiliary cancers is more common than with many other types of cancer (Bruera, 1997). Patients with liver, biliary, and pancreatic cancers often present with anorexia, weight loss, steatorrhea, nausea, vomiting, diarrhea, jaundice, and ascites (James & Kulakowski, 2005; Thomas, 2006). Inadequate nutrition intake can negatively affect performance status, quality of life, and the response to and tolerance of treatment. Malnutrition also contributes to increased healthcare costs, complications of treatment, and morbidity and mortality (McMahon, Decker, & Ottery, 1998; Ottery, 1996b). However, weight loss may be stabilized or reversed in 50%–88% of patients with cancer with early nutrition intervention (NCI, 2011).

Even in the absence of malnutrition, altered nutrient needs, or impaired gastrointestinal (GI) function, many patients and family members will seek guidance regarding nutritional issues. They are often interested in symptom management using nutrition and food choices to help improve tolerance of treatment, quality of life, and healing after completion of therapy.

Screening and Assessment

All patients undergoing treatment for cancer should have regular nutrition screening. Screening allows for the quick identification of patients at risk for malnutrition. Once identified, those patients at risk may be more formally assessed and undergo appropriate intervention (Ottery, 1996a).

Although several different nutrition screening tools exist, only the Malnutrition Screening Tool (MST) (Ferguson, Capra, Bauer, & Banks, 1999) and the Patient-Generated Subjective Global Assessment (PG-SGA) (McCallum, 2006) have been validated for use in the oncology population (Huhmann & August, 2008; Kubrak & Jensen, 2007). A summary of these tools is provided in Table 8-1. The MST was tested in outpatients receiving radiotherapy (Ferguson, Bauer, et al., 1999) and outpatients receiving chemotherapy (Isenring, Cross, Daniels, Kellett, & Koczwara, 2006). The PG-SGA was tested in

Table 8-1. Nutrition Screening Tools Validated for Use in Oncology		
Tool	**Source**	**Components**
Patient-Generated Subjective Global Assessment (PG-SGA)	McCallum, 2006; Ottery, 1996a	Four sections completed by patient: • Weight history • Food intake • Symptoms • Activities and function Three sections completed by clinician: • Relevant diagnosis • Metabolic demand • Physical exam
Malnutrition Screening Tool (MST)	Ferguson, Capra, et al., 1999	Two sections completed by patient: • Weight history • Food intake

hospitalized patients with cancer with therapy not specified (Bauer, Capra, & Ferguson, 2002). Screening before the start of treatment can help to identify patients who are susceptible to nutritional compromise (McCallum, 2006). Interventions to improve nutritional status or prevent deficiency may be initiated early to prevent severe deterioration, which often is irreversible (Ottery, 1996a).

Individual nutrient requirements are based on age, gender, anthropometric measurements (e.g., height, weight), and physical activity (Hurst & Gallagher, 2006). Nutritional status may also be affected by overall health status at the time of cancer diagnosis, the type or location of cancer, and the type of treatments. Additionally, nutrition needs may change over the course of treatment and with progression of disease (Hurst & Gallagher, 2006). Ideally, these patients will meet with a registered dietitian, preferably a board-certified Specialist in Oncology Nutrition (CSO). Patients with poor nutrition are less able to tolerate their prescribed dose and schedule of cancer treatments and, therefore, may have less-favorable outcomes from treatment (Petree, 2005). Nutrition therapy requires a multidisciplinary approach with nurses playing a large role in screening patients and, often, providing education (Ottery, 1996a).

Macronutrient (calorie, protein, and fluid) requirements are generally calculated taking into account weight, height, obesity, age, activity level, and disease factors. Nurses may quickly estimate the energy needs of a patient based on kilocalories per kilogram (kcal/kg) of body weight. For patients with cancer, the needs are generally estimated at 25–35 kilocalories per kilogram per day. (Nurses should use ideal body weight if patients are obese.) Needs for patients who are inactive are generally estimated at the lower end of the aforementioned kcal/kg range, with those being hypermetabolic estimated at the higher end (Hurst & Gallagher, 2006). Patients with pancreatic cancer have been found to be hypermetabolic, both those newly diagnosed and those with cancer cachexia (Cao et al., 2010; Falconer, Fearon, Plester, Ross, & Carter, 1994). Indirect calorimetry is a more precise way to measure energy needs but requires special equipment and training to perform (Hurst & Gallagher, 2006).

Protein needs are elevated in patients with cancer. These too are generally calculated using an estimate based on body weight (1–2 g/kg per day). Again, those patients under less stress have needs at the lower end of the estimate (1–1.2 g/kg), and those with hypercatabolism or severe stress have protein needs estimated near the higher end of the above estimate. If a patient has renal or hepatic insufficiency or failure, estimated needs will likely need to be adjusted. Nitrogen balance studies may be performed to aid with more precise assessment of protein provision (Hurst & Gallagher, 2006).

Fluid needs may be estimated using body surface area, based on a certain volume per kilogram of body weight with stratifications by age, or using the recommended daily allowance of 1 ml/kcal intake per day. Depending on cancer treatment side effects or disease-related symptoms such as vomiting, diarrhea, or fistula drainage, needs may require adjustment to accommodate additional fluid losses (Hurst & Gallagher, 2006).

Assessment of micronutrient (vitamin and mineral) status is more difficult, and patient needs vary depending on the adequacy of food intake. It is therefore important that clinicians monitor patients for the signs and symptoms of vitamin and mineral deficiency (Hurst & Gallagher, 2006). See Table 8-2 for a list of common vitamin and mineral deficiencies in patients with pancreatic and hepatobiliary cancers and the signs and symptoms of these deficiencies. This topic will be discussed in more depth in the section of this chapter about malabsorption.

Table 8-2. Common Micronutrient Deficiencies and Associated Symptoms of Deficiency	
Nutrient	**Deficiency Symptoms**
Calcium	Osteomalacia, tetany
Folate	Megaloblastic anemia, impaired immunity, glossitis, pallor, diarrhea
Iron	Hypochromic microcytic anemia, malabsorption, irritability, anorexia, pallor, lethargy, tachycardia, cold intolerance
Magnesium	Muscle tremors, convulsions, irritability, tetany, hyper- or hyporeflexia, nausea, vomiting
Selenium	Myalgia, muscle tenderness, cardiac myopathy, increased fragility of red blood cells, degeneration of pancreas
Vitamin A	Night blindness, Bitot's spots, dry eyes, dry skin, dry mucous membranes, impaired resistance to infection, papillary hyperkeratosis of the skin
Vitamin B_{12}	Pernicious anemia, neurologic deterioration, glossitis, peripheral neuropathy
Vitamin D	Rickets, osteomalacia
Vitamin E	Hemolytic anemia, retinal degeneration, muscle weakness, edema, irritability
Vitamin K	Prolonged bleeding and prothrombin time, hemorrhagic manifestations
Zinc	Decreased wound healing, hypogonadism, mild anemia, decreased taste acuity, hair loss, diarrhea, skin changes

Note. Based on information from Hurst & Gallagher, 2006; Morley, 2007.

Special Considerations

Impact of Surgery

Pancreaticoduodenectomy (PD), also known as the Whipple procedure, and total pancreatectomy (TP) have greater nutritional implications than distal or central pancreatectomy. Surgery for cholangiocarcinoma often requires PD because of the proximity of the bile duct to the pancreas and liver (Thomas, 2006). Nutritional implications of pancreatic surgery include weight loss, dumping syndrome, gastroparesis, diabetes mellitus, lactose intolerance, and nutrient deficiencies. Symptoms often result from surgical reconstruction or pancreatic exocrine insufficiency (malabsorption). Weight loss and postoperative nutrition parameters appear to be similar in both traditional PD and pylorus-preserving PD (DiMagno, Reber, & Tempero, 1999). Regardless of the site of cancer or type of surgery, individuals who are malnourished at the time of surgery are at risk for poor wound healing as well as an increase in other morbidities and mortality (Thomas, 2006). In addition to the information regarding side effect management discussed later in this chapter, refer to Tables 8-3 and 8-4 and Figure 8-1 for ideas for nutritional reinforcement.

Supportive Care and End-of-Life Issues

At the end of life, dietary restriction is usually not necessary as the quantity of food intake is generally low. The focus should be on ensuring that eating is an enjoyable experience. As death becomes imminent, oral intake of food decreases. At this stage, patients often cease consumption of solid foods. Decisions about artificial nutrition and hydration should be guided by the patient's advance directive or living will as well as the guidelines discussed later in the nutritional support section of this chapter (NCI, 2011). A soft, low-fiber diet with aggressive laxative care is recommended for patients who are at high risk for developing a bowel obstruction. McCallum, Walsh, and Nelson (2002) instruct patients to
- Chew food thoroughly
- Not eat raw fruit or vegetables—only canned or cooked
- Not eat green peas or cooked dry beans, peas, or lentils
- Not eat nuts, popcorn, seeds, or whole spices. (p. 174)

Seventeen patients with advanced pancreatic cancer were given the above instructions; none of them developed bowel obstruction prior to their death. However, 12 of 17 patients who were not given prophylactic education developed an obstruction (McCallum et al., 2002). In addition to these recommendations, patients should also be instructed to avoid high-fiber cereals (such as bran) and to remove any thick skins or peels from fruits and vegetables before cooking and eating them (NCI, 2011).

Table 8-3. Ways to Increase Calories

Food	Suggested Uses
Cheese*	Melt on top of casseroles, potatoes, and vegetables. Add to omelets. Add to sandwiches.
Dried fruits (raisins, prunes, apricots, dates, figs)	Hydrate them in warm water, and eat for breakfast, dessert, or snack. Add to • Muffins • Breads • Rice and grain dishes • Cereals • Puddings • Stuffing • Cooked vegetables (such as carrots, sweet potatoes, yams, and acorn or butternut squash). Combine with nuts or granola for snacks.
Eggs	Add chopped hard-boiled eggs to salads, salad dressings, vegetables, casseroles, and creamed meats. Add extra hard-boiled yolks to deviled egg filling. Beat eggs into mashed potatoes, pureed vegetables, and sauces. (Make sure to keep cooking these dishes after adding the eggs because raw eggs may contain harmful bacteria.) Add extra eggs or egg whites to • Custards • Puddings • Quiches • Scrambled eggs • Omelets • Pancake or French toast batter.
Granola	Use in muffin and bread batters. Sprinkle on • Vegetables • Yogurt • Pudding • Custard • Fruit. Layer with fruits and bake. Mix with dried fruits and nuts for a snack. Use in pudding recipes instead of bread or rice.
Milk*	Pour on hot or cold cereal. Pour on chicken and fish while baking. Mix in hamburgers, meatloaf, and croquettes. Make hot chocolate with milk.

*May need to limit fat content if experiencing pancreatic insufficiency

Note. Based on information from National Cancer Institute, 2011.

Table 8-4. Ways to Increase Protein

Food	Suggested Uses
Beans, legumes, and tofu	Add to casseroles, pasta, soup, salad, and grain dishes. Mash cooked beans with cheese and milk.
Cheese*	Hard or semisoft: Melt on • Sandwiches • Bread • Muffins • Tortillas • Hamburgers • Meats and fish • Vegetables • Eggs • Stewed fruit • Pies. Grate and add to • Soups • Sauces • Casseroles • Vegetable dishes • Mashed potatoes • Rice • Noodles • Meatloaf. Cottage or ricotta cheese: Mix with or use to stuff fruits and vegetables, or add to • Casseroles • Spaghetti • Noodles • Egg dishes (such as omelets, scrambled eggs, and soufflés).
Eggs	Add chopped hard-boiled eggs to salads, vegetables, casseroles, and creamed meats. Add extra hard-boiled yolks to deviled egg filling. Beat eggs into mashed potatoes, pureed vegetables, and sauces. (Make sure to keep cooking these dishes after adding the eggs because raw eggs may contain harmful bacteria.) Add extra eggs or egg whites to • Custard • Puddings • Quiches • Scrambled eggs • Omelets • Pancake or French toast batter.
Meal replacements, supplements, and protein powder	Use "instant breakfast" powder in milk drinks and desserts. Mix with milk and fruit flavoring for a high-protein shake.
Meat, poultry, and fish	Add chopped, cooked meat or fish to • Vegetables • Salads • Casseroles • Soups • Sauces • Biscuit dough • Omelets • Soufflés • Quiches • Sandwich fillings • Chicken and turkey stuffing. Wrap in pie crust or biscuit dough as turnovers. Add to stuffed baked potatoes.

(Continued on next page)

Table 8-4. Ways to Increase Protein *(Continued)*	
Food	**Suggested Uses**
Milk*	Use milk instead of water in drinks and in cooking. Use in hot cereal, soups, cocoa, and pudding.
Nonfat instant dry milk	Add to milk and milk drinks (such as pasteurized eggnog and milkshakes). Use in • Casseroles • Meatloaf • Breads • Muffins • Sauces • Cream soups • Mashed potatoes • Macaroni and cheese • Pudding • Custard • Other milk-based desserts.
Nuts, seeds, and wheat germ*	Add to • Casseroles • Breads • Muffins • Pancakes • Waffles. Sprinkle on • Fruit • Cereal • Yogurt • Vegetables • Salads • Toast. Use in place of breadcrumbs in recipes. Blend with parsley, spinach, or herbs and milk to make a sauce for noodle, pasta, or vegetable dishes. Roll bananas in chopped nuts.
Peanut butter and other nut butters*	Spread on • Sandwiches • Toast • Muffins • Crackers • Waffles • Pancakes • Fruit slices. Use as a dip for raw vegetables. Blend with milk and other drinks. Swirl through frozen yogurt.
Yogurt and frozen yogurt*	Add to • Carbonated drinks • Milk drinks (such as milkshakes*) • Cereal • Fruit • Gelatin • Pies. Mix with soft or cooked fruits. Make a sandwich of frozen yogurt between graham crackers. Mix with breakfast drinks and fruit, such as bananas.

*May need to limit fat content if experiencing pancreatic insufficiency

Note. Based on information from National Cancer Institute, 2011.

Figure 8-1. Medical Food Supplement Drinks

Standard (per serving: 250 calories, 9–11 grams protein)
- Boost®
- Ensure®

High-Calorie, High-Protein (per serving: 350 calories, 13–15 grams protein)
- Boost Plus®
- Ensure Plus®

Carbohydrate-Controlled (per serving: 350 calories, 10–14 grams protein)
- Boost Glucose Control®
- Glucerna®

Fat-Free, Protein-Containing, Clear Liquid (per serving: 180–250 calories, 7–9 grams protein)
- Ensure Clear®
- Ensure Enlive®
- Resource Breeze®

Note. All of the above are lactose free.

Common Nutrition Symptoms and Management Strategies

Although evidence is available indicating that poor nutrition may negatively affect cancer treatments or outcomes, very little is in the literature regarding evidence-based practices for nutritional treatment of symptoms. Therefore, in this chapter, many of the tips for nutrition management of symptoms are largely practice based. It is very important to educate patients and to recognize that nutrition intervention is an adjunct to other medical interventions. Nutrition strategies should be implemented in combination with medical therapies for side effect management.

Nutrition therapy can empower patients to play a more active role in their treatment and recovery. The overall goals for nutrition therapy are to prevent or reverse poor nutrition, support immune function, manage side effects, aid with successful completion of therapy, and optimize quality of life (NCI, 2011). Even in advanced stages of disease, nutrition can play a role in comfort and symptom relief. Good nutrition remains important for survivors who have completed treatment, as it can help to prevent or manage other comorbidities such as diabetes. For each of the common symptoms discussed in the following sections, additional nutrition strategies are provided in Table 8-5.

Resources for diet information and free patient education materials include the Pancreatic Cancer Action Network's *Diet and Nutrition* booklet, NCI's *Eating Hints for Cancer Patients* booklet, and the American Cancer Society's *Nutrition for the Person With Cancer During Treatment*. This is, of course, not an all-inclusive list of resources, but these publications provide comprehensive, reliable, and disease-specific information. Contact information for these organizations is easily accessible online.

Weight Loss, Anorexia, and Cancer Cachexia

Although common in patients with pancreatic cancer, not all weight loss is caused by cachexia (Holmes, 2009). Anorexia is a loss of appetite and a decrease in food intake, whereas cachexia is a multifaceted process that, in addition to anorexia symptoms, involves metabolic alterations, release of cytokines, and other catabolic factors that lead to muscle wasting (Berendt & D'Agostino, 2005). Weight loss in patients with pancreatic and hepatobiliary cancers may be caused by or exacerbated by additional factors. Patients with GI cancers often have to limit intake of food or fluids for diagnostic and staging tests, which may contribute to weight loss (Berendt & D'Agostino, 2005). Often weight loss may be caused by malabsorption rather than anorexia or cachexia (Perez, Newcomer, Moertel, Go, & Dimagno, 1983). Treatment of malabsorption will be further explored later in this chapter.

Anorexia

Anorexia may be caused by physiologic (e.g., nausea, alterations in taste), psychological (e.g., anxiety, depression), and social (e.g., eating environment) factors (Berendt & D'Agostino, 2005). Treatment of anorexia often requires behavioral and diet modifications as well as pharmacologic management (Ottery, 1996b). Exercise may help to improve appetite (Holmes, 2009). Planning meals in advance and keeping ready-to-eat foods easily accessible are also helpful in combating poor appetite. When nutrition strategies have had less than the desired effect, initiation of an appetite-enhancing medication may be helpful (Von Roenn, 2006).

Cachexia

Circulating cytokines are known to contribute to nutritional deterioration of patients (Ottery, 1996b). Cytokines may be released by the tumor itself or the host immune system as a response to the tumor (Berendt & D'Agostino, 2005). Characterized by significant involuntary weight loss, anorexia, early satiety, anemia, and fatigue, cachexia results in loss of weight and lean body mass (Guy & Smith, 2005; Holmes, 2009). Cachexia-related weight loss differs from starvation in that weight loss in starvation is generally associated with fat loss, whereas weight loss in cachexia is the result of fat and skeletal muscle loss (Holmes, 2009). Weight loss in starvation can generally be reversed, but a patient with cachexia may consume 3,000–4,000 kcal per day (about 200% of normal) and not be able to halt weight loss (Holmes, 2009). Cachexia has been described as similar to a parasite—the tumor draws nutrients from the host. If food intake does not meet the needs of the host and the tumor, then the body stores will begin to break down in order for the tumor to continue to receive nutrients (Holmes, 2009).

Table 8-5. Nutrition Interventions for Nutrition Impact Symptoms

Symptom	Interventions
Anorexia Delayed gastric emptying Ascites	Plan a daily menu in advance. Eat small, frequent, high-calorie meals (every 2 hours). Arrange for help in preparing meals. Add extra protein and calories to food. Prepare and store small portions of favorite foods. Consume one-third of daily protein and calorie requirements at breakfast. Snack between meals. Seek foods that appeal to the sense of smell. Be creative with desserts. Experiment with different foods. Perform frequent mouth care to relieve symptoms and decrease aftertastes.
Constipation	Drink plenty of fluids each day: water, warm juices, prune juice, etc. Take walks regularly. Eat more fiber-containing foods (when fluid intake is adequate).
Diarrhea	Limit gas-forming foods and beverages such as soft drinks, cruciferous vegetables, legumes and lentils, and chewing gum. Limit the use of sugar-free candies or gum made with sugar alcohol (sorbitol). Drink at least 1 cup of liquid after each loose bowel movement. Limit milk to 2 cups or eliminate milk and milk products until the source of the problem is determined.
Nausea	Eat dry foods such as crackers, breadsticks, or toast throughout the day. Sit up or recline with a raised head for 1 hour after eating. Eat bland, soft, easy-to-digest foods rather than heavy meals. Avoid eating in a room that has cooking odors or is overly warm; keep the living space comfortable but well ventilated. Rinse out the mouth before and after eating. Suck on hard candies such as peppermints or lemon drops if the mouth has a bad taste.
Lactose intolerance	Prepare your own low-lactose or lactose-free foods. Choose lactose-free or low-lactose milk products. Most grocery stores have products (such as milk and ice cream) labeled "lactose-free" or "low-lactose." Try products made with soy or rice (such as soy or rice milk and ice cream). These products do not have any lactose. Choose dairy products that are naturally lower in lactose. Hard cheeses (such as cheddar) and yogurt are less likely to cause problems. Try using lactase tablets when consuming dairy products. Lactase is an enzyme that breaks down lactose.
Taste changes	Eat small, frequent meals and healthy snacks throughout the day. Be flexible. Eat when hungry rather than at set mealtimes. Use plastic utensils and do not drink directly from metal containers if foods taste metallic. Try favorite foods, if not nauseated. Plan to eat with family and friends. Have others prepare meals. Try new foods when feeling best. Substitute poultry, fish, eggs, and cheese for red meat. Consult a vegetarian or Chinese cookbook for meatless, high-protein recipes. Use sugar-free lemon drops, gum, or mints when experiencing a metallic or bitter taste in the mouth. Add spices and sauces to foods. Eat meat with something sweet, such as cranberry sauce, jelly, or applesauce. Choose foods that look and smell appealing. Marinate foods. Try tart foods and drinks. Sweeten foods. If tastes are dull but not unpleasant, chew food longer to allow more contact with taste receptors.

Note. Based on information from Elliott et al., 2006; Morley, 2007; National Cancer Institute, 2011.

Nutritional interventions for cancer cachexia are limited. Although studies in HIV-related wasting showed that a nutritional supplement containing beta-hydroxy beta-methylbutyrate, L-glutamine, and L-arginine (Juven®) may decrease lean body mass breakdown, studies in cancer-induced cachexia have not been as promising. Berk and colleagues (2008) conducted a double-blind, placebo-controlled trial of Juven but were unable to show preservation of lean body mass. Additionally, patient compliance was an issue, as only 37% of patients completed the trial. A 45% dropout rate was associated with issues related to product acceptance: 38% refused to complete the treatment, and 7% complained of GI side effects. Additionally, supplemental use of arginine is of concern in patients receiving treatment with curative intent for pancreatic adenocarcinoma and hepatocellular carcinoma because arginine deprivation has been demonstrated to inhibit tumor growth (Bowles et al., 2008; Glazer et al., 2010).

The only known way to stop cachexia is to achieve treatment response and control of the cancer (Holmes, 2009). Appetite-stimulating medication has been shown to be helpful in decreasing cachexia-related weight loss (Von Roenn, 2006). Nutrition intervention in the setting of cancer cachexia may decrease the rate of weight loss but it does not lead to recovery of nutritional status (Ellison, Chevlen, Still, & Dubagunta, 2002).

Appetite Stimulants

If nutrition strategies alone do not lead to improved appetite or oral intake, the use of an appetite-stimulating medication may be beneficial. For dosage, prescribing, and side effect information, please refer to the manufacturer's full prescribing information for each medication used. The most common medications for appetite are discussed in the following sections. Medications should be tried for a few weeks before determining efficacy for each individual patient and medication (Von Roenn, 2006).

Corticosteroids

Corticosteroids, such as dexamethasone, may be used to increase appetite, but the effect may be transient (Berendt & D'Agostino, 2005; Ellison et al., 2002; Ottery, 1996b; Von Roenn, 2006). Patients who are not diabetic should be monitored for hyperglycemia while on steroids. Patients who have preexisting diabetes may need adjustments to their blood glucose management, oral medications, and insulin while on steroids (Wilkes & Barton-Burke, 2010).

Dronabinol

A synthetic tetrahydrocannabinol, dronabinol has been shown to be of benefit in appetite stimulation (Ottery, 1996b; Von Roenn, 2006). If a patient is intolerant of daytime dosing, it may be effective to try one dose (per 24 hours) at bedtime (Wilkes & Barton-Burke, 2010). Side effects can include changes in mood, cognition, and memory, as well as nervousness, dizziness, euphoria, and somnolence. Because it is a synthetic derivative of cannabis, caution needs to be exercised if administered to people with a substance abuse history (Wilkes & Barton-Burke, 2010). It may also be best to avoid use of dronabinol if the patient has a history of unpleasant experience with recreational marijuana use.

Megestrol Acetate

Megestrol acetate has been shown to be effective in appetite enhancement (Ottery, 1996b; Von Roenn, 2006). It is important to note that the effective dose is delivered as a suspension. The individual pill dose is so low (40 mg per pill) that an excessive amount of pills would be needed to reach the effective dose of 400–800 mg per day (Wilkes & Barton-Burke, 2010), whereas an 800 mg dose of megestrol acetate is 20 cc of oral suspension.

Some reports indicate that weight gain with megestrol acetate may be a gain of fat mass rather than lean body mass (Guy & Smith, 2005). Side effects from megestrol acetate include deep vein thrombosis or pulmonary emboli occurring in 6% of patients; therefore, it may not be the best choice for patients who are not ambulatory or who have a poor performance status (Wilkes & Barton-Burke, 2010). Additionally, megestrol acetate may cause hyperglycemia (Wilkes & Barton-Burke, 2010).

Mirtazapine

Mirtazapine is an antidepressant that is commonly used off label for its appetite-enhancement properties (Riechelmann, Burman, Tannock, Rodin, & Zimmermann, 2009; Theobald, Kirsh, Holtsclaw, Donaghy, & Passik, 2002). Effectiveness may not be apparent until after four to six weeks of use (Wilkes & Barton-Burke, 2010). Mirtazapine may not be appropriate for use in patients with hepatobiliary cancers because it may have altered drug metabolism in the case of hepatic insufficiency and should be discontinued if the patient becomes jaundiced (Wilkes & Barton-Burke, 2010).

Changes in Taste and Smell

Taste changes may be either a loss or reduction of taste (hypogeusia) or actual or perceived changes in taste (dysgeusia). Alterations in taste may occur as a result of chemotherapy or other supportive medications (Berendt & D'Agostino, 2005). Patients who receive platinum-based chemotherapy often complain of a "metallic" taste (Ottery, 1996b). Food aversions or anorexia may result from taste changes. Patients experiencing taste changes often lose their desire for animal proteins, such as fish, poultry, and red meat. These consequences of dysgeusia may result in weight loss and malnutrition. Table 8-4 includes a list of primary protein sources, including those that may be used as alternatives to animal proteins.

Taste changes may result from a deficiency of zinc. Steatorrhea, diarrhea, or inadequate intake may cause zinc deficiency. Zinc therapy for taste changes may be given for a short time with little concern for side effects or interference with absorption of other nutrients. Evaluation of serum zinc is often inaccurate but may be followed for trends if supplementing. If the patient's diet is adequate in animal protein, a course of 25–100 mg of elemental zinc may be sufficient to improve taste changes (Heyneman, 1996; Prasad, 1985; Takaoka et al., 2010). A dose of 220 mg of zinc sulfate will provide 50 mg of elemental zinc (Office of Dietary Supplements, 2011).

Nausea and Vomiting

Nausea or vomiting may be induced by disease or treatment. Anticipatory nausea may also be situational (Berendt & D'Agostino, 2005). Nutrition interventions can help a patient to maintain nourishment when experiencing nausea, but nausea control is best with antiemetic medications. Patients should be instructed to administer antiemetics on a scheduled basis for the length of the nausea cycle (Berendt & D'Agostino, 2005). It is also important to reinforce the need for adequate hydration, especially fluids with electrolytes, to prevent dehydration.

Constipation

Constipation may be caused or exacerbated by decreased activity, use of narcotic pain medication, inadequate fluid intake, and cancer therapy (Elliott, Molseed, McCallum, & Grant, 2006; Ottery, 1996b). In addition to medicinal therapies such as stool softeners and laxatives, diet modifications may be helpful to prevent constipation or discomfort when experiencing constipation. Gas-forming foods should be limited. Patients should be encouraged to increase fluid intake, especially hot liquids, to help stimulate the bowels. When adequate fluid is being consumed, high-fiber foods can be added to help with regularity. Fiber should be added gradually to the diet (Elliott et al., 2006; NCI, 2011).

Diarrhea

Loose or frequent stooling may be a result of one or several factors, including cancer therapy, pancreatic exocrine insufficiency and malabsorption, lactose intolerance, and bacterial overgrowth (*Clostridium difficile*). Regardless of the cause of diarrhea, when diarrhea is occurring, dietary modification can help mitigate the symptoms. Strategies include limiting or avoiding products with lactose (i.e., dairy), foods high in insoluble fiber, foods sweetened with sugar alcohol (e.g., sorbitol, maltitol), sugar-sweetened beverages, and hot liquids. Patients may be encouraged to increase use of soluble-fiber foods and fluids with electrolytes (Elliott et al., 2006). See Table 8-5 for more details.

Other nutritional strategies for diarrhea management include use of probiotics or medicinal fiber. Probiotics from food (e.g., yogurt, buttermilk, tempeh, and other products with live active cultures) and supplements appear to be beneficial in management or prevention of diarrhea (Natural Medicines Comprehensive Database, 2012b). Medicinal fiber (psyllium or methylcellulose) has been found to be beneficial in decreasing the frequency and severity of diarrhea. Suggested dosage is 1 teaspoon psyllium powder (or dose to provide 3.4 g psyllium) or 1 teaspoon methylcellulose powder mixed with 2 oz of water taken once a day after a meal and gradually increased as needed up to four times per day (Murphy, Stacey, Crook, Thompson, & Panetta, 2000; Singh, 2007).

Supplementation with L-glutamine has been investigated for treatment or prevention of diarrhea, but results are inconclusive. A study by Kozelsky and colleagues (2003) investigated use of glutamine during pelvic radiation and found no effect. Studies of oral glutamine used in patients receiving fluorouracil-based chemotherapy have shown mixed results of effectiveness (Bozzetti et al., 1997; Daniele et al., 2001). Because it is possible that these studies did not test what is thought to be the effective dose (30 g per day in two or three divided doses), use of glutamine to prevent or treat diarrhea should not be fully ruled out but should be recommended on a case-by-case basis with guidance from a registered dietitian (Savy, 2002).

Pancreatic Exocrine Insufficiency and Malabsorption

Pancreatic exocrine insufficiency (PEI) may be observed in patients upon diagnosis or during nonsurgical treatment for pancreatic cancer (Ottery, 1996b). It is often recognized because patients have frequent or loose bowel movements. Such bowel movements may be masked by narcotic use that slows gut motility, but other symptoms of insufficiency may be present (see Figure 8-2) (Ellison et al., 2002; Ottery, 1996b). Unfortunately, malabsorption is frequently not diagnosed or treat-

---

Figure 8-2. Signs and Symptoms of Pancreatic Exocrine Insufficiency

- Abdominal bloating
- Cramping after meals
- Excessive gas (burping or flatulence)
- Fatty stools
- Frequent stools
- Foul-smelling stools or gas
- Floating stools
- Indigestion
- Loose stools
- Unexplained weight loss

Note. Based on information from Elliott et al., 2006; Guy & Smith, 2005; Layer et al., 2001; Ottery, 1996b.

ed (Ottery, 1996b). Symptoms of malabsorption are generally observed in patients who have endogenous pancreatic enzyme output below 10% of normal rate (DiMagno et al., 1999). For patients with severe PEI, it may be impossible to eliminate steatorrhea completely, but it can be reduced by 60%–70% (Sarner, 2003). Malabsorption is also related to bile salts, so a biliary obstruction can lead to weight loss even if exocrine activity is sufficient (Layer, Keller, & Lankisch, 2001). Biliary obstruction symptoms may be reduced by following a low-fat diet and avoiding gas-producing foods (Thomas, 2006).

The effect of pancreatic surgery on PEI has been evaluated in patients having undergone distal pancreatectomy or pancreaticoduodenectomy. Stool elastase testing of patients with normal pancreatic function preoperatively showed that 12% of patients had PEI three months following an extended resection of the distal pancreas (Speicher & Traverso, 2010). By 24 months after distal pancreatectomy, all patients who experienced PEI at three months regained adequate exocrine function (Speicher & Traverso, 2010). The results of pancreaticoduodenectomy lead to more patients developing postoperative PEI. Matsumoto and Traverso (2006) found that 50% of patients who had normal exocrine function before Whipple surgery experienced PEI as a long-term side effect of surgery.

Nutrition strategies for management of malabsorption include the use of supplemental pancreatic enzymes and limiting high-fat foods (DiMagno et al., 1999; Ottery, 1996b; Thomas, 2006). Medium-chain triglyceride (MCT) oil may be substituted for other fats because MCTs do not require enzymatic action or bile salts for digestion or absorption (Babayan, 1985; Sarner, 2003). MCT oil is commercially available over the counter. Side effects can include diarrhea, vomiting, nausea, stomach discomfort, and intestinal gas; use of MCT oil as a patient's only source of fat can lead to essential fatty acid deficiency (Sarner, 2003). Palatability of MCT oil may affect patient compliance, but recipes are available from some manufacturers. Although coconut oil does not provide MCTs exclusively, it is very high in MCTs and may be substituted for other fat sources in the regular diet.

Pancreatic Enzymes (Pancrelipase)

When pancreatic exocrine function is compromised, not only are digestive enzymes inadequate, but bicarbonate production and transport to the small intestine also could be impaired. A more physiologic basic environment is needed not only for enzyme function but also for bile acids to be able to transport fatty acids into the blood. Sarner (2003) suggested the use of an H_2-receptor antagonist or proton pump inhibitor for all patients utilizing pancreatic enzyme supplements. Dosing suggestions for pancreatic enzyme replacement in pancreatic cancer vary from 10,000–40,000 lipase units per meal and 5,000–25,000 per snack (Ellison et al., 2002; Layer et al., 2001; Ottery, 1996b; Sarner, 2003). Refer to the manufacturers' full prescribing information for details of maxi-

mum dose for each product; it is rare that a patient with pancreatic cancer will reach this dose. Enzymes should be taken just after the start of the meal (with the first bite of food) and spread through the meal to ensure that the appropriate amount of enzyme is delivered with the food (Sarner, 2003).

Fat-Soluble Vitamins

Patients may be at risk for several micronutrient deficiencies after surgery because of uncontrolled adverse effects of the surgery or anatomic changes. Patients who do not utilize adequate enzyme supplementation may become deficient in vitamin B_{12} because of an inadequate amount of protease to cleave B_{12} from its carrier protein. Patients who continue to have fat malabsorption may become deficient in the fat-soluble vitamins A, D, E, and K (Thomas, 2006). Vitamin K deficiency may be brought out by coexisting liver disease (Sarner, 2003). In this case, the patient should supplement with water-miscible forms of the fat-soluble vitamins (Thomas, 2006). However, patients who have achieved adequate enzyme supplementation and therefore are absorbing fat adequately should be able to absorb fat-soluble vitamins and B_{12}. Table 8-2 contains common nutrient deficiencies associated with pancreatic and hepatobiliary cancers as well as signs and symptoms of nutrient deficiency.

Diabetes

Diabetes may be preexisting, develop because of the cancer, or be induced by surgery (Sarner, 2003). Because the diet is often already limited as a result of side effects of treatment or poor appetite, diabetes in the setting of active anticancer treatment or postoperative recovery is best treated with insulin or other diabetes medications. Beyond recovery from surgery, diet alone is not generally sufficient to control blood glucose concentrations (Sarner, 2003), but in patients who have no evidence of disease and have completed cancer treatment, diet modification should play a role in blood glucose management. If total pancreatectomy is planned, preoperative nutrition and diabetes education is recommended (Guy & Smith, 2005). Patients should be referred to a diabetes center and receive education about diet management by a certified diabetes educator.

Delayed Gastric Emptying

Delayed emptying is shown to occur in 60% of patients with pancreatic cancer absent of gastroduodenal involvement or obstruction (DiMagno et al., 1999). Use of prokinetic agents should be considered (DiMagno et al., 1999; Leung & Silverman, 2009; Ottery, 1996b). Currently only two are available in the United States—metoclopramide and erythromycin. Diet modifications may also be implemented to help prevent excessive feelings of early satiety (see Table 8-5 for more details). Patients will likely benefit from consuming small, low-fiber, and low-fat meals more frequently (six to eight times per day). They should be instructed to avoid eating two to three hours before bedtime and to keep the head and shoulders elevated above the stomach at all times (Thomas, 2006).

Gastric Outlet or Duodenal Obstruction

Although typically a late-onset effect, 15%–20% of patients experience gastric outlet or duodenal obstruction (DiMagno et al., 1999; Gaidos & Draganov, 2009). Symptoms of obstruction are nausea, vomiting (often characterized by retained food), abdominal distention, or pain. It can lead to dehydration and weight loss as well as poor quality of life. Treatment for outlet obstruction may be performed surgically with a gastrojejunostomy (gastric bypass) or endoscopy with placement of a metallic stent in the duodenum to prevent obstruction (Gaidos & Draganov, 2009; Guy & Smith, 2005). If stenting or gastric bypass is not possible, a gastrostomy tube (g-tube) for drainage and a jejunostomy tube (j-tube) for feeding may be placed.

Little information is published regarding appropriate diet after duodenal stent, but the literature indicates that diet is resumed first as liquids and then a few days later transitioned to a soft-solid (i.e., low-residue) diet as tolerated. Patients should be instructed to chew all foods well and to drink plenty of liquids with meals to ensure a liquid food bolus (Adler & Baron, 2002; Dormann, Meisner, Verin, & Lang, 2004; Ly, O'Grady, Mittal, Plank, & Windsor, 2009).

Dumping Syndrome

Patients who have undergone a classic pancreaticoduodenectomy (pylorus removed) may have symptoms of dumping syndrome (see Figure 8-3) when consuming an oral diet (Thomas, 2006). Dietary modifications include avoiding foods containing high amounts of refined sugars, hot liquids, and any other foods the individual believes contributes to symptoms of dumping as well as not drinking liquids with or within one hour of meals (Thomas, 2006).

Biliary Obstruction

Steatorrhea is a common symptom in hepatocellular cancers. It may be related to underlying liver disease or caused by biliary obstruction. Treatment for obstruction is often bile duct stent placement (James & Kulakowski, 2005). Biliary obstruction symptoms may be reduced by following a low-fat diet and avoiding gas-producing foods (Thomas, 2006). Methods for managing steatorrhea are discussed in the earlier section about malabsorption.

Hepatic Insufficiency

Postoperative liver failure is reported to occur in 20%–70% of patients having undergone hepatectomy (Hassanain et al., 2008). This may be short term or long term. Some patients may develop hepatic encephalopathy. Historically, a low-protein diet has been recommended for patients with encephalopathy, but current literature suggests against restricting protein. Recommended protein intake in patients with mild encephalopathy is 1–1.5 grams protein per kilogram. In cases of severe encephalopathy, diet should not be restricted any less than 0.5 grams protein per kilogram of body weight and when possible, this should be increased to at least 1 gram per kilogram per day (Schulz, Campos, & Coelho, 2008). Adequate protein intake is important to promote visceral protein synthesis and to prevent breakdown of lean body mass. The use of branched-chain amino acids for treatment of encephalopathy remains a debate. Nutritional supplementation with vegetable proteins may also be helpful in achieving adequate protein intake in patients with liver disease (James & Kulakowski, 2005; Schulz et al., 2008). Patients with hepatic insufficiency should be followed by a registered dietitian to assist with detailed planning of protein content of diet and monitoring of signs and symptoms of encephalopathy.

Ascites

The accumulation of fluid in the abdomen may be related to malignancy or malnutrition. It may lead to discomfort, early satiety, nausea, and vomiting. Often, therapy for ascites involves paracentesis. Repeated paracentesis depletes protein. Strategies for coping with ascites are the same as the strategies for dealing with delayed gastric emptying (see Table 8-5) and additionally following a sodium-restricted, high-protein diet (Berendt & D'Agostino, 2005).

Specialized Nutrition Support

Even with the modifications described in this chapter, pancreatic and hepatobiliary cancers and treatments for these cancers can limit the functional ability to intake and absorb adequate food and fluids. The American Society for Parenteral and Enteral Nutrition (A.S.P.E.N.) Guidelines for the Use of Parenteral and Enteral Nutrition recommend against routine use of tube feeding or parenteral nutrition (i.e., specialized nutrition support [SNS]), for patients with cancer (A.S.P.E.N. Board of Directors & the Clinical Guidelines Task Force, 2002). However, if patients are receiving anticancer treatment, are malnourished, and expect to

---

Figure 8-3. Signs and Symptoms* of Dumping Syndrome

- Diaphoresis
- Difficulty concentrating
- Faintness
- Fatigue
- Flushing
- Headache
- Hunger
- Loose bowel movements
- Tachycardia

*Symptoms generally occur 15–60 minutes after a meal.

Note. Based on information from Thomas, 2006.

be unable to ingest or absorb nutrition adequately for an extended period of time, A.S.P.E.N. suggests that SNS may be appropriate. Additionally, SNS may be appropriate for patients who are preoperative and moderately to severely malnourished and will be able to receive SNS for at least seven days preoperatively.

Tube Feeding (Enteral Nutrition)

Unless malabsorption is uncontrolled or the GI tract is otherwise impaired, enteral nutrition (EN) infusion should be used. The benefits of EN over parenteral nutrition (PN) are that it stimulates bile flow and prevents cholestasis, it may reduce risk of bacterial translocation, and it carries a lower risk of infection than PN (Robinson, 2006). Tube feeding may be administered via several routes (e.g., nasogastric, gastrostomy, and jejunostomy tubes) and continuously or intermittently by pump, gravity drip, or syringe bolus. Some contraindications for enteral feeding include intractable vomiting, ileus, and intractable diarrhea (Robinson, 2006). Tube feeding should be considered when adequate oral intake is limited because of a mechanical obstruction from the tumor, such as gastric outlet obstruction (Luthringer, 2006).

Parenteral Nutrition

PN is appropriate in the case of significant GI impairment. As discussed previously, PN may be considered in the preoperative setting or if a patient is undergoing cancer treatment and not expected to be able to tolerate adequate oral intake for a prolonged period. A study by Pelzer and colleagues (2010) found a positive effect on nutritional status in patients with stage IV pancreatic cancer who received PN infusion; overall survival and quality of life were not assessed. Only patients with acceptable performance status who were expected to die from starvation prior to cancer progression received PN (Pelzer et al., 2010).

Complementary Nutrition Therapies

In a survey completed by Richardson, Sanders, Palmer, Greisinger, and Singletary (2000), 80% of respondents reported using complementary and alternative medicine therapies. Two specific nutrients have gained the attention of patients with pancreatic cancer, although this is not an exhaustive list.

Curcumin

Curcumin is found in turmeric, a spice commonly used in Asian and East Indian curry dishes (Natural Medicines Comprehensive Database, 2012c). It has been used for thousands of years in traditional Asian medicine to treat GI upset, arthritis, and other inflammatory conditions. Because of its antioxidant, anti-inflammatory, and antiproliferative properties, curcum-

in is being studied for its use in cancer treatment and cancer prevention. It has been used for thousands of years in certain cultures as an herbal medicine (Natural Medicines Comprehensive Database, 2012c). It has limited bioavailability when consumed orally. Despite this, early studies in animals have shown promising results. A few small studies have been conducted in humans with pancreatic cancer. Curcumin has been found to be safe with no systemic toxic effects; however, it is contraindicated in patients with biliary obstructions, gallstones, and gastric or duodenal ulcers (Dhillon et al., 2008). The most commonly described side effect is GI upset (Natural Medicines Comprehensive Database, 2012c). The dose studied was 8 grams per day divided into two daily doses. In some patients, curcumin has been found to stabilize disease. One patient in the study by Dhillon and colleagues (2008) actually had tumor regression. Although curcumin in combination with gemcitabine has been studied for feasibility, additional studies are being conducted to determine the safety and efficacy of combining curcumin with current chemotherapeutic agents (Bar-Sela, Epelbaum, & Schaffer, 2010).

Fish Oil

Supplementation with fish oil has been of particular interest for use in the pancreatic cancer population. Although early studies showed promise that high doses of eicosapentaenoic acid (EPA) may mitigate cancer cachexia syndrome, other studies have refuted this information (Natural Medicines Comprehensive Database, 2012a). Many of the early studies were nonrandomized, noncontrolled studies of small subject pools. Moses, Slater, Preston, Barber, and Fearon (2004) conducted a randomized, double-blind trial of 24 patients (50% consumed a supplement enriched with EPA and 50% consumed an isocaloric isonitrogenous supplement without EPA) and found no significant changes from baseline weight, lean body mass, or physical activity in either the experimental or control group. An evaluation of plasma EPA concentration showed that four of the control subjects had high levels of EPA, suggesting intake from another source. Ad hoc analysis showed the high-EPA group (including the four control subjects) to have an increase in physical activity level but still no significant increase in weight or lean body mass (Moses et al., 2004). Jatoi and colleagues (2004) found no improvement in weight, survival, or quality of life when EPA was supplemented alone or in combination with megestrol acetate compared with the use of megestrol acetate alone.

Survivorship

For patients who have completed curative therapy and have no evidence of disease, it is important to address additional nutrition issues that may occur as long-term consequences of cancer therapy, including surgery.

Additional Nutrient Deficiency Risks

In addition to the fat-soluble vitamin deficiencies related to malabsorption discussed earlier, other nutrient deficiencies may be related to alterations in the GI tract after some surgeries for pancreatic and hepatobiliary cancers. Because calcium generally is absorbed by the duodenum, patients may be at higher risk for calcium malabsorption and subsequent osteoporosis after undergoing a Whipple procedure. Zinc and iron may also be deficient after such a surgery. Zinc, similar to calcium, is generally absorbed in the duodenum. Iron may not be converted to an active form in the stomach because of the reduction in stomach acid (Thomas, 2006). Although calcium, zinc, and iron may be deficient because of anatomic changes, there is no suggestion in the current literature for prophylactic oral replacement of these minerals beyond the dietary reference intakes as determined by the Food and Nutrition Board of the Institute of Medicine (2001). It is reasonable to monitor patients for serum deficiencies (or patterns of deficiency) of zinc and iron and for radiographic evidence of abnormalities in bone mineral density and to treat as necessary.

Diet and Physical Activity

After completion of treatment and recovery, it is recommended that survivors follow the same guidelines for cancer prevention as are recommended for those who have never had cancer. Following these guidelines may help to prevent secondary cancers or recurrent disease. Minimizing the known lifestyle risk factors by following a plant-based diet and being physically active is ideal (World Cancer Research Fund & American Institute for Cancer Research, 2007).

Summary

Although the prognosis for patients with pancreatic or hepatobiliary cancers is poor, nutrition interventions can improve treatment outcomes and empower patients and families to play an active role in their care. For those patients who do survive long term, the nutrition implications of the disease and treatments are likely to endure for the rest of their lives. Nurses, dietitians, and other healthcare providers should expect to help patients cope with nutrition issues throughout the course of treatment and survivorship.

References

Adler, D.G., & Baron, T.H. (2002). Endoscopic palliation of malignant gastric outlet obstruction using self-expanding metal stents: Experience in 36 patients. *American Journal of Gastroenterology, 97,* 72–78. doi:10.1111/j.1572-0241.2002.05423.x

A.S.P.E.N. Board of Directors & the Clinical Guidelines Task Force. (2002). Guidelines for the use of parenteral and enteral nutrition in adult and pediatric patients. *Journal of Parenteral and Enteral Nutrition, 26*(Suppl. 1), 1SA–138SA.

Babayan, V.K. (1987). Medium chain triglycerides and structured lipids. *Lipids, 22,* 417–420. doi:10.1007/BF02537271

Bar-Sela, G., Epelbaum, R., & Schaffer, M. (2010). Curcumin as an anticancer agent: Review of the gap between basic and clinical applications. *Current Medicinal Chemistry, 17,* 190–197.

Bauer, J., Capra, S., & Ferguson, M. (2002). Use of the scored Patient-Generated Subjective Global Assessment (PG-SGA) as a nutrition assessment tool in patients with cancer. *European Journal of Clinical Nutrition, 56,* 779–785. doi:10.1038/sj.ejcn.1601412

Berendt, M., & D'Agostino, S. (2005). Alterations in nutrition. In J.K. Itano & K.N. Taoka (Eds.), *Core curriculum for oncology nursing* (4th ed., pp. 277–317). St. Louis, MO: Elsevier Saunders.

Berk, L., James, J., Schwartz, A., Hug, E., Mahadevan, A., Samuels, M., ... Kachnic, L. (2008). A randomized, double-blind, placebo-controlled trial of a beta-hydroxyl beta-methyl butyrate, glutamine, and arginine mixture for the treatment of cancer cachexia (RTOG 0122). *Supportive Care in Cancer, 16,* 1179–1188. doi:10.1007/s00520-008-0403-7

Bowles, T.L., Kim, R., Galante, J., Parsons, C.M., Virudachalam, S., Kung, H.J., ... Bold, R.J. (2008). Pancreatic cancer cell lines deficient in argininosuccinate synthetase are sensitive to arginine deprivation by arginine deiminase. *International Journal of Cancer, 123,* 1950–1955. doi:10.1002/ijc.23723

Bozzetti, F., Biganzoli, L., Gavazzi, C., Cappuzzo, F., Carnaghi, C., Buzzoni, R., ... Baietta, E. (1997). Glutamine supplementation in cancer patients receiving chemotherapy: A double-blind randomized study. *Nutrition, 13,* 748–751. doi:10.1016/S0899-9007(97)83038-9

Bruera, E. (1997). ABC of palliative care. Anorexia, cachexia, and nutrition. *BMJ, 315,* 1219–1222. doi:10.1136/bmj.315.7117.1219

Cao, D.X., Wu, G.H., Zhang, B., Quan, Y.J., Wei, J., Jin, H., ... Yang, Z.A. (2010). Resting energy expenditure and body composition in patients with newly detected cancer. *Clinical Nutrition, 29,* 72–77. doi:10.1016/j.clnu.2009.07.001

Daniele, B., Perrone, F., Gallo, C., Pignata, S., De Martino, S., De Vivo, R., ... D'Agostino, L. (2001). Oral glutamine in the prevention of fluorouracil induced intestinal toxicity: A double blind, placebo controlled, randomised trial. *Gut, 48,* 28–33. doi:10.1136/gut.48.1.28

Dhillon, N., Aggarwal, B.B., Newman, R.A., Wolff, R.A., Kunnumakkara, A.B., Abbruzzese, J.L., ... Kurzrock, R. (2008). Phase II trial of curcumin in patients with advanced pancreatic cancer. *Clinical Cancer Research, 14,* 4491–4499. doi:10.1158/1078-0432.CCR-08-0024

DiMagno, E.P., Reber, H.A., & Tempero, M.A. (1999). AGA technical review on the epidemiology, diagnosis, and treatment of pancreatic ductal adenocarcinoma. *Gastroenterology, 117,* 1464–1484. doi:10.1016/S0016-5085(99)70298-2

Dormann, A., Meisner, S., Verin, N., & Lang, A. (2004). Self-expanding metal stents for gastroduodenal malignancies: Systematic review of their clinical effectiveness. *Endoscopy, 36,* 543–550. doi:10.1055/s-2004-814434

Elliott, L., Molseed, L.L., McCallum, P.D., & Grant, B. (2006). Appendix A. In L. Elliott, L.L. Molseed, P.D. McCallum, & B. Grant (Eds.), *The clinical guide to oncology nutrition* (2nd ed., pp. 241–245). Chicago, IL: American Dietetic Association.

Ellison, N.M., Chevlen, E., Still, C.D., & Dubagunta, S. (2002). Supportive care for patients with pancreatic adenocarcinoma: Symptom control and nutrition. *Hematology/Oncology Clinics of North America, 16,* 105–121.

Falconer, J.S., Fearon, K.C., Plester, C.E., Ross, J.A., & Carter, D.C. (1994). Cytokines, the acute-phase response, and resting energy expenditure in cachectic patients with pancreatic cancer. *Annals of Surgery, 219,* 325–331. Retrieved from http://www.ncbi.nlm.nih.gov/pmc/articles/PMC1243147/?tool=pubmed

Ferguson, M.L., Bauer, J., Gallagher, B., Capra, S., Christie, D.R., & Mason, B.R. (1999). Validation of a malnutrition screening tool for patients receiving radiotherapy. *Australasian Radiology, 43,* 325–327. doi:10.1046/j.1440-1673.1999.433665.x

Ferguson, M.L., Capra, S., Bauer, J., & Banks, M. (1999). Development of a valid and reliable malnutrition screening tool for adult acute hospital patients. *Nutrition, 15,* 458–464. doi:10.1016/S0899-9007(99)00084-2

Gaidos, J.K., & Draganov, P.V. (2009). Treatment of malignant gastric outlet obstruction with endoscopically placed self-expandable metal stents. *World Journal of Gastroenterology, 15,* 4365–4371. doi:10.3748/wjg.15.4365

Glazer, E.S., Piccirillo, M., Albino, V., Di Giacomo, R., Palaia, R., Mastro, A.A., ... Izzo, F. (2010). Phase II study of pegylated arginine deiminase for nonresectable and metastatic hepatocellular carcinoma. *Journal of Clinical Oncology, 28,* 2220–2226. doi:10.1200/JCO.2009.26.7765

Guy, J.L., & Smith, T.R. (2005). Pancreatic cancer. In V.J. Kogut & S.L. Luthringer (Eds.), *Nutritional issues in cancer care* (pp. 139–152). Pittsburgh, PA: Oncology Nursing Society.

Hassanain, M., Schricker, T., Metrakos, P., Carvalho, G., Vrochides, D., & Lattermann, R. (2008). Hepatic protection by perioperative metabolic support? *Nutrition, 24,* 1217–1219. doi:10.1016/j.nut.2008.05.019

Heyneman, C.A. (1996). Zinc deficiency and taste disorders. *Annals of Pharmacotherapy, 30,* 186–187.

Holmes, S. (2009). A difficult clinical problem: Diagnosis, impact and clinical management of cachexia in palliative care. *International Journal of Palliative Nursing, 15,* 320, 322–326.

Huhmann, M.B., & August, D.A. (2008). Review of American Society for Parenteral and Enteral Nutrition (ASPEN) Clinical Guidelines for Nutrition Support in Cancer Patients: Nutrition screening and assessment. *Nutrition in Clinical Practice, 23,* 182–188. doi:10.1177/0884533608314530

Hurst, J.D., & Gallagher, A.L. (2006). Energy, macronutrient, micronutrient, and fluid requirements. In L. Elliott, L.L. Molseed, P.D. McCallum, & B. Grant (Eds.), *The clinical guide to oncology nutrition* (2nd ed., pp. 54–71). Chicago, IL: American Dietetic Association.

Institute of Medicine. (2001). Dietary reference intakes: Elements. Retrieved from http://www.iom.edu/Global/News%20Announcements/~/media/48FAAA2FD9E74D95BBDA2236E7387B49.ashx

Isenring, E., Cross, G., Daniels, L., Kellett, E., & Koczwara, B. (2006). Validity of the Malnutrition Screening Tool as an effective predictor of nutritional risk in oncology outpatients receiving chemotherapy. *Supportive Care in Cancer, 14,* 1152–1156. doi:10.1007/s00520-006-0070-5

James, H.C., & Kulakowski, K.P. (2005). Hepatobiliary cancer. In V.J. Kogut & S.L. Luthringer (Eds.), *Nutritional issues in cancer care* (pp. 117–125). Pittsburgh, PA: Oncology Nursing Society.

Jatoi, A., Rowland, K., Loprinzi, C.L., Sloan, J.A., Dakhil, S.R., MacDonald, N., ... Christensen, B. (2004). An eicosapentaenoic acid supplement versus megestrol acetate versus both for patients with cancer-associated wasting: A North Central Cancer Treatment Group and National Cancer Institute of Canada collaborative effort. *Journal of Clinical Oncology, 22,* 2469–2476. doi:10.1200/JCO.2004.06.024

Kozelsky, T.F., Meyers, G.E., Sloan, J.A., Shanahan, T.G., Dick, S.J., Moore, R.L., ... Martenson, J.A. (2003). Phase III double-blind study of glutamine versus placebo for the prevention of acute diarrhea in patients receiving pelvic radiation therapy. *Journal of Clinical Oncology, 21,* 1669–1674. doi:10.1200/JCO.2003.05.060

Kubrak, C., & Jensen, L. (2007). Critical evaluation of nutrition screening tools recommended for oncology patients. *Cancer Nursing, 30,* E1–E6. doi:10.1097/01.NCC.0000290818.45066.00

Layer, P., Keller, J., & Lankisch, P.G. (2001). Pancreatic enzyme replacement therapy. *Current Gastroenterology Reports, 3,* 101–108.

Leung, J., & Silverman, W. (2009). Diagnostic and therapeutic approach to pancreatic cancer-associated gastroparesis: Literature review and our experience. *Digestive Diseases and Sciences, 54,* 401–405. doi:10.1007/s10620-008-0354-3

Luthringer, S.L. (2006). Nutritional implications of radiation therapy. In L. Elliott, L.L. Molseed, P.D. McCallum, & B. Grant (Eds.), *The clinical guide to oncology nutrition* (2nd ed., pp. 88–93). Chicago, IL: American Dietetic Association.

Ly, J., O'Grady, G., Mittal, A., Plank, L., & Windsor, J.A. (2009). A systematic review of methods to palliate malignant gastric outlet obstruction. *Surgical Endoscopy, 24,* 290–297. doi:10.1007/s00464-009-0577-1

Matsumoto, J., & Traverso, L.W. (2006). Exocrine function following the Whipple operation as assessed by stool elastase. *Journal of Gastrointestinal Surgery, 10,* 1225–1229. doi:10.1016/j.gassur.2006.08.001

McCallum, P.D. (2006). Nutrition screening and assessment in oncology. In L. Elliott, L.L. Molseed, P.D. McCallum, & B. Grant (Eds.), *The clinical guide to oncology nutrition* (2nd ed., pp. 44–53). Chicago, IL: American Dietetic Association.

McCallum, P.D., Walsh, D., & Nelson, K.A. (2002). Can a soft diet prevent bowel obstruction in advanced pancreatic cancer? *Supportive Care in Cancer, 10,* 174–175. doi:10.1007/s005200100307

McMahon, K., Decker, G., & Ottery, F.D. (1998). Integrating proactive nutritional assessment in clinical practices to prevent complications and cost. *Seminars in Oncology, 25*(2, Suppl. 6), 20–27.

Morley, J.E. (2007, July). Nutrition: General considerations. *The Merck manual online.* Retrieved from http://www.merck.com/mmpe/sec01/ch001/ch001b.html?qt=nutrition&alt=sh

Moses, A.W., Slater, C., Preston, T., Barber, M.D., & Fearon, K.C. (2004). Reduced total energy expenditure and physical activity in cachectic patients with pancreatic cancer can be modulated by an energy and protein dense oral supplement enriched with n-3 fatty acids. *British Journal of Cancer, 90,* 996–1002. doi:10.1038/sj.bjc.6601620

Murphy, J., Stacey, D., Crook, J., Thompson, B., & Panetta, D. (2000). Testing control of radiation-induced diarrhea with a psyllium bulking agent: A pilot study. *Canadian Oncology Nursing Journal, 10,* 96–100.

National Cancer Institute. (2011, November 30). Nutrition in cancer care (PDQ®) [Health professional version]. Retrieved from http://www.cancer.gov/cancertopics/pdq/supportivecare/nutrition/Health Professional

Natural Medicines Comprehensive Database. (2012a). Fish oil. Retrieved from http://naturaldatabase.therapeuticresearch.com/nd/Search.aspx?cs=&s=ND&pt=100&id=993&ds=&lang=0

Natural Medicines Comprehensive Database. (2012b). Lactobacillus. Retrieved from http://naturaldatabase.therapeuticresearch.com/nd/Search.aspx?cs=&s=ND&pt=100&id=790&ds=&name=LACTOBACILLUS&lang=0&searchid=35371890

Natural Medicines Comprehensive Database. (2012c). Turmeric. Retrieved from http://naturaldatabase.therapeuticresearch.com/nd/Search.aspx?cs=&s=ND&pt=100&id=662&ds=&name=TURMERIC&lang=0&searchid=35371890

Office of Dietary Supplements. (2011, September 20). Dietary supplement fact sheet: Zinc [Health professional version]. Retrieved from http://ods.od.nih.gov/factsheets/zinc.asp

Ottery, F. (1996a). Definition of standardized nutritional assessment and interventional pathways in oncology. *Nutrition, 12*(Suppl. 1), S15–S19. doi:10.1016/0899-9007(95)00067-4

Ottery, F. (1996b). Supportive nutritional management of the patient with pancreatic cancer. *Oncology, 10*(Suppl. 9), 26–32. Retrieved from http://www.cancernetwork.com/display/article/10165/98628

Pelzer, U., Arnold, D., Gövercin, M., Stieler, J., Doerken, B., Riess, H., ... Oettle, H. (2010). Parenteral nutrition support for patients with pancreatic cancer: Results of a phase II study. *BioMed Central Cancer, 10,* 86. doi:10.1186/1471-2407-10-86

Perez, M.M., Newcomer, A.D., Moertel, C.G., Go, V.L., & Dimagno, E.P. (1983). Assessment of weight loss, food intake, fat metabolism, malabsorption, and treatment of pancreatic insufficiency in pancreatic cancer. *Cancer, 52,* 346–352. doi:10.1002/1097-0142(19830715)52:2<346::AID-CNCR2820520228>3.0.CO;2-Z

Petree, J.M. (2005). Supportive care: Support therapies and procedures. In J.K. Itano & K.N. Taoka (Eds.), *Core curriculum for oncology nursing* (4th ed., pp. 137–160). St. Louis, MO: Elsevier Saunders.

Prasad, A.S. (1985). Clinical manifestations of zinc deficiency. *Annual Review of Nutrition, 5,* 341–363. doi:10.1146/annurev.nu.05.070185.002013

Richardson, M.A., Sanders, T., Palmer, J.L., Greisinger, A., & Singletary, S.E. (2000). Complementary/alternative medicine use in a comprehensive cancer center and the implications for oncology. *Journal of Clinical Oncology, 18,* 2505–2514.

Riechelmann, R.P., Burman, D., Tannock, I.F., Rodin, G., & Zimmermann, C. (2009). Phase II trial of mirtazapine for cancer-related cachexia and anorexia. *American Journal of Hospice and Palliative Care, 27,* 106–110. doi:10.1177/1049909109345685

Robinson, C.A. (2006). Enteral nutrition in adult oncology. In L. Elliott, L.L. Molseed, P.D. McCallum, & B. Grant (Eds.), *The clinical guide to oncology nutrition* (2nd ed., pp. 138–155). Chicago, IL: American Dietetic Association.

Sarner, M. (2003). Treatment of pancreatic exocrine deficiency. *World Journal of Surgery, 27,* 1192–1195. doi:10.1007/s00268-003-7237-8

Savy, G.K. (2002). Glutamine supplementation: Heal the gut, help the patient. *Journal of Infusion Nursing, 25,* 65–69. doi:10.1097/00129804-200201000-00010

Schulz, G.J., Campos, A.C., & Coelho, J.C. (2008). The role of nutrition in hepatic encephalopathy. *Current Opinion in Clinical Nutrition and Metabolic Care, 11,* 275–280. doi:10.1097/MCO.0b013e3282f9e870

Singh, B. (2007). Psyllium as therapeutic and drug delivery agent. *International Journal of Pharmaceutics, 334,* 1–14. doi:10.1016/j.ijpharm.2007.01.028

Speicher, J.E., & Traverso, L.W. (2010). Pancreatic exocrine function is preserved after distal pancreatectomy. *Journal of Gastrointestinal Surgery, 14,* 1006–1011. doi:10.1007/s11605-010-1184-0

Takaoka, T., Sarukura, N., Ueda, C., Kitamura, Y., Kalubi, B., Toda, N., … Takeda, N. (2010). Effects of zinc supplementation on serum zinc concentration and ratio of apo/holo-activities of angiotensin converting enzyme in patients with taste impairment. *Auris Nasus Larynx, 37,* 190–194. doi:10.1016/j.anl.2009.07.003

Theobald, D.E., Kirsh, K.L., Holtsclaw, E., Donaghy, K., & Passik, S.D. (2002). An open-label, crossover trial of mirtazapine (15 and 30 mg) in cancer patients with pain and other distressing symptoms. *Journal of Pain and Symptom Management, 23,* 442–447. Retrieved from http://www.jpsmjournal.com/article/S0885-3924(02)00381-0/fulltext

Thomas, S. (2006). Nutritional implications of surgical oncology. In L. Elliott, L.L. Molseed, P.D. McCallum, & B. Grant (Eds.), *The clinical guide to oncology nutrition* (2nd ed., pp. 94–109). Chicago, IL: American Dietetic Association.

Von Roenn, J.H. (2006). Pharmacological management of nutrition impact symptoms associated with cancer. In L. Elliott, L.L. Molseed, P.D. McCallum, & B. Grant (Eds.), *The clinical guide to oncology nutrition* (2nd ed., pp. 165–179). Chicago, IL: American Dietetic Association.

Wilkes, G.M., & Barton-Burke, M. (2010). *2010 oncology nursing drug handbook.* Burlington, MA: Jones and Bartlett.

World Cancer Research Fund & American Institute for Cancer Research. (2007). *Food, nutrition, physical activity, and the prevention of cancer: A global perspective.* Retrieved from http://www.dietandcancerreport.org/cancer_resource_center/downloads/Second_Expert_Report_full.pdf

CHAPTER 9

Advance Care Planning

Peter Miller, RN, BSN, PHN

Introduction

Patients with unresectable pancreatic or hepatobiliary cancers have a poor prognosis (National Cancer Institute [NCI], 2011). Anatomic location of the tumor and progression, recurrence, and relapse after treatment make palliative and hospice care an early necessity (NCI, 2011). Once patients are diagnosed with one of these cancers, it is important to initiate advance care planning discussions with them and their families.

Advance care planning is the process of planning for and carrying out advance directives, which document who will make decisions for the patient if he or she cannot and what types of care the patient would choose or decline in specific health situations. Advance care planning includes information about advance directives and making decisions about goals of care, extent of treatments, advanced life support, resuscitation, when to forgo treatments, and where to die. These discussions need to continue as the disease progresses and treatment goals change. Finally, the bereavement needs for those who will be left behind should be discussed.

Recommendations

The National Comprehensive Cancer Network (NCCN, 2012) palliative care guidelines list topics that should be discussed at least one year before the patient needs a definitive advance plan of care, including

- Fears and anxieties about the process of dying
- Palliative and hospice care
- The need for a surrogate decision maker based on the patient's decision-making capacity
- The patient's values and preferences for end-of-life care, including cardiopulmonary resuscitation, mechanical ventilation, and artificial nutrition and hydration, and congruence with the family's and health team's values and preferences
- Advance directives and do not resuscitate (DNR) options

- The need for the patient to discuss his or her wishes with the family
- The need for appointing a healthcare proxy or durable power of attorney for health care (dependent on the state in which the patient resides)
- The patient's wishes for organ donation or autopsy.

These discussions should be expanded as time progresses to address the patient's and family's preferences for the location of the patient's death; specific directives regarding the use of blood products, dialysis, and antibiotics; and reaching agreement to settle conflicts between the patient's and family's goals and wishes (NCCN, 2012). Alano and colleagues (2010) interviewed 200 individuals older than age 65 about advance directives and reported that 63% (125) had completed an advance directive. Five factors were associated with completing advance directives, including

- Belief that the advance directive would help to lessen suffering at end of life
- A personal request to complete the advance directive or receiving instruction on how to complete it
- Having major surgery
- Female gender
- Increasing age.

Ray et al. (2006) reported that 17.5% of the terminally ill patients (n = 280) with advanced cancer they studied expressed feeling peaceful while completely aware of their disease status and prognosis. When compared to patients who were peacefully aware, those who were not experienced more psychological distress and had lower rates of advance care planning. In postmortem assessments, survivors of peacefully aware patients reported better quality of death outcomes for the family member who died.

Ideally, advance care planning would take place and be documented years before the plan needs to be used, or at the time of diagnosis of any illness that is life threatening or debilitating (NCCN, 2012; National Consensus Project for Quality Palliative Care, 2009; Zoeller, 2011). Patients find relief in knowing that family members will not experience the additional stress and burden of having to make end-of-life care decisions for them (NCCN, 2012).

Barriers

Unfortunately, physicians frequently have difficulty discussing end-of-life issues, such as prognosis, DNR status, hospice, and preferred site of death with asymptomatic patients who have a four- to six-months' life expectancy (Keating et al., 2010). Keating and colleagues (2010) reported on a survey of 4,074 physicians in the United States, noting that 65% said they would discuss prognosis and possible additional treatments right away, although discussing prognosis does not guarantee that the patient will begin to discuss end-of-life issues. Forty-four percent of the physicians surveyed would discuss DNR status, 26% would discuss hospice, and only 21% would discuss where the patient would like to die (e.g., home, hospice). Younger physicians, surgeons, and oncologists were more apt to initiate the discussions. Most of the physicians confirmed their preference to wait to initiate end-of-life discussions until the patient became symptomatic or all possible treatments had been tried and proved unsuccessful (Keating et al., 2010). As a result, advance care planning discussions may fall to the nurse, social worker, or clergy. They may initiate discussions with patients and their families and coach them about talking with the physician.

Barriers to advance care planning discussions identified by Keating and colleagues (2010) include unrealistic patient expectations, lack of physician training in end-of-life care discussions, and lack of understanding of patients' wishes for their care at the end of their life. For example, patients who continue or insist on treatment for advanced cancer may have unrealistic expectations of remission or cure despite successive poor responses to treatment. Physicians who have not received training in end-of-life discussions may be uncomfortable initiating those discussions and put them off.

Fine, Reid, Shengelia, and Adelman (2010) conducted a descriptive thematic analysis of 20 articles that used direct observation techniques such as audiotaping or videotaping to record physician-patient discussions at the end of life. Four themes were revealed, including (a) physicians focused on technical topics and avoided emotional and quality-of-life (QOL) issues, (b) physicians correctly perceived sensitive topics to take longer to discuss, (c) physicians dominated the discussions, and (d) patient and family satisfaction was associated with supportive physician behaviors, such as participation and support (Fine et al., 2010). Desharnais, Carter, Hennessy, Kurent, and Carter (2007) cited additional reasons that physicians may not engage in end-of-life care discussions, including (a) physicians may be in denial about the patient dying, (b) physicians may not be aware of hospice resources in the community to which they can refer the patient, (c) physicians may not know the patient well and erroneously believe that the patient will not find end-of-life care options acceptable, thereby electing to avoid the discussion completely, and (d) physicians may believe they do not have the time to engage the patient and family in a lengthy conversation about end-of-life care. Research testing the agreement between physicians and terminally ill patients during end-of-life care discussions revealed discrepancies regarding patients' preferences for pain control and place of death and the understanding of religious and financial issues that affect other patient preferences (Desharnais et al., 2007).

Not being able to talk with a patient about stopping treatment and providing end-of-life care will result in a lack of understanding of the patient's hopes and expectations and may create a situation where the patient's wishes are not followed. Healthcare professionals need to be able to share information in a developmentally appropriate and effective manner that includes shared decision making and use of communication skills such as active listening (Mohan, Alexander, Garrigues, Arnold, & Barnato, 2010; National Consensus Project for Quality Palliative Care, 2009; Weiner & Cole, 2004). It is imperative for physicians to receive assistance in overcoming emotional, cognitive, and skill barriers; to employ the multidisciplinary collaboration of social workers, nurses, psychiatrists, psychologists, and clergy; and to provide information in a sensitive, therapeutic manner so patients can maintain hope while receiving full support with advance care planning (Thorne, Oglov, Armstrong, & Hislop, 2007; Weiner & Cole, 2004). Referrals to multidisciplinary team members can be particularly beneficial to the physician and patient in the absence of a bona fide palliative care program.

Initiating Advance Planning

Beginning advance planning starts with finding common ground. What are the goals of treatment? What life activities does the patient want to complete? The Oregon Health and Science University (2011) guide for professionals and the Coalition for Compassionate Care of California (2009) conversation guides offer some suggestions to initiate the conversation with loved ones, including sharing an article or recent broadcast on the subject and inquiring about their emotional reaction to it or talking to them about the recent death of someone they knew and asking: Is that the kind of care you would like? Figure 9-1 lists additional questions for loved ones that might be helpful in determining preferences for end-of-life care.

The Agency for Healthcare Research and Quality (AHRQ) recognized that healthcare providers may not be certain about when to initiate advance care planning, aware of the presence of a living will or durable power of attorney in the patient's medical record, or know when to update these documents (Kass-Bartelmes, Hughes, & Rutherford, 2003). Kass-Bartelmes and colleagues (2003) developed a five-step plan to help physicians start—and continue—talking with their pa-

---

> ### Figure 9-1. Questions to Ask a Loved One About Advance Care Planning
>
> - What are your hopes and ideas about the end of life?
> - What are your fears and concerns regarding dying?
> - Have you thought about the care you would like to have or not have in a serious illness or as you are dying?
> - Have you thought about what kind of funeral arrangements you would like?
> - Do you believe life should be preserved at all costs? Or do you think there are situations where life-prolonging treatments should be restricted, such as experiencing severe pain or being unable to recognize important relationships?
> - Is there someone who could speak for you if you became unable that you would trust to follow your wishes?
> - Why not make decisions now when you are healthy enough to make them?
>
> *Note.* From "Advance Care Planning—Conversation Guide," by the Coalition for Compassionate Care of California, 2009, retrieved from http://www.coalitionccc.org/_pdf/Conversation_Guide.pdf. Adapted with permission.

tients about end-of-life care. The first step is to *start with a guided discussion* of the patient's illness where the physician could share hypothetical outcomes of treatment. The physician could then ascertain the patient's preferences to treat or not treat in the hypothetical outcomes and begin to develop a sense of the patient's personal preferences and values. It is important for the physician to help the patient understand the actual chances of a positive outcome with particular circumstances, for example, survival once artificial ventilation or nutrition is initiated. The second step is to *introduce the subject of advance care planning and offer information.* The physician should review the patient's preferences with the patient and his or her loved ones, ensuring that all of the patient's and family's questions about life-sustaining treatment are answered. The physician should *verify that the patient has an advance directive and power of attorney form to review and complete*, which is the third step; assistance in completing the forms is available through social services or clergy. Additional information about advance planning forms will be discussed later. The fourth step is to *review the patient's preferences on a regular basis and update documentation.* Patients have the right to change their decisions, and the advance directives may be revised at any time or as the situation changes. Last, *apply the patient's desires to the actual circumstances* that lead to the patient's death (Kass-Bartelmes et al., 2003).

The National Consensus Project for Quality Palliative Care (2009) developed *Clinical Practice Guidelines for Quality Palliative Care* to give physicians a preplanned process for addressing specific elements of palliative care for patients at the end of life when a structured palliative care program is not established or available. Topics in the guidelines are divided into the following domains (National Consensus Project for Quality Palliative Care, 2009).

- Structure and process of care
- Physical aspects of care
- Psychosocial and psychiatric aspects of care
- Social aspects of care
- Spiritual, religious, and existential aspects of care
- Cultural aspects of care
- Care of the imminently dying patient
- Ethical and legal aspects of care

Additional information about the *Clinical Practice Guidelines for Quality Palliative Care* may be found at www.nationalconsensusproject.org/guidelines_download.asp.

Forms for Advance Planning

Once the patient's wishes are known, it is important to get the information onto a legal form. Several forms are currently used, including the following.

- *Living wills* or *advance directives* are legal documents in which individuals can exercise their autonomy by specifying what types of health care they want and do not want in the event they cannot make decisions or are incapacitated at the time they need care. Each state has documents specifically authorized for individuals to record those instructions for care. The forms are shared with both the family and physician (Coalition for Compassionate Care of California, 2009). Living wills/advance directives may also include a durable power of attorney (Kass-Bartelmes et al., 2003). Although an advance directive appoints a surrogate decision maker for the patient, it is not automatically translated into a physician's order (see POLST that follows).
- *Durable power of attorney for health care* (DPAHC) or healthcare proxy is a form where individuals can designate who they want to voice treatment decisions for them in the event they become incapacitated and cannot speak those decisions (Coalition for Compassionate Care of California, 2009). DPAHC forms can be very simple or very complex. The simple ones only require signatures of a notary public or witnesses who are not family members or caregivers. The more complex ones require a lawyer because these documents can become a part of larger power of attorney statement including financial assignments.
- *Advance healthcare directive* (AHCD) is a legal form in California that essentially combines the advance directive and DPAHC forms previously described. It enables residents in this state to specify instructions for future healthcare decisions and appoint a power of attorney for health care; either or both may be stipulated on the form (Coalition for Compassionate Care of California, 2005).

Newer forms include the *physician orders for life-sustaining treatments* (POLST) and the Five Wishes form. The selection of forms depends on laws in the state of the patient's home.

The POLST paradigm is the term developed by the Oregon Health and Science University to describe programs, forms, and policies nationwide that translate a patient's wishes for end-of-life care into portable and easily implemented physician's orders (Oregon Health and Science University, 2008). The POLST forms (sample forms are available at www.ohsu .edu/polst/programs/sample-forms.htm) were designed to help healthcare professionals discuss and develop patients' end-of-life wishes with them and to clearly state those wishes so physicians, rapid response, emergency department, and other healthcare personnel can know and implement those wishes (Oregon Health and Science University, 2008). POLST forms, however, do not replace an advance directive or DPAHC (California POLST, n.d.). The POLST forms have existed since the mid-1990s but are not available in all states. Various state coalitions have received state sanctioning. Currently, 21 states have no POLST programs. Each state individualizes its forms; for example, New York uses the term *medical orders for life-sustaining treatment* (or MOLST) that is based on Oregon's original paradigm (Oregon Health and Science University, 2010).

Five Wishes is a living will form that was introduced in 1997 and originally distributed with support from a grant by the Robert Wood Johnson Foundation. It is similar to the AHCD form used in California in that it stipulates care wishes and who can make healthcare decisions for the patient. The five wishes addressed in this comprehensive living will include (Aging with Dignity, 2011a)

- Identification of the person who will make decisions for the patient if the patient cannot
- Types of medical treatment the patient wants or does not want
- How comfortable the patient wants to be kept
- How the patient wants to be treated
- What the patient wants loved ones to know.

The Five Wishes form meets legal requirements in all but eight states: Alabama, Indiana, Kansas, New Hampshire, Ohio, Oregon, Texas, and Utah. In those states, statutory forms for advance care are available to use in tandem with the Five Wishes form. Skilled nursing facilities and mental hygiene facilities may require an addendum (Aging with Dignity, 2011b).

Advance care planning forms reflect the wishes of individuals who can change their mind at any time about previously made designations, revoke the old forms, and create new ones. It is important, therefore, for healthcare providers to discuss the forms with each patient on a regular basis to be certain that the most current version is being used.

Treatment

AHRQ (2003) reported that

Predicting what treatments patients will want at the end of life is complicated by the patient's age, the nature of the illness, the ability of medicine to sustain life, and the emotions families endure when their loved ones are sick and possibly dying.

When seriously ill patients are nearing the end of life, they and their families sometimes find it difficult to decide on whether to continue medical treatment and, if so, how much treatment is wanted and for how long. In these instances, patients rely on their physicians, or other trusted health professionals for guidance. (p. 1)

Medical culture is geared toward treating illness, and the intent of treatment must be discussed with the patient. The patient and his or her family should have a clear understanding of the status of the disease and the goals, risks, and benefits of treatment including how it will affect the patient's QOL (NCCN, 2012). A number of factors play a role in the delivery of treatments to patients who are likely to die in the months ahead. Patient incentives range from the possibility of prolonged survival, symptom improvement, the preservation of hope, or simply not wanting to "give up." Treatment might seem appealing if the physician assures the patient that side effects will be closely monitored and managed.

In the course of a life-threatening illness such as cancer, the need for life-prolonging treatments decreases as the need for palliative care increases (National Consensus Project for Quality Palliative Care, 2009). Advanced hepatobiliary and pancreatic cancers have a poor prognosis. Therapies to ease symptoms can greatly affect a patient's QOL. Chemotherapy or less-toxic targeted therapies, radiation, surgery, stent placement, ablation, or nerve blocks may offer some benefit; the patient must be able to make informed decisions based on risk versus benefit. Patients should be instructed as to what distinguishes aggressive treatments aimed at cure from those that provide comfort care. For example, chemotherapy in certain advanced-stage cancers is deemed better than the best supportive care and may prolong survival (NCCN, 2012). Aggressive treatments at life's end must involve a sophisticated oncologic assessment that includes a review of the patient's goals of care; a discussion of the meaning of the treatment to the patient and family; an evaluation of the patient's vital organs, performance status, and serious comorbid conditions; and balancing the perspective of the patient and the oncologist (Mohammed & Peter, 2009; NCCN, 2012). Advance care planning involves keeping patients apprised of their situation so they can choose the best options available with symptom management and QOL always a reachable goal.

Treatment decisions may become difficult when determining whether the treatment is too great of a burden on the patient is a source of conflict between the physician and patient. Some institutions have devised futility-of-care policies for their ethics committees to intervene in such cases (Center for Practical Bioethics, 2006).

Kasman (2004) defined *medical futility* as "a clinical action serving no useful purpose in attaining a specified goal for a given patient with a threshold for success of less than 1%–5%" (p. 1055). It can also be defined using physiologic, benefit-centered, and utility terms. Is there physiologic benefit? Will the treatments benefit the patient? Will costs, money, or living situation requirements exceed measurable benefits? Many physicians feel that if they do not offer aggressive treatment, they are abandoning the patient (Keating et al., 2010) or will "diminish the patient's hope" (Escalante, Martin, Elting, & Rubenstein, 1997, p. 276). The healthcare provider can instead initiate a discussion of possible options such as focusing on comfort rather than cure and completing advance directives if that has not been done.

Another potential decision with administering treatment is where a person would want the treatments and where the treatments could be given. Palliative care and hospice care can be delivered in many different settings. As palliative care becomes more complex, inpatient settings become more likely as palliative care uses more intense therapies such as certain infusion therapies. Related issues are the patient's ability to pay for the different settings and treatments, support systems available to the patient, available services, and tolerance to the treatments. Tamir, Singer, and Shvartzman (2007) found that

> Death at home occurred for 80.3% of the patients with access to homecare and 20.5% of those without access, that caring for a loved one at home was a greater financial and emotional burden, but there was a greater overall satisfaction with the caring experience of those whose loved ones died at home and had access to the homecare program. (p. 541)

In 2008, pancreatic cancer was the 16th top hospice diagnosis, including 21,944 patients, each with an average length of stay (LOS) in hospice of 38 days; in 1998 the total number of patients was 17,962 with an LOS of 43 days. Liver cancer was the 18th top diagnosis with an LOS of 37 days (Centers for Medicare and Medicaid Services, 2009). Hospice care is delivered in skilled nursing facilities, residential facilities, and homes, with some hospices owning hospice house facilities. The hospices of the Veterans Administration, Kaiser Permanente, and other institutions are associated with use of inpatient hospital services.

Akin to the decision of where to receive treatments is the patient's decision about where to die. According to NCCN (2012), most patients with cancer would prefer to die at home with hospice care, although some elect to receive end-of-life care as an inpatient at a hospital. Regardless of where patients wish to die, it is important for their wishes to be discussed and documented in an advance directive. This is particularly important to discuss and verify with the patient when it becomes evident that the patient has only months to weeks to live (NCCN, 2012) or at the point of disease progression or stopping treatment.

Stubenrauch (2010) interviewed Dr. Janet Abrahm of Harvard Medical School and Dana-Farber Cancer Institute about initiating or continuing aggressive treatment at the end of a patient's life. Abrahm noted that "the deeper issue is hope" (p. 4) and most physicians would do better to tell patients that

they are aware of and understand their hopes. From there, physicians can say that additional treatment would cause more distress than improvement and offer to help patients to focus their energy on accomplishing what is important to them in the time that remains.

Reframing Hope

Hope is a beneficial and very individualized part of coping. It has been linked to subjective psychosocial factors rather than physical factors (Rustøen et al., 2003; Utne et al., 2008). Hope for cure is very different from the hope that is a symbol for life in a dying patient (NCCN, 2012; Olsson, Östlund, Strang, Grassman, & Friedrichsen, 2011). Research has shown that hope helped patients to continue to live when they were close to death (Olsson et al., 2011). However, it can extend the dying process if false (Center for Practical Bioethics, 2006). Therefore, as the patient's condition changes, so should the healthcare goals and hope for specific outcomes. Reframing hope involves helping the patient understand the status of the disease, identifying priorities that are meaningful to the patient, and reflecting on how the disease has changed his or her focus in life. It is a process that should continue as the disease progresses, despite treatment.

Although discussions of healthcare goals and hope should always start at diagnosis, they also need to be held at critical junctures. Healthcare providers and patients must agree ahead of time when that will be (at recurrence, progression, end of treatment), how the patient's previous healthcare wishes compare to the current situation, what patient values may be affected with the current treatment options, and how the process has met the patient's needs to the present time (Mohammed & Peter, 2009; NCCN, 2011).

Tools to Predict Prognosis

Knowing the signs of disease progression is critical in initiating additional advance care planning discussions with the patient and family. Providing them with clear prognostic information will empower them to make informed and appropriate decisions about end-of-life care (NCCN, 2012). Although no universally accepted prognostic marker or scale for pancreatic/hepatobiliary cancer exists, many methods are available to predict prognosis. Anatomic and nonanatomic patient variables that can help clinicians to determine prognosis include the health status of the patient (known as performance status [PS]), QOL, the specific biologic properties of the cancer, serum markers, and bioimpedance spectroscopy (Crawford, Robinson, Hunt, Piller, & Esterman, 2009; FACIT.org, 2010b).

The Karnofsky and Eastern Cooperative Oncology Group (ECOG) PS scales are most commonly used in clinical practice, and PS is known to affect a patient's prognosis and treatment (Viale, 2009). Ongoing evaluation of the patient's PS and response to treatment can help the healthcare provider predict prognosis to an even greater degree.

The Functional Assessment of Cancer Therapy–Hepatobiliary (FACT-Hep) form is a QOL questionnaire developed for patients with hepatobiliary cancers based on the original Functional Assessment of Chronic Illness Therapy (FACIT) form (FACIT.org, 2010a). Questions are divided into four primary QOL domains of well-being: physical, social and family, emotional, and functional, as well as addressing disease-specific symptoms. Symptoms assessed in the questionnaire for hepatobiliary and pancreatic cancers include abdominal cramping, anorexia, fatigue, pain, bowel issues, itch, jaundice, taste changes, dry mouth, and weight loss. Higher scores are indicative of a poorer patient prognosis. Steel, Eton, Cella, Olek, and Carr (2006) reported that an alkaline phosphate level greater than 147 U/L and a hemoglobin count less than 12 g/dl were associated with poor FACT-Hep results and a poorer patient prognosis.

Jamieson, Carter, McKay, and Oien (2011) conducted a systematic review and meta-analysis of the literature for possible immunohistochemistry-based biomarkers that might predict the prognosis of patients with pancreatic ductal adenocarcinoma who have undergone pancreaticoduodenectomy. More than 100 proteins, including BAX, Bcl-2, survivin, Ki-67, COX-2, and E-cadherin, appeared promising for the prediction of overall survival in patients with pancreatic ductal adenocarcinoma and met the reporting recommendations for tumor marker prognostic studies. However, more research is necessary.

Tissue factor (TF) is a transmembrane glycoprotein whose primary function is to trigger the blood coagulation cascade (Kasthuri, Taubman, & Mackman, 2009; Nitori et al., 2005). It is associated with normal physiologic functions such as intracellular signaling and a variety of pathophysiologic conditions such as inflammation, atherosclerosis, and cancer (Nitori et al., 2005). It is common knowledge that patients with cancer are prone to hypercoagulation and that patients with pancreatic cancer have one of the highest rates of venous thromboembolic events (VTE) (Nitori et al., 2005; Zwicker et al., 2009). Research in the last decade has expanded that knowledge. It is now known that TF expressed by tumors is reported to have a key role in thrombosis, tumor growth, metastasis, and tumor angiogenesis (Kasthuri et al., 2009; Khorana et al., 2007; Nitori et al., 2005; Zwicker et al., 2009). Specifically, in patients with pancreatic cancer, TF expression is strikingly increased when compared to normal epithelium and has been found to play a role in modulating the biologic behavior of cancer cells (Nitori et al., 2005). High TF expression is associated with a 26% VTE rate compared with low TF expression and a 4.5% VTE rate (Khorana et al., 2007). Few deaths are related to VTE; therefore, poor prognosis is associated with high TF expression independent of thrombo-

sis (Nitori et al., 2005), and TF occurs early in neoplastic development and is associated with vascular endothelial growth factor expression, increased microvessel density, and possibly tumor angiogenesis (Khorana et al., 2007). Essentially, TF expression predicts poor survival in patients with resected pancreatic cancer. This is vital information in identifying patients who might benefit from aggressive treatment or molecular targeting therapy (Nitori et al., 2005).

Tanaka and colleagues (2008) identified the following six factors as closely associated with longer survival in Japanese patients with advanced pancreatic cancer treated with single-agent gemcitabine as first-line therapy: (a) stage III or less of the cancer, (b) Karnofsky PS of 90 and 100, (c) serum hemoglobin level greater than 10 g/dl, (d) serum C-reactive protein level less than 5.0 mg/dl, (e) a serum carcinoembryonic antigen level less than 10 ng/ml, and (f) serum CA 19-9 level less than 10,000 U/ml. The Corridor Group, Inc. (2006) identified guidelines for access to hospice care, including advanced liver disease (serum albumin level less than 2.5 g/dl with ascites or hepatorenal syndrome) and renal failure (elevated blood urea nitrogen and creatinine, less than 400 cc urine/24 hours, urine sodium concentration less than 10 mEq/L), which indicate poor prognosis. Viganò, Dorgan, Buckingham, Bruera, and Suarez-Almazor (2000) performed a literature review and reported a correlation between several factors and poor patient survival: a poor Karnofsky score, and the presence of edema, anorexia, weight loss, cognitive impairment, xerostomia, and dysphagia. Goebel (2010) reported that anorexia-cachexia syndrome, which is characterized by unintentional weight loss and wasting of body tissues (cachexia), decreased appetite (anorexia), and weakness, is associated with physical and emotional distress, poor QOL, and increased mortality in patients with advanced cancer.

Bioimpedance spectroscopy is a tool that evaluates body composition and has been assessed for its usefulness in predicting prognosis. Bioimpedance spectroscopy examines the drop in voltage when a constant alternating current flows through the human body (Crawford et al., 2009). The impedance or opposition to the current is composed of resistance, which is the opposition to the current flow in body fluids, and reactance, which is the opposition to current flow due to cell membranes and tissues. Bioimpedance spectroscopy can identify fluid and fat composition and rates of change in different parts of the body up to 10 months before they are evident in physical examination (Crawford et al., 2009). This is helpful to determine what kind of weight loss has occurred: minerals, fat, muscle, fluids, or a combination of each. Measurements are based on specific body parts, the limbs, and the trunk. The Crawford et al. (2009) study did not demonstrate a linear change for predicting patient prognosis but identified what the authors referred to as *tipping points* where clinical progression would be expected to occur much more rapidly (i.e., basal metabolism greater than 1,600 kcal/day, an extracellular to intracellular fluid ratio greater than 1 to 1.67). They did not find a tipping point for changes in fat, protein, or mineral composition but concluded that more research was indicated. Bioimpedance is seen in some of the newer home scales, and the more complete tests are no more uncomfortable than an electrocardiogram.

Reframing Hope

Several methods are available to reframe or redefine hope, including helping the patient to define meaning in life, develop a legacy, and conduct a life review. To fully implement these methods, a psychotherapist or psychiatrist should be consulted. It is essential to create a relaxed, accepting environment, assure the patient of confidentiality, and have the patient's symptoms controlled before he or she can focus well on the past. The first method is to find out what gives meaning to the patient and how cancer has or has not changed it. The patient is encouraged to "relax and name three things that [he or she is] responsible for, three things that are beautiful, and three or four things that still make [him or her] laugh" (Breitbart & Heller, 2003, p. 982). Time is provided for the patient to reflect on these things, share what about them gives meaning to the patient, and if or how the cancer has changed that meaning.

Dignity therapy or developing a legacy can be helpful, documenting the patient's history, or story (Breitbart & Heller, 2003; Stetka & Irwin, 2011).

> Dignity therapy is a brief psychotherapy where the therapist asks the patient a series of questions such as: When did you feel most alive? What are things you would like people to learn from your life? What are some times that weren't so great for you? What were your brushes with fame? (Stetka & Irwin, 2011, p. 5)

The patient's answers are recorded and written out and then compiled and returned to the patient for editing. The patient then adds a title and a concluding or summary statement; the finished booklet is given to the patient to keep. Patients who have participated in dignity therapy report experiencing a greater sense of dignity and self-esteem. They rekindle an increased will to live and report fewer symptoms of depression (Stetka & Irwin, 2011). Some patients will express their story in religious terms and may need a chaplain or clergy to help with the process. Others may use this to look beyond themselves and their current situation in useful ways that they wish to share with others (Breitbart & Heller, 2003). Stetka and Irwin (2011) reported that the family of a patient in their care elected to display the booklet at a memorial service.

Verbal life review is another technique to help reframe hope that does not involve documentation of the patient's story. It offers the patient an opportunity to verbalize problems experienced, how he or she dealt with the problems, what worked and what did not, what emotions he or she experienced while dealing with the problems, and which were helpful and which were not. This gives the patient a chance to reexamine how he or she solved old problems and acknowledge feelings and

difficulties in dealing with them. Life review also allows the patient to recall things he or she wishes to share with family, even if those experiences were not good for the patient. It may be difficult for the patient to discuss past failures or mistakes without feeling depressed, as forgiveness of others and self can seem overwhelming. Jenko, Gonzalez, and Seymour (2009) noted that once patients accept their own mortality, their physical, emotional, and spiritual energy can be redirected to hope and goals.

Cultural and Religious Sensitivity

Nurses and healthcare providers should be culturally sensitive in advance care planning discussions with patients and families. Culturally sensitive advance care planning covers a wide range of topics right up to and encompassing the death of the patient and includes decision-making preferences and styles, customs and beliefs, the concept of a good death, after-death interventions, and bereavement support (NCCN, 2012).

Western culture generally accepts the view that individual patient autonomy is paramount for ethical decision making and problem solving. However, some cultures, such as those in Greece, Italy, China, and Ethiopia, view autonomy as isolating and burdensome to a patient who may be too sick and uninformed about his or her condition to be able to make meaningful choices (Johnstone & Kanitsaki, 2009). In these cultures, family decisions take precedence over individual decisions (NCCN, 2012). Therefore, a patient's individual decision would be viewed as causing disharmony in the family and would bring shame on the patient (Johnstone & Kanitsaki, 2009). Mohammed and Peter (2009) described cross-cultural, self-limiting autonomy in some cultures, such as Greek, Italian, Chinese, and Ethiopian, as heavily guided by the social practices and moral codes within that specific culture. The nurse will better understand what is important and of value to a patient if he or she is aware of the patient's cultural accountability in social networks and personal relationships. The physician or nurse needs to be sensitive to and identify for each patient who is making healthcare decisions, what information they would like the patient to have about his or her illness, or if that even is an issue (Johnstone & Kanitsaki, 2009; NCCN, 2012).

Similarly, a survey of 236 physicians (53% White; 28% Asian; 17% Black) revealed that 72% believed that ethnic groups have diverse views about advance directives and 58% were not familiar with the end-of-life preferences of African American patients (Wallace et al., 2007). Williams and colleagues (2010) used focus group interviews to explore cultural perceptions and expectations of 42 African American participants (50% patients with cancer and 50% caregivers). Results identified effective physician communication with the patient and decision making as important QOL indicators. Participants believed that it was the physician's responsibility to know the patient and family and customize to the communication of medical information accordingly. They also revealed that crucial to decision making was the patient and family having control over treatment selection.

Implementing culturally sensitive advance care plans as death approaches includes respecting the cultural customs and beliefs of the patient directly or through a cultural liaison such as a pastoral care counselor, professional translator, the patient's personal clergy, or representatives from the patient's cultural community. Culturally meaningful rituals should be encouraged and supported by healthcare providers as well as encouraging visits by children if that is culturally acceptable (NCCN, 2012).

NCCN (2012) describes a "good death" as "one where patients, families, and caregivers do not experience avoidable distress and suffering; that follows the patient's and family's wishes; and is consistent with clinical, cultural, and ethical standards" (p. PAL-31).

It is important for family members to witness and nurses to administer culturally sensitive, respectful treatment of the patient's body immediately after death. Family members should be provided time with the body in a private setting. Family concerns about autopsy or organ donations should be addressed and, if an autopsy is not to be done, implanted devices may need to be removed. At that time, it will be essential to support the family as they arrange funeral and memorial services in accordance with the patient's personal values and cultural beliefs (NCCN, 2012).

A question that may come up in some cultures is where to place the "blame of death" when medical treatment fails. In particular, tension may be created among family members about whether to allow death to occur naturally, which would allow the family to attribute the cause of death to a failure of the patient's body, or hastening death through withholding or withdrawing treatment, which may shift the "blame" to the family member who made the decision or the doctor (Mohammed & Peter, 2009). Helping the patient and family understand that withholding or withdrawing treatment will allow the body to progress to death naturally may decrease some tension and help the patient to make culturally acceptable healthcare decisions as the disease progresses (Mohammed & Peter, 2009).

When considering a patient's culture, it is important to explore the individual's spiritual beliefs about the end of life. Not all patients are associated with organized religions, but spiritual concerns should not be neglected. Religion can sometimes affect healthcare decisions. Babgi's (2009) study of Saudis and the Muslim religion revealed beliefs that life cannot be ended without Allah's permission, illness is a trial or a test of faith from Allah, and illness is intended as a cleansing by Him, not as a punishment. The Saudis believed that they were obligated to seek treatment and to not terminate their life early and that an afterlife awaits them. In Islam, death is a natural process and "a truth that everyone will taste" (Babgi, 2009, p. 122).

A useful assessment tool is the FICA Spiritual History Tool that uses structured questions to obtain the spiritual history of a person (George Washington Institute for Spirituality and Health, n.d.). Domains assessed include faith and belief (F), importance (I), community (C), and address in care (A). Examples of questions used include: What gives you meaning in your life (F)? Do you have spiritual or religious beliefs that help you cope with stresses (F)? What importance do these beliefs have in regaining health (I)? Is there a group of people that are important to you (C)? Is there a group that gives you support (C)? How would you like your healthcare providers to deal with these beliefs and people? (A) (George Washington Institute for Spirituality and Health, n.d.). The George Washington Institute for Spirituality and Health (n.d.) recommends that healthcare providers who perform assessments on others use this tool for themselves as well. More information on taking a spiritual history, self-assessment, and FICA plastic pocket cards for professionals may be found at www .gwumc.edu/gwish/clinical/fica-spiritual/index.cfm.

Bereavement

Grief and bereavement interventions such as making information on loss and grief available and assessing family members for signs of complicated grief, when a person is "essentially frozen or stuck in a state of chronic mourning"(Zhang, El-Jawahri, & Prigerson, 2006, p. 1191), should begin before the death of a loved one (Grassi, 2007). NCCN (2012) and the National Consensus Project for Quality Palliative Care (2009) guidelines foster bereavement services as part of palliative care. When death finally comes, the family and caregivers are faced with dealing with loss, grief, and bereavement. Bereavement services should be available to the families for at least one year so as not to interfere with the natural grieving process and should include community bereavement support programs and referral to a psychologist or psychiatrist, if necessary. Cherlin and colleagues (2007) followed 161 family caregivers of patients with cancer and found that of the 30% who used bereavement services in the year after the death of a loved one, most were in the first six months. Bereavement interventions should be developmentally appropriate and culturally sensitive to those who feel they need it and request it in order to maximize the outcome of helping an individual return his or her life to a satisfactory state (NCCN, 2012; National Consensus Project for Quality Palliative Care, 2009; Schut & Stroebe, 2005; Shear et al., 2011).

Although only a small portion of the bereaved need intervention after the death of a family member, some individuals may be at higher risk for developing complicated grief, also known as *pathological* or *traumatic grief* (Schut & Stroebe, 2005; Shear et al., 2011; Wittouck, Van Autreve, De Jaegere, Portzky, & van Heeringen, 2011). Complicated grief may be described as a prolongation of the intense suffering and extreme, persistent, negative mental and physical effects of bereavement (Schut & Stroebe, 2005). Complicated grief and bereavement are associated with depression in older adults (National Consensus Project for Quality Palliative Care, 2009). Rates of complicated grief are higher in spouses than in other loved ones of patients with a terminal illness and in individuals with a history of psychological illness before the death of the patient, previous loss, and exposure to trauma (Lobb et al., 2010; Schut & Stroebe, 2005).

Complicated grief is a universal phenomenon that affects people of all nations and cultures. Chiu and colleagues (2009) interviewed 668 caregivers in Taiwan about nine months after the patient with cancer that they were caring for died to evaluate factors that influenced complicated grief. They determined that, in addition to the risk factors listed previously, female gender, parents-children relationship, lack of religious belief, and unavailable family support would increase one's chances for developing complicated grief. Conversely, caregivers who experienced a longer duration of caring or had a history of a medical disease were not predisposed to complicated grief. Caregivers of patients cared for in hospice also did not experience complicated grief. Weise et al. (2007) conducted interviews of 50 family caregivers of 50 patients receiving palliative care. Thirty percent exhibited signs of complicated grief even though 97% of the caregiving families expressed satisfaction with the care provided by the palliative care team. In a qualitative study of 24 widows with children in Iran, Khosravan, Salehi, Ahmadi, Sharif, and Zami (2010) reported that hopelessness related to the death of a spouse adversely affected the health of the women. The authors call on nurses to identify widows at risk and provide hope therapy to assist with positive bereavement outcomes. Another technique in bereavement is "the Seven Levels of Healing," which include (a) education, (b) connection, (c) the body as a garden, (d) emotional healing, (e) nature of the mind, (f) life assessment, and (g) nature of the spirit (Geffen, 2010).

A recent meta-analysis of the prevention and treatment of complicated grief demonstrated inconsistent support for the effectiveness of preventive grief interventions (Wittouck et al., 2011). Wittouck and colleagues (2011) also reported that treatment interventions for complicated grief successfully improved both short- and long-term symptoms.

Nursing Implications

Nurses have an essential, albeit delicate, role in advance care planning. They collaborate with patients, physicians, and families, focusing on understanding patients' values, priorities, and specific wishes for end-of-life care (Cohen & Nirenberg, 2011). Nurses also collaborate with social workers, clergy, and other members of the healthcare team to educate patients and families about advance directives and living wills and encourage patients to complete them.

Nurses will enhance the health outcomes and the QOL of patients if they incorporate supportive care and treatment early in the course of an incurable disease such as a hepato-

biliary cancer (Cohen & Nirenberg, 2011). They are vital in helping patients and families maintain hope and achieve their wishes at the end of life.

Summary

Conversations about advance care planning should be frequent, ongoing, open discussions with patients and families about treatment options, defining goals for treatment, end-of-life care, and the planning of bereavement. Advance care planning is a conversation that should be repeated with the collaboration of physicians and nurses and the assistance of multidisciplinary team members. Knowing the expected course of hepatic, pancreatic, and biliary cancers with the signposts of progression, nurses are prepared to guide the discussion. Working with patients' cultural and spiritual beliefs will allow the most personal growth possible for the patients and those around them as the end of life approaches.

I wonder if it hurts to live—
And if They have to try—
And whether—could They choose between—
It would not be—to die—

I note that Some—gone patient long—
At length, renew their smile—
An imitation of a Light
That has so little Oil—

I wonder if when Years have piled—
Some Thousands—on the Harm—
That hurt them early—such a lapse
Could give them any Balm

Emily Dickinson, "I Measure Every
Grief I Meet," stanzas 3–5

References

Aging with Dignity. (2011a). Five wishes. Retrieved from http://www.agingwithdignity.org/five-wishes.php

Aging with Dignity. (2011b). Five wishes: Forms, information, and states using the forms. Retrieved from http://www.agingwithdignity.org/five-wishes-states.php

Alano, G.J., Pekmezaris, R., Tai, J.Y., Hussain, M.J., Jeune, J., Louis, B., … Wolf-Klein, G.P. (2010). Factors influencing older adults to complete advance directives. *Palliative and Supportive Care, 8,* 267–275. doi:10.1017/S1478951510000064

Babgi, A. (2009). Legal issues in end of life care: Perspectives from Saudi Arabia and the United States. *American Journal of Hospice and Palliative Medicine, 26,* 119–127. doi:10.1177/1049909108330031

Breitbart, W., & Heller, K.S. (2003). Reframing hope: Meaning-centered care for patients near the end of life. *Journal of Palliative Medicine, 6,* 979–988. doi:10.1089/109662103322654901

California POLST. (n.d.). Honoring patients' end-of-life wishes: A provider's guide to POLST (physician orders for life-sustaining treatment). Retrieved from http://coalitionccc.org/_pdf/POLST_Provider _Brochure.pdf

Center for Practical Bioethics. (2006, November). Recommended policy guidelines regarding medical futility. Retrieved from http://www.practicalbioethics.org/documents/guidelines/19-Futility-web-2008.pdf

Centers for Medicare and Medicaid Services. (2009). Hospice statistics, 1998–2008. Retrieved from http://www.cms.gov/Hospice/Downloads/Hospice_Data_1998-2008.zip

Cherlin, E.J., Barry, C.L., Prigerson, H.G., Schulman-Green, D., Johnson-Hurzeler, R., Kasl, S.V., & Bradley, E.H. (2007). Bereavement services for family caregivers: How often used, why, and why not? *Journal of Palliative Medicine, 10,* 148–158. doi:10.1089/jpm.2006.0108

Chiu, Y.-W., Huang, C.-T., Yin, S.-M., Huang, Y.-C., Chien, C.-I., & Chuang, H.-I. (2009). Determinants of complicated grief in caregivers who cared for terminal cancer patients. *Supportive Care in Cancer, 18,* 1321–1327. doi:10.1007/s00520-009-0756-6

Coalition for Compassionate Care of California. (2005, March 31). Health care decisions law fact sheet for professionals. Retrieved from http://coalitionccc.org/_pdf/Healthcare_Decisions_Law _factsheet.pdf

Coalition for Compassionate Care of California. (2009, October). Advance care planning—conversation guide. Retrieved from http://coalitionccc.org/_pdf/Conversation_Guide.pdf

Cohen, A., & Nirenberg, A. (2011). Current practices in advance care planning: Implications for oncology nurses. *Clinical Journal of Oncology Nursing, 15,* 547–553. doi:10.1188/11.CJON.547-553

Corridor Group, Inc. (2006). *Hospice Quickflips: The Corridor Guide for Hospice Clinicians* [NGS version]. San Francisco, CA: Author.

Crawford, G.B., Robinson, J.A., Hunt, R.W., Piller, N.B., & Esterman, A. (2009). Estimating survival in patients with cancer receiving palliative care: Is analysis of body composition using bioimpedance helpful? *Journal of Palliative Medicine, 12,* 1009–1014. doi:10.1089/jpm.2009.0093

Desharnais, S., Carter, R.E., Hennessy, W., Kurent, J.E., & Carter, C. (2007). Lack of concordance between physician and patient: Reports on end-of-life care discussions. *Journal of Palliative Medicine, 10,* 728–739. doi:10.1089/jpm.2006.2543

Dickinson, E. (1896). I measure every grief I meet. Retrieved from http://www.americanpoems.com/poets/emilydickinson/10513

Escalante, C.P., Martin, C.G., Elting, L.S., & Rubenstein, E.B. (1997). Medical futility and appropriate medical care in patients whose death is thought to be imminent. *Supportive Care in Cancer, 5,* 274–280. doi:10.1007/s005200050074

FACIT.org. (2010a). Cancer Therapy–General (FACT-G) questionnaire. Retrieved from http://www.facit.org/FACITOrg/Questionnaires

FACIT.org. (2010b). Overview. Retrieved from http://www.facit.org/FACITOrg/Overview

Fine, E., Reid, M.C., Shengelia, R., & Adelman, R.A. (2010). Directly-observed patient-physician discussions in palliative and end-of-life care: A systematic review of the literature. *Journal of Palliative Medicine, 13,* 595–603. doi:10.1089/jpm.2009.0388

George Washington Institute for Spirituality and Health. (n.d.). FICA spiritual history tool. Retrieved from http://www.gwumc.edu/gwish/clinical/fica-spiritual/index.cfm

Geffen, J.R. (2010). Integrative oncology for the whole person: A multidimensional approach to cancer care. *Integrative Cancer Therapies, 9,* 105–121. doi:10.1177/1534735409355172

Goebel, M. (2010). Anorexia-cachexia syndrome in advanced cancer. *Journal of Palliative Medicine, 13,* 627–628. doi:10.1089/jpm.2010.9828

Grassi, L. (2007). Bereavement in families with relatives dying of cancer. *Current Opinion in Supportive and Palliative Care, 1,* 43–49. doi:10.1097/SPC.0b013e32813a3276

Jamieson, N.B., Carter, C.R., McKay, C.J., & Oien, K.A. (2011). Tissue biomarkers for prognosis in pancreatic ductal adenocarcinoma: A systematic review and meta-analysis. *Clinical Cancer Research, 17,* 3316–3331. doi:10.1158/1078-0432.CCR-10-3284

Jenko, M., Gonzalez, L., & Seymour, M.J. (2007). Life review with the terminally ill. *Journal of Hospice and Palliative Nursing, 9,* 159–167.

Johnstone, M.J., & Kanitsaki, O. (2009). Ethics and advance care planning in a culturally diverse society. *Journal of Transcultural Nursing, 20,* 405–416. doi:10.1177/1043659609340803

Kasman, D.L. (2004). When is medical treatment futile? A guide for students, residents, and physicians. *Journal of General Internal Medicine, 19,* 1053–1056. doi:10.1111/j.1525-1497.2004.40134.x

Kass-Bartelmes, B.L., Hughes, R., & Rutherford, M.K. (2003, March). Advance care planning: Preferences for care at the end of life. *Research in Action, 2003*(12). AHRQ Pub No. 030018. Retrieved from http://www.ahrq.gov/RESEARCH/endliferia/endria.pdf

Kasthuri, R.S., Taubman, M.B., & Mackman, N. (2009). Role of tissue factor in cancer. *Journal of Clinical Oncology, 27,* 4834–4838. doi:10.1200/JCO.2009.22.6324

Keating, N.L., Landrum, M.B., Rogers, S.O., Baum, S.K., Virnig, B.A., Huskamp, H.A., … Kahn, K.L. (2010). Physician factors associated with discussions about end-of-life care. *Cancer, 116,* 998–1006. doi:10.1002/cncr.24761

Khorana, A.A., Ahrendt, S.A., Ryan, C.K., Francis, C.W., Hruban, R.H., Hu, Y.C., … Taubman, M.B. (2007). Tissue factor expression, angiogenesis, and thrombosis in pancreatic cancer. *Clinical Cancer Research, 13,* 2870–2875. doi:10.1158/1078-0432.CCR-06-2351

Khosravan, S., Salehi, S., Ahmadi, F., Sharif, F., & Zami, A. (2010). Experiences of widows with children: A qualitative study about spousal death in Iran. *Nursing and Health Sciences, 12,* 205–211. doi:10.1111/j.1442-2018.2010.00522.x

Lobb, E.A., Kristjanson, L.J., Samar, M.A., Monterosso, L., Halkett, G.K.B., & Davies, A. (2010). Predictors of complicated grief: A systematic review of empirical studies. *Death Studies, 34,* 673–698. doi:10.1080/07481187.2010.496686

Mohammed, S., & Peter, E. (2009). Rituals, death, and the moral practice of medical futility. *Nursing Ethics, 16,* 292–302. doi:10.1177/0969733009102691

Mohan, D., Alexander, S.C., Garrigues, S.K., Arnold, R.M., & Barnato, A.E. (2010). Communication practices in physician decision-making for an unstable critically ill patient with end-stage cancer. *Journal of Palliative Medicine, 13,* 949–956. doi:10.1089/jpm.2010.0053

National Cancer Institute. (2011, August 19). Extrahepatic bile duct cancer treatment (PDQ®): General information about extrahepatic bile duct cancer [Health professional version]. Retrieved from http://www.cancer.gov/cancertopics/pdq/treatment/bileduct/HealthProfessional/#Section_1

National Comprehensive Cancer Network. (2012). *NCCN Clinical Practice Guidelines in Oncology: Palliative care* [v.2.2012]. Retrieved from http://www.nccn.org/professionals/physician_gls/pdf/palliative.pdf

National Consensus Project for Quality Palliative Care. (2009). *Clinical practice guidelines for quality palliative care* (2nd ed.). Retrieved from http://www.nationalconsensusproject.org/guideline.pdf

Nitori, N., Ino, Y., Nakanishi, Y., Yamada, T., Honda, K., Yanagihara, K., … Hirohashi, S. (2005). Prognostic significance of tissue factor in pancreatic ductile adenocarcinoma. *Clinical Cancer Research, 11,* 2531–2539. doi:10.1158/1078-0432.CCR-04-0866

Olsson, L., Östlund, G., Strang, P., Grassman, E.J., & Friedrichsen, M. (2011). The glimmering embers: Experiences of hope among cancer patients in palliative home care. *Palliative and Supportive Care, 9,* 43–54. doi:10.1017/S1478951510000532

Oregon Health and Science University. (2008). History of the POLST paradigm initiative. Retrieved from http://www.ohsu.edu/polst/developing/history.htm

Oregon Health and Science University. (2010). POLST, Oregon's physician orders for life-sustaining treatment paradigm. Retrieved from http://www.ohsu.edu/polst/programs/oregon-details.htm

Oregon Health and Science University. (2011). Using the POLST form, guidance for healthcare professionals. Retrieved from http://www.ohsu.edu/polst/resources/documents/POSTUsersGuide2011.pdf

Ray, A., Block, S.D., Friedlander, R.J., Zhang, B., Maciejewski, P.K., & Prigerson, H.G. (2006). Peaceful awareness in patients with advanced cancer. *Journal of Palliative Medicine, 9,* 1359–1368. doi:10.1089/jpm.2006.9.1359

Rustøen, T., Wahl, A.K., Hanestad, B.R., Lerdal, A., Miaskowski, C., & Moum, T. (2003). Hope in the general Norwegian population, measured using the Hearth Hope Index. *Palliative and Supportive Care, 1,* 309–318.

Schut, H., & Stroebe, M.S. (2005). Interventions to enhance adaption to bereavement. *Journal of Palliative Medicine, 8*(Suppl. 1), S140–S147. doi:10.1089/jpm.2005.8.s-140

Shear, M.K., Simon, N., Wall, M., Zisook, S., Neimeyer, R., Duan, N., … Keshaviah, A. (2011). Complicated grief and related issues for DSM-5. *Depression and Anxiety, 28,* 103–117. doi:10.1002/da.20780

Steel, J.L., Eton, D.T., Cella, D., Olek, M.C., & Carr, B.I. (2006). Clinically meaningful changes in health-related quality of life in patients diagnosed with hepatobiliary carcinoma. *Annals of Oncology, 17,* 304–312. doi:10.1093/annonc/mdj072

Stetka, B., & Irwin, S.A. (2011). What is palliative care psychiatry? *Medscape Psychiatry.* Retrieved from http://www.medscape.com/viewarticle/741903_print

Stubenrauch, J.M. (2010). Study: Few physicians discussing end-of-life options with advanced-stage patients. *Oncology Times, 32,* 26–29. doi:10.1097/01.COT.0000370073.55788.2a

Tamir, O., Singer, Y., & Shvartzman, P. (2007). Taking care of terminally ill patients at home: The economic perspective revisited. *Palliative Medicine, 21,* 537–541. doi:10.1177/0269216307080822

Tanaka, T., Ikeda, M., Okusaka, T., Ueno, H., Morizane, C., Hagihara, A., … Kojima, Y. (2008). Prognostic factors in Japanese patients with advanced pancreatic cancer treated with single-agent gemcitabine as first-line therapy. *Japanese Journal of Clinical Oncology, 38,* 755–761. doi:10.1093/jjco/hyn098

Thorne, S., Oglov, V., Armstrong, E.A., & Hislop, T.G. (2007). Prognosticating futures and the human experience of hope. *Palliative and Supportive Care, 5,* 227–239. doi:10.1017/S1478951507000399

Utne, I., Miaskowski, C., Bjordal, K., Paul, S.M., Jakobsen, G., & Rustøen, T. (2008). The relationship between hope and pain in a sample of hospitalized oncology patients. *Palliative and Supportive Care, 6,* 327–334. doi:10.1017/S1478951508000527

Wallace, M.P., Weiner, J.S., Pekmezaris, R., Almendral, A., Cosiquien, R., Auerbach, C., & Wolf-Klein, G. (2007). Physician cultural sensitivity in African American advance care planning: A pilot study. *Journal of Palliative Care, 10,* 721–727. doi:10.1089/jpm.2006.0212

Weiner, J.S., & Cole, S.A. (2004). Three principles to improve clinician communication for advance care planning: Overcoming emotional, cognitive, and skill barriers. *Journal of Palliative Medicine, 7,* 817–829. doi:10.1089/jpm.2004.7.817

Wiese, C.H.R., Morgenthal, H.C., Bartels, U.E., Vossen-Wellmann, A., Graf, B.M., & Hanekop, G.G. (2010). Post-mortal bereavement of family caregivers in Germany: A prospective interview-based investigation. *Weiner Klinische Wochenschrift, 122,* 384–389. doi:10.1007/s00508-010-1396-z

Williams, S.W., Hanson, L.C., Boyd, C., Green, M., Goldmon, M., Wright, G., & Corbie-Smith, G. (2008). Communication, decision making, and cancer: What African Americans want physicians to know. *Journal of Palliative Medicine, 11,* 1221–1226. doi:10.1089/jpm.2008.0057

Wittouck, C., Van Autreve, S., De Jaegere, E., Portzky, G., & van Heeringen, K. (2011). The prevention and treatment of complicated grief: A meta-analysis. *Clinical Psychology Review, 31,* 69–78. doi:10.1016/j.cpr.2010.09.005

Viale, P. (2009). Cancer diagnosis and staging. In B.H. Gobel, S. Triest-Robertson, & W.H. Vogel (Eds.), *Advanced oncology nursing certification review and resource manual* (pp. 77–147). Pittsburgh, PA: Oncology Nursing Society.

Viganò, A., Dorgan, M., Buckingham, J., Bruera, E., & Suarez-Almazor, M.E. (2000). Survival prediction in terminal cancer patients: A systematic review of the medical literature. *Palliative Medicine, 14,* 363–374.

Zhang, B., El-Jawahri, A., & Prigerson, H.G. (2006). Update on bereavement research evidence-based guidelines for the diagnosis and treatment of complicated bereavement. *Journal of Palliative Medicine, 9,* 1188–1203. doi:10.1089/jpm.2006.9.1188

Zoeller, L.S. (2011, August 11). Dr. Larry Cripe: Palliative care throughout the cancer continuum. Retrieved from http://oncologystat.com/viewpoints/interviews/Dr_Larry_Cripe_Palliative_Care_Throughout_the_Cancer_Continuum.html

Zwicker, J.I., Liebman, H.A., Neuberg, D., Lacroix, R., Bauer, K.A., Furie, B.C., & Furie, B. (2009). Tumor-derived tissue factor-bearing microparticles are associated with venous thromboembolic events in malignancy. *Clinical Cancer Research, 15,* 6830–6840. doi:10.1158/1078-0432.CCR-09-0371

CHAPTER 10

Economic and Social Challenges

Neal R. Niznan, MSW, LCSW

Introduction

Sometimes, nurses who provide care to patients with hepatobiliary or pancreatic cancers may become so focused on the medical concerns of symptom management, chemotherapy administration, diagnostic results, and other functions of the job that they may miss experiencing the person behind the issues. In order to treat the whole patient, the healthcare team needs to have an understanding of the psychosocial impact the illness has in the patient's life. Nurses need to take a moment and ask themselves: What other areas in patients' lives are affected by the cancer? What does it feel like to be in their shoes? How do they cope with all these challenges?

The purpose of this chapter is to consider the economic and social challenges patients encounter from diagnosis through treatment and survivorship. This chapter will highlight the impact on employment and financial considerations of leaving work; the issue of maintaining adequate medical and prescription coverage and the potential problems this poses for the patient and treatment team; locating adequate housing and care outside the patient's home; finding available community resources for educational, financial, and emotional support; the emotional effects of living with cancer; and how patients and their families cope with all the practical and logistical challenges of medical care. The more nurses understand the whole patient—physically, emotionally, and socially—and see their world from their vantage point, the better they can provide comprehensive holistic care at a crucial time in these patients' lives.

Cost of Care

Current cancer treatment is a cutting-edge science with new targeted chemotherapeutic agents, proton beam radiation therapy, robotic surgical excisions, and pharmaceutical interventions for the management of treatment side ef-

fects. The direct medical cost associated with cancer in 2007 was estimated at $103.8 billion (American Cancer Society [ACS], 2012). Different cancer sites are associated with certain treatment modalities, but in general, surgery, chemotherapy, and radiation are the standard of care for pancreatic and hepatobiliary cancers. In a study analyzing Medicare claims from 2000 to 2007 for patients with pancreatic cancer, the median direct medical cost of care was $65,500 (O'Neill et al., 2012).

Both initial and ongoing costs are associated with diagnosis and monitoring treatment effectiveness. Blood work and scans comprise most of these costs. Each treatment or follow-up appointment to the specialist includes billable events. Homecare expenses, durable medical equipment, home infusion, and enteral nutritional support are also common expenses.

Many of these major expenses can be covered by patients' insurance. However, subtle costs not covered by insurance are constant throughout treatment—transportation, parking, child care on treatment days, and nutritional supplements, to name a few. All of these costs accumulate over time. Patients may not have the financial reserve to handle these recurrent expenses, not to mention mortgage, utilities, and normal family expenses that also continue to accrue throughout the treatment process. How do patients pay all of their bills while on a reduced short-term disability salary or missing income of family caregivers? With all of the costs ongoing from diagnosis through treatment and beyond, the ability of patients to maintain their jobs for income and insurance benefits is paramount.

Employment

Both on a practical and an emotional level, maintaining employment is the key to reducing one of the major stressors in cancer treatment. Many people feel increased stress over financial issues. Increased financial burden associated with treatment and decreased income through reduced work hours or job loss creates a recipe for greater stress. The psychological loss of feeling unproductive when one cannot work can place the patient at risk for depression.

One of the best things patients can do is to continue to work as long as they can during their treatment. Maintaining a full salary and benefits will help reduce financial stress and foster a healthy sense of self-esteem (Brown, Owens, & Bradley, 2011). The patients can explore options through the human resources department at their place of employment to see if flex-time schedules, reduced work schedule, or even working from home are options to maintain employment. Many of these options have enabled patients to keep up with their treatment schedule and allow time for rest. Patients should have a frank conversation with their employer once they know the demands of their treatment and the probable impact it will have on their work performance. Exploring all options is beneficial for patients. It never hurts to ask what reasonable accommodations the employer can make to enable the patient to maintain his or her job. Another issue to explore with human resources is short-term disability benefits and the Family and Medical Leave Act (FMLA) (U.S. Department of Labor, Wage and Hour Division, n.d.). The patient has to consider when it is best to elect to receive short-term disability benefits and how long they will continue. Questions to consider are whether short-term disability can be followed by long-term private policy or, if an individual will be out for more than one year, whether he or she will be eligible for Social Security Disability Insurance (SSDI).

FMLA enables patients and family caregivers to take 12 weeks of unpaid leave within a 12-month period to deal with serious medical conditions. Their health benefits will remain active, but they will not be able to draw a salary during this time. Many times caregivers will use FMLA leave to care for loved ones for a period of time and then return to work (U.S. Department of Labor, Wage and Hour Division, n.d.).

If patients need to terminate their position, they should start COBRA insurance to extend health benefits during treatment. COBRA stands for Consolidated Omnibus Budget Reconciliation Act (U.S. Department of Labor, n.d.). This act protects workers who lost their employment from being uninsured. The coverage maintains the health benefits from their employer for 18 months for the same premium that the employee and employer paid jointly. The premium is paid monthly for as long as it is needed. Individuals can elect to extend coverage past the 18-month period, but the premium cost increases exponentially (U.S. Department of Labor, n.d.).

Some employers, such as Seton Hall University (n.d.), allow coworkers to donate their own extra vacation hours to people who are struggling with a health crisis. This is a good way for coworkers who would like to help an individual in need in some way but do not know what they can do to help. Keeping a record of everyone's time is usually coordinated through the human resources department.

Insurance

In 2010, the number of people without health insurance was 49.9 million, or 16.3% of the U.S. population (U.S. Census Bureau, 2011). Carrying and maintaining both medical and prescription coverage is a necessity for patients with cancer. The three ways an individual can present to a healthcare practice regarding insurance coverage are uninsured, underinsured, or carrying adequate coverage for treatment. Trying to understand everything there is to know about insurance coverage with its myriad plan options is a bit daunting. Having at least a basic knowledge of patients' insurance will help nurses understand some of the financial burdens and stress they may face.

Uninsured Patients

When patients present to a healthcare facility with no insurance coverage, they pose a practical and ethical issue from the beginning. First, unless they are admitted via the emergency department and have received an initial consultation or possible treatment at the facility, someone in the practice should check new patients' coverage status. Clinicians need to know the protocol for their practice, hospital, or treatment facility regarding the treatment of uninsured individuals before setting up the initial appointment. If the practice does not treat uninsured clients, then appropriate referrals need to be made to practices or clinics in the community. This could be in conjunction with a referral to a local branch of the state's Board of Social Services office to help them apply for medical insurance coverage, Medicaid, for low-income individuals and families. Medicaid is federally funded through the U.S. Department of Health and Human Services and administered by each state. Links to each state's Medicaid program requirements and benefits can be found at www.healthcare.gov. Medicaid benefits also include prescription drug coverage.

Many times, however, these individuals are already in the system before they reach the practice. By the time someone realizes they are not insured, the clinicians may be ethically obligated to treat them. A conversation with someone from the billing office will help in navigating this delicate territory. Unfortunately, even with the U.S. Supreme Court's decision to uphold the Affordable Care Act, which enables wider access to healthcare coverage for individuals who currently cannot afford it, there is no provision in the law for undocumented aliens to receive benefits (ProCon.org, 2010).

Underinsured Patients

The next group, underinsured patients, doubled in size from 2009 to 2012 to reach more than 25 million people in the United States (Patterson, 2012). These individuals have medical coverage, but their benefits are less than adequate to meet the financial demands of treatment over time. These plans, although inexpensive, have limited coverage for most long-standing illnesses. These plans have low annual and lifetime caps on the amount they will pay. They may restrict the number and type of diagnostic scans or procedures. This leaves patients in a position of not having coverage when they need it. This is quite unfortunate because the individuals pay monthly premiums for health coverage, but soon realize it does not cover what they need. These individuals also pose a difficulty for the healthcare team if at some point the insurance no longer covers their current treatment because the plan has reached its maximum benefit amount. The medical team may need to rework the treatment plan for a less favorable option that can be covered. Because many of these patients fall within upper- and middle-income families and have some coverage, although inadequate, they may not be eligible for Medicaid or financial assistance from community organizations that help patients who are uninsured (Patterson, 2012). Although having some coverage is better than none, the underinsured find themselves stuck with what they have: not being able to get supplemental coverage or public assistance unless they drop their coverage altogether. It is never advisable to drop coverage unless new insurance can be established first.

Adequately Insured Patients

The last group is people with adequate insurance coverage. Much of this coverage is through insurance plans from their employers, spouses' coverage, or a group, organization, or union of which they are members. It is beyond the scope of this work to examine in detail all of the various plan options patients may have. These traditional insurance plans may have out-of-pocket expenses such as copays for office visits and annual deductibles that the patient needs to reach before the coverage starts. Budgeting for theses out-of-pocket costs can be difficult. It is important to keep in mind what plans require prior authorization from the insurance company for procedures, such as interventional radiology, before they can be completed. Failure to follow insurance preauthorization procedures can delay the treatment process or cause issues with billing.

Medicare

This section on insurance would not be complete without a few words about Medicare. As the Baby Boomer generation reaches retirement age and modern medicine continues to extend the life span, many patients will have let go of their employer-based plans and enrolled in full Medicare coverage.

Medicare is federal government health insurance coverage for individuals who have contributed to the Medicare system over years of employment. Medicare has two basic parts, Medicare A and Medicare B. Medicare A covers medical expenses incurred during inpatient hospitalizations and has a deductible of $1,156 during a hospitalization period. Medicare B covers expenses associated with outpatient doctor vis-

its, procedures, and therapies, which are covered at 80% of the healthcare cost; the patient is responsible for the remaining 20%. Medicare covers the majority of treatments and diagnostic procedures with some exceptions (e.g., home IV hydration, bathtub or shower seats). Part A becomes effective on a person's 65th birthday, and Part B can be elected at age 65 unless the individual chooses to keep insurance coverage through the current employer while continuing to work. Once retired, the individual only has eight months to elect Part B coverage or else be subjected to penalties and a waiting period before coverage is active. The timing of this could be crucial if a person becomes ill outside the enrollment period. Part B has a monthly premium of $99 (at the time of this writing), which is deducted from the individual's Social Security check (Medicare, n.d.-a).

Medigap is a supplemental plan that covers the cost of medical expenses that Medicare Part A and Part B do not. For those who can afford these plans, it is money well spent. It is almost impossible to predict the total cost of one's treatment. The benefit of having the coverage far exceeds the cost of monthly premiums for a patient receiving cancer treatment.

Prescription Drug Coverage

The cost of prescription medications today is overwhelming, and coverage for prescription medications is a must for patients receiving treatment for pancreatic or hepatobiliary cancers. The cost of a monthly supply of a cancer drug averaged more than $1,600 in 2006 and has been rising steadily (ACS, 2011). In addition, patients with cancer are also prescribed myriad antiemetics, pain medications, anticoagulants, and other treatments used to manage the symptoms and side effects of the disease and treatment. Without prescription drug coverage, patients can be financially devastated by the pharmacy bills alone. Again, it is important to know what type of prescription coverage patients have and whether they can afford the copays associated with these prescriptions.

For example, retired adults who receive Social Security benefits and those who receive state welfare benefits usually have more available cash in the beginning of the month. If a prescription is written in the middle of the month, a doctor or nurse practitioner may not discover until the next treatment appointment that the patient did not fill the prescription because he or she could not afford the medication prescribed. This leaves the patient having to endure symptoms longer than needed because he or she did not get the medication in a timely manner.

Knowing patients' prescription coverage also implies knowing what medications require prior authorizations to be filled. For example, clinicians can save patients a few days of waiting for pain medication if they first contact the plan's pharmacy department regarding prior authorization. Most plans have preferred medications in their formulary that are covered under the patients' benefits. If the medication a clinician would like to prescribe is not on the formulary, the clinician will be required to justify its use and show that the preferred medications have been tried and failed to provide the desired effect. This prior authorization process could take 24–72 hours for approval.

It would be close to impossible to know every plan and what the pharmacy policies are, but with experience, clinicians learn which medications always require prior authorization. For example, Medicaid plans will not approve long-acting or sustained-release oxycodone without a prior authorization, and many of the newer medications used in treatment are not on the pharmacy's preferred list and will require authorization for use.

Medicare Part D plans, the prescription coverage for those with Medicare coverage, have a range of options as well as premiums. The biggest drawback to the plans is that the tiers of coverage change as the member utilizes the benefits. A simplification of the plan is as follows. Annually, the members, after meeting an initial deductible, will pay a coinsurance charge per prescription until they and their plan have reached prescription charges of $2,930. They then move into the next tier, or "coverage gap," where they now pay 86% for generic medications and 50% for brand name medication until the total cost paid by the patient reaches $3,727.50. In the third tier, patients pay only 5% of the prescription cost through the remainder of the year. Starting the following January, the three-tier process begins again. Patients who meet annual income requirements may be eligible to receive their prescriptions at a reduced coinsurance cost (Medicare, n.d.-b).

The major financial challenge for patients is to budget money for when they reach the second tier or "coverage gap" to cover the needed prescriptions at full cost. When this happens, symptom management becomes a challenge if patients cannot afford the medication and rely on less effective prescriptions they might be able to afford. At this point in the treatment process, the savvy nurse or social worker can assist patients in locating community organizations, pharmaceutical companies, or state prescription programs to defray some of the cost for prescriptions.

Disability Insurance

Some patients may be eligible for short-term disability through work or hold a private policy. Most short-term disability plans only provide coverage for three to six months at 45%–60% of the employee's current salary. If the need for coverage extends past six months, patients should consider applying for SSDI or activate their long-term disability benefits, if available. SSDI is a federal government program that provides monthly income to patients based on the criteria of being mentally or physically disabled. Patients are considered disabled if they are legally blind, have a physical or mental impairment, or are unable to perform the duties of their job for 12 months or more or have a terminal illness. Patients who

receive SSDI for two consecutive years will be eligible to receive Medicare benefits even if they are younger than age 65 (U.S. Social Security Administration, 2012b).

The process of applying for SSDI should be started early to reduce the gap in income between the end of short-term disability and the start of SSDI. SSDI approval can take up to three months from the date of becoming disabled. A patient with a diagnosis of metastatic or stage IV cancer can be eligible for "compassionate allowance." This is a fast track in the approval process and can take less than one month (U.S. Social Security Administration, 2012a). Once approved, individuals will not receive their first disability check from the government for six weeks. A potential gap in income is reduced as soon as the application is submitted and approved. Patients should consider that the first payment may take upwards of four-and-a-half months from the time of application.

The amount of the first SSDI payment is calculated retroactively to the date of application or disability. The patient's oncologist can establish this date. The amount of the monthly payment is based on the patient's current salary and recorded work history or "credits." According to the U.S. Social Security Administration (2012b), individuals are eligible for disability if they have worked full time for 10 or more years or accrued 40 credits.

A patient can apply online via the Social Security Administration Web site (www.ssa.gov). This application process can be password secured so the patient or family members assisting the patient with the application can complete the application over a period of time. The application can then be sent to the local Social Security office electronically for review. Patients can also apply in person by setting up an appointment at the local Social Security office. With both application processes, patients need to submit documentation regarding proof of age, citizenship, and related medical records to the local office to complete the application for review (U.S. Social Security Administration, 2012b).

The U.S. Social Security Administration obtains patients' medical records when they sign a release and provide the names and contact information for their physicians. A clinician can help patients expedite the application process by providing a set of complete medical records from the treatment team. Patients can include these with the required documentation. This can save the patient a minimum of three weeks off the time they wait for approval. Encourage the patient to complete the application online, print it out, and submit all the required documentation to the local Social Security Administration Office at one time. This keeps the application as one unit and reduces the possibility of paperwork becoming misplaced. The key point here is the sooner the office has all the required paperwork, the sooner it can begin the approval process.

Although the individual is considered "disabled," the recipient is allowed to supplement disability income with part-time employment. The amount individuals can earn while receiving disability income has a cap. They may not earn what their previous position paid, but the opportunity to remain active and feel productive has great psychological benefit (U.S. Social Security Administration, 2012d).

Housing and Care Options

For many patients, staying in the comfort of their own home surrounded by familiar objects and family members may be the best option in managing their cancer (National Cancer Institute, 2009). The impact of the disease is disruptive enough without having to uproot from everything that provides comfort and routine. Being in one's own home also provides daily diversions with light chores or small projects to busy oneself and at the same time gain a sense of accomplishment. Being able to maintain employment by working from home allows them the opportunity to rest when necessary (National Cancer Institute, 2009).

Patients should look at what their needs are and be creative to see how those needs can be met. Sometimes it is necessary for patients to relocate for a period of time during treatment. More consistent care by a family member, a larger space to accommodate a hospital bed, or closer access to the treatment facility to reduce travel time are just a few reasons. A comfortable home environment is also a priority. Many times during treatment, a calm environment where patients can get the rest they need is hard to find. They should be open to exploring options with family and friends to see what choices optimize their care.

As the disease progresses, assistance from outside agencies to provide medical care and equipment in the home helps to maintain the patient's quality of life. Families should develop a good working relationship with their care team to get the services they need to help manage the patient's symptoms at home.

If the family is unable to care for the patient at home, then freestanding and inpatient hospice programs can be considered. The decision to engage in hospice services is often addressed after a patient with pancreatic or hepatobiliary cancer experiences frequent rounds of chemotherapy and hospitalizations (Sheffield et al., 2011). Both the patient and family caregivers may be better served if plans for palliative care are discussed closer to the start of treatment.

If patients need to travel a distance to a treatment facility, they may consider staying closer to the facility, especially for radiation therapy, which is usually five days a week for a number of weeks. The expense of a daily commute is cost-prohibitive, and the trip itself could be physically taxing. Many times, the social worker on the treatment team has resources for local lodging. One suggestion is the ACS Hope Lodge®. This is a freestanding facility open to patients who are actively in treatment. Most are located near large cities

with a number of hospitals providing cancer care. Currently, ACS hosts 31 lodges in 22 states. Patients stay free of charge. Accommodations include a private room and bath, communal kitchen area for meal preparation, and common areas for networking with other patients. The criteria for staying at the lodge are being in active treatment, living more than 40 miles from the treatment facility, and having a "caregiver" stay with the patient for the duration of treatment. Clinicians can contact the local ACS chapter for locations close to their practice (ACS, n.d.).

Joe's House (www.joeshouse.org) is a national clearinghouse of lodging options for patients throughout the United States. It lists free lodging as well as hotels and furnished apartments.

Community Resources

Resources specifically for pancreatic and hepatobiliary cancers are not as abundant as other cancer sites (e.g., breast cancer). Most of the general cancer organizations can provide information and support for both patients and caregivers. The Pancreatic Canter Network (www.pancan. org) was established in 1999 to support people with the disease. It provides detailed information about the illness and its treatment and facilitates educational support seminars across the country.

ACS has a large database of community resources listed by zip code and categorized by type of resource (e.g., financial assistance, support groups). It is always beneficial to contact ACS's local office to see what services and financial resources they may offer. Services vary by state and geographic region. Some ACS regional offices have financial resources in the form of pharmacy grants, transportation reimbursement, and a homemaker grant that covers nonmedical expenses (e.g., housecleaning, babysitting). See Figure 10-1 for contact information for ACS as well as other resources.

CancerCare is another source of cancer information and available community resources. The organization has an archive of numerous teleconferences on a wide range of disease sites, treatments, and symptom management issues. CancerCare also has limited financial assistance for copays and a small stipend for nonmedical expenses. Trained professionals are available to provide counseling and emotional support to patients and their families.

New oral chemotherapies and medications to control symptoms are extremely expensive even with prescription coverage. Many pharmaceutical companies have patient assistance programs to help qualified patients obtain the medications they need. Consult the manufacturer's Web site for information on their patient assistance program. An easy way to obtain that same information is through the Web site NeedyMeds, an information clearinghouse that lists both brand and generic names of medications. Available fi-

Figure 10-1. Patient Resources

American Cancer Society
800-227-2345
www.cancer.org

Cancer and Careers
www.cancerandcareers.org

Cancer*Care*
800-813-HOPE (800-813-4673)
www.cancercare.org

Cancer Legal Resource Center
866-THE-CLRC (866-843-2572)
www.disabilityrightslegalcenter.org/about/cancerlegalresource.cfm

Cancer Support Community
888-793-9355
www.cancersupportcommunity.org

CanLiv: The Hepatobiliary Cancers Foundation
www.canliv.org

Centers for Medicare and Medicaid Services
800-MEDICARE (800-633-4227)
www.medicare.gov

Chronic Disease Fund
877-968-7233
www.cdfund.org

Joe's House
877-563-7468
www.joeshouse.org

Law Help
www.lawhelp.org

National Association of Hospital Hospitality Houses
800-542-9730
www.nahhh.org

NeedyMeds
www.needymeds.com

OncoLink
www.oncolink.org

Pancreatica
+1-831-658-0060
www.pancreatica.org

Pancreatic Cancer Action Network (PANCAN)
877-272-6226
www.pancan.org

Patient Advocate Foundation
800-532-5274
www.patientadvocate.org

U.S. Social Security Administration
800-772-1213
www.ssa.gov

nancial assistance programs are organized by medication. Some programs require patients to meet certain financial criteria, and others only assist patients without prescription coverage. Two other organizations that provide copay assistance for those managing pancreatic cancer and liver disease are the Chronic Disease Fund and the Patient Advocate Foundation.

Ongoing emotional support including programs for caregivers and children can be located through a number of community-based organizations. The Cancer Support Community, formed through a merger of The Wellness Community and Gilda's Club, provides holistic-based care for patients currently undergoing treatment, caregivers, and post-treatment survivors. The organization provides professionally led support groups, individual counseling, creative arts for nurturing self-expression, and stress reduction through mindfulness meditation and Tai Chi. Since its inception, Gilda's Club has been recognized for its psychosocial support of caregivers and family members.

Emotional Impact of Serious Illness

The preceding sections of this chapter have been dedicated to the economic and social challenges that face patients dealing with pancreatic and hepatobiliary cancers. Equally evident is the emotional impact of the illness and the psychological challenges it presents. Dealing with these emotional challenges spans the trajectory of the illness from diagnosis through post-treatment survivorship. With each phase, patients experience changes in their thoughts about themselves, ability to cope with their present situation, mortality, and the meaning this illness has in their lives.

Patients' emotional well-being shifts and changes with each new phase of treatment. The patient that clinicians see on initial presentation may be very different than the patient seen by the end of treatment. As healthcare professionals focused on treating the whole patient, it is important to recognize, understand, and support these emotional changes and provide individual empathy and guidance throughout the treatment trajectory. The more healthcare providers understand what having cancer is like for patients, the better they can support these patients on their journey toward feeling well. Holland and Lewis (2000) stated

> Every person brings unique characteristics to dealing with illness: a particular personality, a way of coping, a set of beliefs and values, a way of looking at the world. The goal is to take these qualities into consideration and make sure that they work in favor of the person at each point along the cancer journey. (p. 3)

The first challenge most patients experience happens with diagnosis or slightly before as they begin to realize their health is changing, and they may not be sure what is happening. Patients experience a change in their *assumptive world-*

view, the personal understanding of how they see their lives. This view is developed over the life of the individual and incorporates an idealized positive model of their world. As with those left to grieve the loss of a loved one who dies unexpectedly, the reality of the experience is incongruent with the model of their assumptive worldview (Janoff-Bolman, 1985). They initially have difficulty assimilating the fact that this is really happening to them—that they actually have cancer. The emotional result is one of shock, anger, or even anxiety. For some patients, this shift in worldview may temporarily lead to disbelief expressed as denial. This at times may be exhibited as an inability to schedule or keep appointments for initial treatment.

Patients' anger about their illness for some may be difficult to keep in check and often spills out inappropriately at family members or the treatment team. Clinicians should keep in mind that this expression of anger, which may be transmitted as complaints about scheduling appointments or discourteous treatment by clinic staff, is a sign of an underlying issue of loss the patient is experiencing. Loss comes from many sources in the patient's life, including tangible losses of one's physical strength or energy level because of fatigue from illness or treatment and the loss of time from work and the corresponding loss of income, as well as the loss of socialization resulting from decreased physical energy or the emotional discomfort of being with others who, despite their best efforts to be supportive, do not really understand what the patient is experiencing. Friends and loved ones may unintentionally say hurtful things that result in the patient avoiding their company. Patients may feel a loss of living their life and the perceived time they have left to accomplish goals and experience future events. This loss of the future coupled with tangible losses leads to decreased self-esteem and frustration, which in turn could foster depression.

For patients to endure pain from disease, decreased energy, and decreased appetite and sleep, to name only a few symptoms, requires not only stamina but also emotional fortitude. What keeps these patients returning for more treatment, even when the very treatment that is helping them makes them feel worse? It may be the support of family and friends or the positive words of encouragement from the treatment team. Ultimately, it comes from within the individual as he or she develops a set of coping skills, adaptive thoughts, and behaviors that allow him or her to endure the hardships of illness (Kneier, 1996). For some patients, it means using a set of skills that were beneficial in past difficulties. Others develop new coping skills and a realization that they can face their worst fears and manage each day, if only at times moment by moment.

Nurses are vital in helping patients to cope not only with the physical challenges but also the emotional ones as well. In this role, by initially providing education and comfort around the physical symptoms of the disease and its treatment, nurses are in the perfect position to educate and support patients with the emotional challenges they face. By listening to how they cope and guiding them to change or adjust what is not working, nurses can help them to achieve psychological adjustment to the illness (American Society of Registered Nurses, 2008).

Nurses can help patients achieve psychological adjustment in several ways. First, nurses can help them feel like part of the treatment team by respecting their input and listening to their desires. Allowing patients input in the decision-making process regarding their treatment fosters a proactive stance about their care. The more they participate in their care, the less they feel victimized by it. Nurses can encourage patients to reach out for support from friends and family and should be prepared to discuss changes they observe in patients' moods that could be indicative of depression or untreated anxiety. Referral to a psychotherapist can enable patients to manage these symptoms in a constructive way. Patients should be encouraged to engage in activities that promote creativity and recreation. Fostering increased attention to one's spiritual nature, either through formalized religious practice or a connection to something greater than themselves, also helps to promote positive psychological adjustment (Kneier, 1996).

One of the biggest emotional challenges that patients dealing with serious illness face is to somehow find meaning in loss and suffering from their cancer experience. This is a difficult concept to explain and put into practice. Looking at their illness in a positive way, as an opportunity for growth, enables them to view themselves differently. Can they use this very difficult experience as a path toward personal growth? By beginning to foster a different attitude toward their illness, patients may begin to decrease their sense of bitterness and anger and possibly reduce their fear of mortality.

Summary

Patients who receive a pancreatic or hepatobiliary cancer diagnosis wrestle with many economic and social challenges over the course of treatment. Changes in their work schedules impact income and could potentially affect insurance coverage needed to defray the cost of health care. Patients will rely more on family and friends to support them with both practical as well as emotional challenges, helping them feel more in control of the ever-changing landscape of the treatment trajectory.

Nurses play a pivotal role in the process by providing education and emotional support. They can be a resource of information pertaining not only to symptom management but also to community support, financial assistance, and insurance and medication coverage. The nursing role helps to foster open dialogue with patients regarding the emotional impact of the illness and helps to tailor their coping skills to provide psychological adjustment. Allotting time to understand the economic and social challenges patients encounter is integral in effectively providing for both their physical and emotional well-being.

References

American Cancer Society. (n.d.). Find support and treatment: Hope Lodge. Retrieved from http:// http://www.cancer.org/Treatment/SupportProgramsServices/HopeLodge/

American Cancer Society. (2011, May 20). The cost of cancer treatment. Retrieved from http://www.cancer.org/Treatment/FindingandPayingforTreatment/ManagingInsuranceIssues/the-cost-of-cancer-treatment

American Cancer Society. (2012, February 9). Economic impact of cancer. Retrieved from http://www.cancer.org/Cancer/CancerBasics/economic-impact-of-cancer

American Society of Registered Nurses. (2008, February 1). Cancer care—Can a caring nurse make a difference? *Journal of Nursing.* Retrieved from http://www.asrn.org/journal-nursing/286-cancer-care-can-a-caring-nurse-make-a-difference.html

Brown, R.F., Owens, M., & Bradley, C. (2011). Employee to employer communication skills: Balancing cancer treatment and employment. *Psycho-Oncology.* Advance online publication. doi:10.1002/pon.2107

Holland, J.C., & Lewis, S. (2000). *The human side of cancer: Living with hope, coping with uncertainty.* New York, NY: HarperCollins.

Janoff-Bolman, R. (1985). The aftermath of victimization: Rebuilding shattered assumptions. In C.R. Figley (Ed.), *Trauma and its wake* (pp. 15–35). New York, NY: Brunner/Mazel.

Kneier, A.W. (1996). The psychological challenges facing melanoma patients. *Surgical Clinics of North America, 76,* 1413–1421. doi:10.1016/S0039-6109(05)70523-5

Medicare. (n.d.-a). Medicare basics. Retrieved from http://www.medicare.gov/navigation/medicare-basics/medicare-basics-overview.aspx

Medicare. (n.d.-b). Medicare prescription drug coverage (Part D). Retrieved from http://www.medicare.gov/navigation/medicare-basics/medicare-benefits/part-d.aspx#CoverageGap

National Cancer Institute. (2009, March 9). Fact sheet: Home care for patients. Retrieved from http://www.cancer.gov/cancertopics/factsheet/Support/home-care

O'Neill, C.B., Atoria, C.L., O'Reilly, E.M., LaFemina, J., Henman, M.C., & Elkin, E.B. (2012). Cost and trends in pancreatic cancer treatment. *Cancer, 118,* 5132–5139. doi:10.1002/cncr.27490

Patterson, S. (2012, April 18). 25 million Americans underinsured including middle and upper income families. Retrieved from http://healthcaresavvy.wbur.org/2012/04/25-million-americans-underinsured-including-middle-and-upper-income-families

ProCon.org. (2010, August 23). Healthcare reform/Obamacare. Retrieved from http://healthcarereform.procon.org/view.answers.php?ID=001480

Seton Hall University. (n.d.). Department of Human Resources—Vacation donation policy. Retrieved from http://www.shu.edu/offices/policies-procedures/human-resources-vacation-donation-policy.cfm

Sheffield, K.M., Boyd, C.A., Benarroch-Gampel, J., Kuo, Y.F., Cooksley, C.D., & Riall, T.S. (2011). End-of-life care in Medicare beneficiaries dying with pancreatic cancer. *Cancer, 117,* 5003–5012. doi:10.1002/cncr.26115

U.S. Census Bureau. (2011, September 14). Health insurance—Highlights: 2010. Retrieved from http://www.census.gov/hhes/www/hlthins/data/incpovhlth/2010/highlights.html

U.S. Department of Labor. (n.d.). Health plans and benefits: Continuation of health coverage—COBRA. Retrieved from http://www.dol.gov/dol/topic/health-plans/cobra.htm

U.S. Department of Labor, Wage and Hour Division. (n.d.). Family and Medical Leave Act. Retrieved from http://www.dol.gov/whd/fmla

U.S. Social Security Administration. (2012a, July 5). Compassionate allowances. Retrieved from http://www.socialsecurity.gov/compassionateallowances

U.S. Social Security Administration. (2012b, May 17). Disability programs: Benefits for people with disabilities. Retrieved from http://www.ssa.gov/disability

U.S. Social Security Administration. (2012c, July 11). Frequently asked questions: Apply for Social Security disability benefits. Retrieved from http://ssa-custhelp.ssa.gov/app/answers/detail/a_id/326

U.S. Social Security Administration. (2012d, January). Working while disabled—How we can help. Retrieved from http://www.socialsecurity.gov/pubs/10095.html#a0=2

Index

The letter f *after a page number indicates that relevant content appears in a figure; the letter* t, *in a table.*